Holes in the Head

The Art and Archaeology of Trepanation in Ancient Peru

· · · · · · · · · · · ·

STUDIES IN PRE-COLUMBIAN ART AND ARCHAEOLOGY · NUMBER 38

Holes in the Head

The Art and Archaeology
of Trepanation in Ancient Peru

John W. Verano

with contributions by
Bebel Ibarra Asencios, David Kushner, Mellisa Lund Valle,
Anne R. Titelbaum, and J. Michael Williams

DUMBARTON OAKS RESEARCH LIBRARY AND COLLECTION

WASHINGTON, D.C.

LIBRARY OF CONGRESS CATALOGING-IN-PUBLICATION DATA

NAMES: Verano, John W., author.

TITLE: Holes in the head : the art and archaeology of trepanation in ancient Peru / John W. Verano, with contributions by Bebel Ibarra Asencios, David Kushner, Mellisa Lund Valle, Anne R. Titelbaum, and J. Michael Williams.

DESCRIPTION: Washington, D.C. : Dumbarton Oaks Research Library and Collection, 2016. | Series: Studies in pre-Columbian art and archaeology ; 38 | Includes bibliographical references and index.

IDENTIFIERS: LCCN 2015033339 | ISBN 9780884024125 (pbk. : alk. paper)

SUBJECTS: LCSH: Indians of South America—Craniology—Peru. | Trephining—Peru—History. | Indians of South America—Peru—Antiquities. | Indians of South America—Peru—Medicine. | Craniology—Peru. | Peru—Antiquities.

CLASSIFICATION: LCC F3429.3.C85 V47 2016 | DDC 617.5/14008998—dc23

GENERAL EDITOR: Colin McEwan

ART DIRECTOR: Kathleen Sparkes

DESIGN AND COMPOSITION: Melissa Tandysh

MANAGING EDITOR: Sara Taylor

COVER PHOTOGRAPH: Adult male from Patallacta with five healed trepanations. Museo Nacional de Antropología, Arqueología, y Historia del Perú, original catalog number 628.

www.doaks.org/publications

CONTENTS

FOREWORDS

MY OWN FIRST, AND ALTOGETHER MEMORABLE, ENCOUNTER WITH PRE-
Columbian trepanned skulls took place in early 1976 in the medical consulting office of
Dr. Pedro Weiss at the home he and his wife Amalia shared for many years.* She was a
talented sculptor and painter, and my visit to their beautiful art deco house in Lima had
been arranged by Pedro's niece Anita Barker de Weiss, whose father I had met on board
the Pacific Steam Navigation Company vessel SS *Ortega* en route from Liverpool to Callao.
With typical generosity, Anita thought that an aspiring young archaeologist recently
arrived in Peru should not miss the opportunity to meet her uncle. Pedro was a renowned
dermatologist who belonged to that erudite circle of medical and other professionals in
Peru whose expertise embraced a passionate interest in, and commitment to, studying
and preserving vestiges of Andean culture past and present. He was the first person to
identify and describe a rare skin cancer, and he kept two or three Peruvian hairless dogs at
home as pets because of their distinctive characteristics. Together with other colleagues,
he contributed significantly to efforts to save this increasingly rare breed from the threat
of extinction.

Pedro Weiss was also an avid pioneer in the study of modified Pre-Columbian skulls,
and I still treasure the gift copy of his small book *Osteologica cultural: Prácticas cefálicas*
(1958). Handling the skulls under Pedro's tutelage left an indelible impression. I was priv-
ileged to watch and listen as he observed and explained the features of several notable
specimens in his personal collection—a masterclass by a trained medical practitioner with
boundless curiosity, enthusiasm, and admiration for the scientific accomplishments of his
Pre-Columbian forebears. Pedro died in 1994, and I cannot help but think of how gratified
and excited he would have been to peruse this monograph and to digest the wealth of new
data it contains. Had it been possible, he would surely have contributed with the fruits of
his own accumulated knowledge and insights.

The present work is the culmination of nearly three decades invested by John Verano
and his colleagues in patiently recording and compiling the information on skulls dispersed far and wide in both public and private collections. The comprehensive, adroit
treatment of the subject from their complementary perspectives fills a long overdue gap
in the field. As the authors themselves note, the history of trepanation in Peru holds a special place, as more evidence of cranial surgery has been found in Andean South America
than everywhere else in the world combined. The inclusion of this title in the recently res-
urrected Studies in Pre-Columbian Art and Archaeology monograph series is, therefore,
particularly welcome for a number of reasons. It is the first devoted primarily to physical

anthropology, something that might not have been considered entirely appropriate as a Dumbarton Oaks title in earlier years. Interdisciplinary advances in the field now demand that an approach to the trepanned skulls encompass everything from the techniques and tools required to conduct such sophisticated and successful surgery on living patients to due consideration of the long-standing native Andean traditions and beliefs within which these practices were embedded. This study offers wide-ranging new perspectives on general issues of health, disease, and curing strategies as well as the traumatic injuries inflicted in the course of warfare. With the publication of this volume, Pre-Columbian trepanned skulls are placed fairly and squarely "on the map." Long the subject of speculative interpretation, the study of the skulls is sure to derive lasting benefit from this substantive and amply illustrated body of comparative material.

Our customary sincere thanks go to the two reviewers, to the Pre-Columbian Studies program coordinator Kelly McKenna, who facilitated transmittal of the manuscript, and, not least, to our stellar colleagues Kathy Sparkes, director of publications, and Sara Taylor, managing editor of art and archaeology publications.

Colin McEwan
Director, Pre-Columbian Studies
Dumbarton Oaks

---

* Dr. Pedro Weiss Harvey was born in 1893 or 1894 and died in 1994, just short of his one hundredth birthday. I am grateful for the recollections and notes kindly supplied by Monica Barnes, whose friendship with Anita Barker de Weiss has endured over the years.

⁝⁝⁝

EXQUISITELY ILLUSTRATED, THIS VOLUME IS AUTHORITATIVE AND engaging in a manner that should attract a broad and enthusiastic readership. John Verano, a physical anthropologist who is well known both for his knowledge of ancient Peruvians and his self-deprecating humor, has produced a monolithic volume on ancient Andean trepanations—surgically induced holes in the head—that will stand as a monument for eons to come. Written for professionals from such fields as archaeology, forensic science, medical history, neuroscience, and neurosurgery, the book will also speak to nonspecialists who wish to learn about the earliest cranial surgeons whose patients commonly recovered—long before Lister and antisepsis.

As Verano notes, cranial surgery is first documented in Neolithic Europe, among farmers who lived seven thousand years before the present. Even so, ancient cranial surgery par excellence developed in South America, first on the coast of present-day Peru approximately 2,500 years ago. Coastal examples then ceased, with trepanations appearing in the northern and central highlands, where the procedure flourished until the conquest.

Overall, the volume is richly contextualized, placing the development of Peruvian cranial surgery within a global setting and then tracing Andean regional examples in remarkable detail. Verano recounts efforts by early collectors, such as Muñiz, Tello, and Hrdlička, to preserve and interpret these early cranial surgeries. After emphasizing the importance of rigorous differential diagnosis in identifying true cases of trepanation, Verano turns to his own massive data set.

Verano has worked on this volume for a quarter-century, amassing data from approximately eight hundred trepanned Peruvian skulls. His analyses overall underscore the remarkable rate of patient survival for ancient Peruvians (>50 percent) when compared to 10–25 percent for nineteenth-century Europe. Multiple trepanations were survived, and Verano's data confirm the association of trepanations with cranial trauma, thus supporting the probable predisposing factor for this surgical intervention. In his regional treatments, Verano carefully details the earliest Peruvian trepanations recovered from the coastal Paracas cemeteries and adjacent areas. Mysteriously, these bold examples disappear on the coast, and the practice then begins, spreads, and flourishes in the northern, central, and southern highlands. Collections surveyed and their histories, data collected, and summarizing analyses are systematically reported.

Noting the dearth of ethnographic or ethnohistoric accounts of trepanation from the Andes, Verano turns to other regions, such as north and east Africa and the South Pacific, for comparative models. He reports these various traditions of skull surgery, frequently following head trauma, with simple instruments and ensuing survival. This discussion is followed by two chapters by guest authors, who consider ancient trepanation from the modern perspectives of neurosurgery and neuropsychology. These essays present medically informed inferences about the neurological, behavioral, and cognitive sequelae of the blunt force trauma and subsequent surgery. Two examples from near the turn of the twentieth century illuminate this discussion, followed by a narrative interpretation of an ancient Peruvian example from the southern highlands, wherein two large trepanations followed severe blunt force trauma to the temporal bone. These underscore the need for postoperative care, frequently over an extended period, following cranial surgery, an aspect often overlooked in studies of trepanation.

This is indeed a marvelously rich volume on an engaging subject. The illustrations are superb, enhanced by the use of color images. Although Verano states in closing that the "final chapter on trepanation in ancient Peru has yet to be written," the scholarship represented here will not be surpassed for a very long time.

Jane E. Buikstra
Regent's Professor of Bioarchaeology
School of Human Evolution and Social Change
Arizona State University

PREFACE

THIS IS A BOOK ABOUT HOLES IN THE HEAD. MORE SPECIFICALLY, IT IS A book about the art of cranial surgery (trepanation) and the archaeological record of its practice in ancient Peru. The book is the culmination of a research project begun in 1989 in collaboration with neuropsychologist J. Michael Williams. The idea for doing such a study grew out of Mike's interest in the neuropsychology of head injury and my own research focus on paleopathology and medical practices in ancient Peru. Indeed, trepanation is a subject of interest to a broad range of scholars, including archaeologists and biological anthropologists, medical historians, psychologists, neurologists, and neurosurgeons. It is a subject of some fascination to the general public as well, as we have come to appreciate as we conducted this research. In the history of trepanation, Peru holds a special place, as more evidence of ancient cranial surgery has been found here than everywhere else in the world combined.

Over the past two decades, with the kind permission of directors and staff of natural history and anthropology museums in Peru and the United States, Williams and I have photographed and recorded detailed information on hundreds of Peruvian trepanned skulls. We are grateful to the following museums for providing access to their collections and archives: in Peru, the Museo Nacional de Antropología, Arqueología, y Historia del Perú, Museo de la Nación, Museo de Arqueología y Antropología de la Universidad Nacional Mayor de San Marcos, Museo Arqueológico Rafael Larco Herrera, Museo Inka de la Universidad Nacional de San Antonio Abad del Cuzco, and the Museo Regional de Ica; and in the United States, the National Museum of Natural History (Smithsonian Institution), the American Museum of Natural History, the Peabody Museum of Archaeology and Ethnology (Harvard University), the Phoebe A. Hearst Museum of Anthropology (University of California, Berkeley), the Field Museum of Natural History, Chicago, the San Diego Museum of Man, and the Mütter Museum (College of Physicians, Philadelphia). I am grateful to many students and volunteers who assisted with data collection, but in particular would like to thank my Peruvian colleague Mellisa Lund Valle, who worked with me recording trepanned skulls at multiple museums in Peru, and John McClelland, who volunteered at the National Museum of Natural History to help organize and standardize the mass of data we accumulated in this study. J. Michael Williams and I would also like to thank A. Rand Coleman and Kelli S. Williams for their assistance with this project, and Lane Beck for her patience during several research visits we made to the Peabody Museum. I am grateful to Valerie Andrushko and Danielle Kurin for permission to publish their photographs of trepanned crania from their own research projects (Chapter 7), to Michael Mueller for permission to publish his photographs of a modern Kisii trepanation (Chapter 8), and to David Hunt of the National Museum of Natural History for seeking out and photographing several crania in their collections for the differential diagnosis chapter. Finally, I thank Mike Williams, David Kushner, Anne Titelbaum, Mellisa Lund Valle, and Bebel Ibarra Asencios for their collaboration and excellent contributions to this book. At Dumbarton Oaks, I am grateful for the support and encouragement of Jan Ziolkowski (director), Colin McEwan (director of Pre-Columbian Studies), and the Pre-Columbian Studies Senior Fellows committee. I especially wish to thank Kathleen Sparks (publications director) and Sara Taylor (managing editor of art and archaeology publications) for producing such a beautiful volume. Finally, I thank the two external reviewers for their very helpful comments and suggestions.

My travel to museums and archaeological sites was made possible by Fulbright Lectureships in Peru (1989, 1996) funded by the Council for the International Exchange of Scholars and travel grants from the Research Opportunities Fund of the National Museum of Natural History (1992) and the Roger Thayer Stone Center for Latin American Studies at Tulane University (2002). Library research, data analysis, and writing were done while I was a fellow in Pre-Columbian studies at Dumbarton Oaks (2006–2007) and during sabbatical leave from Tulane University (2012–2013).

Unless otherwise noted, all photographs are by the author.

John W. Verano

Define your terms.
—Voltaire

TREPANATION, OR TREPHINATION, IS THE SCRAPING, CUTTING, OR DRILLING of an opening (or openings) into the skull. It is the oldest form of surgery known from the archaeological record, extending back more than five thousand years in Europe and to at least the fifth century BC in the New World. Global surveys of the practice reveal that a surprising number of ancient cultures experimented with cranial surgery, and that in some areas these surgeries continued into modern times (Arnott et al. 2003; Lisowski 1967). Ancient trepanation continues to be a topic of considerable interest to scholars and the general public as well. According to one recent estimate, more than a thousand journal articles and many books have been published on the subject (Rose 2003).

The word *trepanation* comes from the ancient Greek word *trypanon*, meaning a drill or borer. *Trephination* is a later variant generally attributed to John Woodall, a British barber-surgeon, who in 1639 described and illustrated a circular drill with a T-shaped handle that he called a "Trafine" (trephine): a tool with "three ends" (Figure 1.1). According to Charles Gross (2003), Woodall was not the inventor of the three-ended trephine: in the previous century, Fabricus ab Aquapendente developed a cranial drill with three arms that he named "tres fines" (Latin for "three ends"). In 1563, Croce also illustrated a cylindrical drill with a T-shaped handle, although he called it by another name (Kirkup 2003). Through time, *tres fines* became *trafine*, and later *trephine* (Gross 2003).

The terms *trepanation* and *trephination* both continue in general use, and there has been some debate over which is preferable. Paleopathologist Della Collins Cook wrote an entertaining piece in the *Paleopathology Newsletter* documenting her attempt to clarify the issue by consulting medical dictionaries, where she found more confusion than clarity. Cook discovered the most consistent etymology in the *Oxford English Dictionary*, supporting the primacy (and Greek origin) of the terms *trepanation* and *trepan* (Cook 2000). In this book, I will use *trepanation* to describe ancient cranial surgery, and *trephination* to refer to surgery performed with the "crown" trephine, which was developed by the ancient

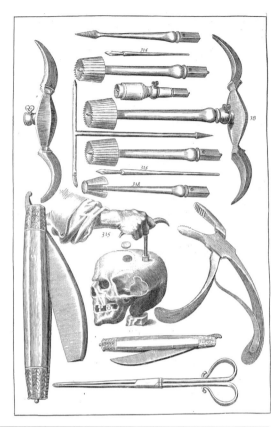

Figure 1.1
Illustration of various instruments for cranial surgery (Woodall 1639:26, pl. 1). Courtesy of Wellcome Images.

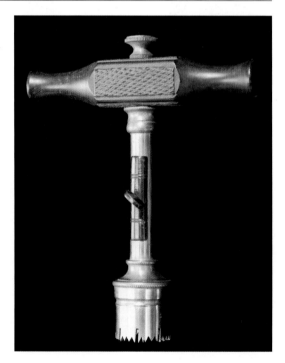

Figure 1.2
Nineteenth-century trephine. Courtesy of the Mütter Museum, Philadelphia, 1069-misc.

HOLES IN THE HEAD

Greeks and went on to become the most widely used tool for drilling holes in the skull through the end of the nineteenth century (Figure 1.2). In modern neurosurgery, the terms *burr hole*, *craniotomy*, and *craniectomy* are used to describe procedures for making holes in skulls and removing portions of bone (see Chapter 9).

TREPANATION AND BRAIN SURGERY

It must be clarified from the start that trepanation is *not* brain surgery. Unless done under sterile conditions, penetrating the dura mater, a thick membrane that covers and protects the brain (Figure 1.3), puts a patient at high risk of infection (e.g., meningitis or brain abscess). Prehistoric trepanners no doubt learned to avoid the dura mater and its attendant complications. Historically, Western surgeons since the time of Hippocrates abstained from cutting the dura unless it was deemed necessary to drain a subdural accumulation of fluid (Ruisinger 2003). Given the risk of infection, bleeding, and physical damage to the brain, exploratory surgery of the cranial contents by ancient trepanners seems most unlikely. Instead, trepanation appears to have originated in the practical treatment of head

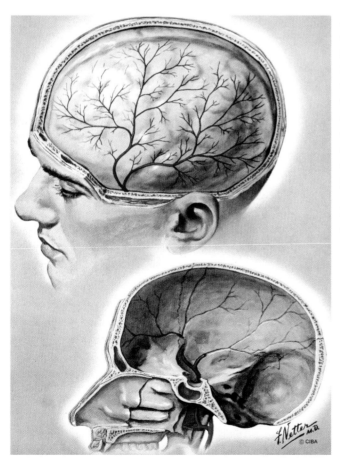

Figure 1.3
Cut-away illustrations, showing the dura mater and middle meningeal artery exposed after removal of a portion of the skull vault (above) and a mid-sagittal section of the skull with the path of the artery (below). Illustration by Frank Netter © 2015 NetterImages.

injuries, perhaps beginning at the most simple level as a means of cleaning wounds by removing bone fragments and smoothing broken edges, and for relieving pressure on the brain from swelling and depressed bone.

THE ORIGINS OF MODERN CRANIAL SURGERY: A BRIEF HISTORY

The Hippocratic Corpus—a series of medical texts attributed to Hippocrates (460–377 BC)—includes the important treatise *On Injuries [Wounds] of the Head* (Adams 1886). The work, regardless of whether it was actually written by Hippocrates or by his students (Lloyd 1975; Martin 2000), is a classic in medical history because of the detailed information it presents on the diagnosis and treatment of head wounds, including recommendations for when trepanation is appropriate.

On Injuries of the Head begins with a description of cranial anatomy, including details such as the variations in the form of cranial sutures and the thickness of different cranial bones and their susceptibility to fracture. It then provides a guide to the assessment and treatment of head injuries, starting with collecting a patient history, still a doctor's first step today. The text recommends that head wounds first be examined visually, then palpated and carefully probed to assess the nature of the injury. It classifies and describes six distinct types of skull fracture: (1) fissured (linear); (2) contused but not visibly fractured; (3) depressed; (4) *hedra* (a fracture that presents an impact scar from a weapon but does not visibly affect the surrounding bone); (5) fractures distant from the point of impact (*contrecoup* fractures); and (6) wounds above cranial sutures. Each of these types is described in terms of its diagnostic features, prognosis, and method of treatment. Trepanation is recommended for four of the six: fissured, contused, hedra, and wounds above sutures (although trepanation is not to be done through the sutures themselves, but adjacent to them). Interestingly, the Hippocratic treatise does not recommend trepanation for depressed fractures (Adams 1886; Panourias et al. 2005). Apparently, an attempt to elevate or drill broken fragments of bone was considered dangerous, and since depressed fractures often created an open wound from which fluids could drain, trepanation was not necessary for this purpose.

Surgical Instruments

Tools for treating head wounds described in the Hippocratic Corpus include a probe to examine bone surfaces and determine the depth of injuries, a rasp for scraping tissues from the surface of cranial bones, pointed drills for making small holes, and a serrated trepan (*prion charactos* or *terebra serrata*) for creating a larger circular hole to allow the removal of a plug of bone (Bakay 1985). While no Greek serrated trepans have survived, Roman examples are known, and these presumably were derived from original Greek designs (Brothwell 1974; Jackson 1988, 1990; Künzl et al. 1983; Tullo 2010).

Roman Medical Texts

The early treatises of the Hippocratic School were incorporated and expanded by Celsus and Galen, both of whom wrote in the first century AD. Aulus Aurelius Cornelius Celsus

(25 BC–AD 50) was not a physician himself, but rather a gatherer of practical medical information, including the evaluation and treatment of head injuries (Goodrich 1997). Although his principal work *De re medicina* was lost until 1443, it gained renewed notoriety in 1478, when it became the first medical book to be printed and widely distributed in Europe, thanks to the invention of moveable type. Celsus was conservative about trepanation, advising against the immediate trepanning of patients with head wounds unless their condition was deteriorating. Unlike Hippocrates, he recommended treating depressed skull fractures first by removing bone fragments and then cutting away overriding bone pieces by chiseling the broken edge, or by elevating the fragment though a perforation placed adjacent to the fracture (Bakay 1985). Celsus made a number of important contributions to the evaluation of head wounds, including observations on intracranial bleeding and the diagnostic value of localized pain as a guide to where to trepan the skull. He is credited with inventing a crown trepan with a center pin to stabilize it, and was the first to describe a drilling and cutting method of trepanation, where multiple drilled holes were connected by chiseling the bone between them, allowing a bone flap to be removed (Bakay 1985; Goodrich 1997).

Galen of Pergamum (ca. AD 129–210) was a disciple of the Hippocratic School and a prolific writer and compiler of medical information. Appointed as physician to the gladiator school of Pergamum, he gained extensive practical experience treating combat injuries, including head wounds (Rocca 2003). Galen favored prompt surgical treatment of skull fractures and gave detailed recommendations on the safe use of the trepan (Goodrich 1997). To perfect trepanation techniques and to study the anatomy of the brain, Galen experimented on monkeys (dissection of cadavers was not permitted in ancient Greece or Rome), oxen, and other mammals (Rocca 2003). Galen's death in AD 210 led to the decline of neuroanatomy as a scientific pursuit, and few advances were made in the study of skull fractures and their treatment, with the exception of the later writings of Paul of Aegineta (AD 625–690), considered the last of the great Byzantine physicians (Goodrich 1997).

The Islamic and Medieval Periods

From AD 800 to 1200, the Islamic school of physicians was the principal reservoir for classical Greek and Roman medical knowledge. Trepanation for skull fractures continued, although there were relatively few new advances (Bakay 1985). Medical scholarship in Europe during this time was largely quiescent, only awakening when classical texts were translated from Arabic into Latin during the thirteenth century.

By the end of the fifteenth century, a new medical practitioner emerged in Europe: the wound surgeon, who specialized in treating battlefield injuries (Bakay 1985; Goodrich 1997). With limited education and training primarily via apprenticeship, barber-surgeons specialized in the practical treatment of war wounds, many of which involved the head (Dobson and Walker 1979; Pelling 1998). During this time, trepanation was a practical treatment for head injury, but some also considered it a method for treating epilepsy and mental illness.

Epilepsy and the "Stones of Madness"

The origins of trepanation as a treatment for epilepsy may be traced to Hippocrates, who noted that convulsions resulting from head injury tend to appear on the opposite side of the body, and that prompt trepanation should be done in those cases (Meador et al. 1989). Later literary and artistic references to epilepsy and its treatment by cautery or trepanation are known from the late twelfth century (Ladino et al. 2013). At about the same time (ca. 1170), Roger of Parma recommended trepanation to release vapors that were causing neurological symptoms. He wrote: "For mania or melancholy the skin at the top of the head should be incised in a cruciate fashion and the skull perforated to allow matter to escape" (Valenstein 1997:500). Nearly five hundred years later, Robert Burton made a similar recommendation: "Tis not amiss to bore the skull with an instrument, to let out the fuliginous vapors. . . . Guinerius cured a nobleman in Savoy by drilling alone, leaving the hole open a month together by means of which, after two year's melancholy and madness he was delivered" (Gross 1999:430).

Thus, in the Middle Ages, trepanation was recommended not only for head injury but also for epilepsy and mood disorders. In the sixteenth century, a number of paintings depict the treatment of a novel "illness" by trepanation: the removal of "stones of madness" or "folly." The most famous of these was painted around 1475 by the Flemish artist Hieronymus Bosch, and is known variously as *The Cure for Madness* (or *Folly*) and the *Extraction of the Stone of Madness* (or *Insanity*) (Gross 1999; Ladino et al. 2013). Whether this and similar paintings by Jan Sanders Van Hemessen, Pieter Brueghel, Pieter Huys, David Teniers the Younger, Jacob Cats, and others depict purely imaginary scenarios or examples of medical quackery has been discussed extensively by historians of art and medicine alike. Gross, in a review of the topic, emphasizes that regardless of whether these paintings depict sheer quackery, trepanation was certainly practiced in Europe at the time, not only for practical treatment of head injuries but also for neurological symptoms (Gross 1999). Unfortunately, relatively few trepanned skulls are known from Europe during this period. An exception is a report by Per Holck on two cases of incomplete trepanation from a medieval cathedral in Norway, one of which he suggests might represent a case of medical "swindle" by a remover of "stones" (Holck 2008).

Unfortunately, medieval Europe's experimentation with trepanation as a treatment for mental illness has led to the popular notion that trepanation in other parts of the world was done primarily to release "demons" or for other magical or ritual purposes, rather than being a practical treatment for head wounds. Introductory psychology textbooks frequently include a photo of a trepanned skull (often from Peru) as an example of such "psychosurgery." While this may have been true in medieval Europe, there is little or no evidence of this elsewhere in the world (see Chapter 8).

Peru

In the early sixteenth century, trepanation was practiced on both sides of the Atlantic (Di Matteo et al. 2013; Figure 1.4). Although one can imagine that Europeans would have found Inca trepanation quite interesting, there is no evidence that they ever witnessed an operation, as no written documents from this time period mention it. Nevertheless, at the time of European contact, Peru was the epicenter of trepanation in the New World, with skull surgery common throughout the highland areas of the Inca Empire (Figures 1.5 and 1.6).

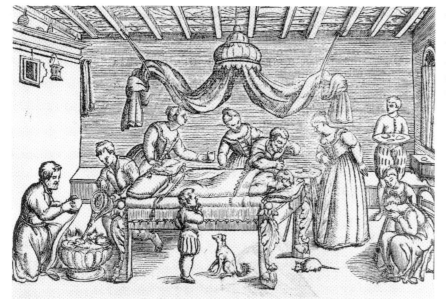

Figure 1.4
Sixteenth-century woodcut of cranial surgery being done in the home (Della Croce 1596).

While it is unclear why trepanation was so common in prehistoric Peru, advances have been made in documenting its geographic and temporal distribution, as well as in understanding the possible motivations for the practice. Most previous studies have been limited, however, to collections from a single geographic area or time period (MacCurdy 1923; Stewart 1958; Tello 1913) or to skulls of unknown provenance and antiquity (Lastres and Cabieses 1960; Rifkinson-Mann 1988; Weiss 1958). These limitations make it difficult to examine such issues as temporal and regional variation in techniques, survival rates, and possible motivations for the procedure. Clearly there is a need for a comprehensive study of Peruvian trepanation across space and time if we are to understand the origins and development of this surgical art.

The objective of this study is to overcome the limitations of previous investigations by systematically recording all large collections of Peruvian trepanned skulls (Verano and Williams 1992). Based on the examination of more than eight hundred trepanned skulls from Peru, this book provides a detailed regional and temporal survey of cranial surgery in ancient Peru, along with background on the history of collectors and their interpretations of trepanned skulls. The following chapter describes how prehistoric trepanation was first recognized by anthropologists and neurosurgeons of the mid-nineteenth century, and how initial skepticism about ancient surgery was overcome by careful argumentation and the presentation of physical evidence. Chapter 3 examines the importance of distinguishing openings in the skull created by surgical procedures from those produced by other mechanisms, such as developmental defects, disease, or taphonomic damage. Chapters 4 through 7 detail the history of discoveries of trepanned skulls from ancient Peru, beginning with early exploration of burial caves in the central highlands (Chapter 4), followed by the discovery of the earliest evidence of trepanation on the south coast of Peru (Chapter 5), and later examples from the northern highlands and cloud forest (Chapter 6) and the

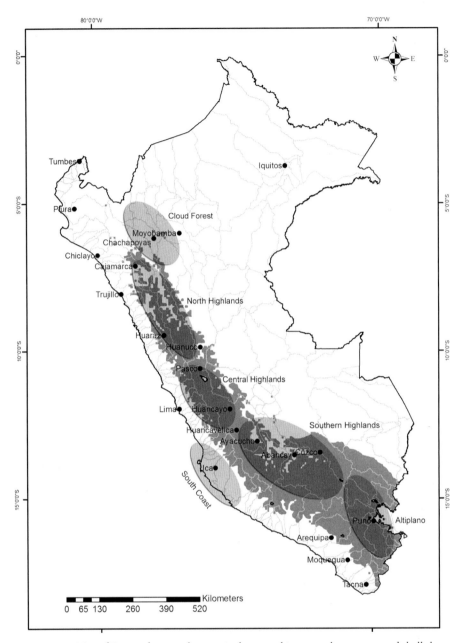

Figure 1.5 Map of Peru, indicating the principal geographic areas where trepanned skulls have been found (northern, central, and southern highlands; northern cloud forest; Altiplano; and the south coast). Map by Bebel Ibarra Asencios.

Figure 1.6 Trepanation in ancient Peru and Bolivia: Chronological chart.

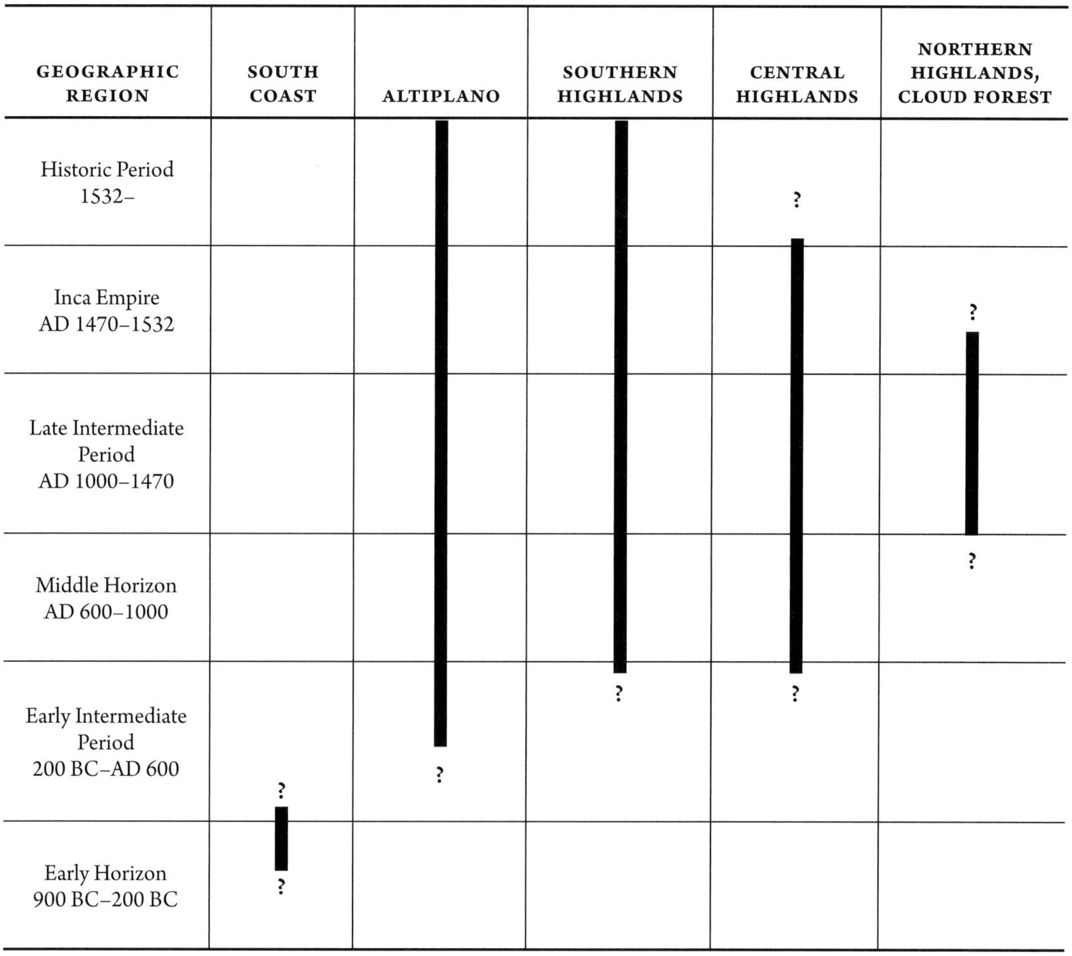

GEOGRAPHIC REGION	SOUTH COAST	ALTIPLANO	SOUTHERN HIGHLANDS	CENTRAL HIGHLANDS	NORTHERN HIGHLANDS, CLOUD FOREST
Historic Period 1532–		▌	▌	?	
Inca Empire AD 1470–1532		▌	▌	▌	?
Late Intermediate Period AD 1000–1470		▌	▌	▌	▌
Middle Horizon AD 600–1000		▌	▌	▌	?
Early Intermediate Period 200 BC–AD 600	?	▌ / ?	?	?	
Early Horizon 900 BC–200 BC	? / ?				

southern highlands and Altiplano of southern Peru and Bolivia (Chapter 7). Chapter 8 examines ethnographic accounts of traditional cranial surgery in the South Pacific and north and east Africa and explores their potential as comparative models for understanding the origins and development of trepanation in ancient Peru. It goes on to describe two unusual cases of modern surgery using ancient tools, and recent movements promoting self-trepanation as a means of enhancing consciousness. Chapters 9 and 10 provide modern clinical perspectives on trepanation in ancient Peru, from the viewpoints of modern neurosurgery (Chapter 9) and neuropsychology (Chapter 10). In Chapter 11, the archaeological record of trepanation in ancient Peru is compared with that of other regions in the Americas and beyond, examining questions of where and when trepanation was practiced and why it may have evolved independently in different parts of the world. For readers who may not be familiar with cranial anatomy, illustrations of the major bones of the skull, cranial sutures, and select anatomical landmarks are provided in the Appendix.

It has often been said that the two oldest living professions are prostitution and neurosurgery.

—James Goodrich (1999)

IN 1867, PAUL BROCA, ONE OF THE MOST PROMINENT NEUROSURGEONS and anthropologists of his day, presented a prehistoric skull found near Cuzco, Peru, to the Société d'Anthropologie de Paris (Figure 2.1). The skull had been brought from South America by Ephraim George Squier (Figure 2.2), an American diplomat and anthropologist, and delivered to Broca for his expert opinion. What makes this skull unusual is a rectangular hole in the frontal bone made by four intersecting linear incisions (Figure 2.3). The incisions were clearly made by human hands, but Broca went on to make a most surprising claim: that the opening was evidence of surgery performed on a living patient in prehistoric times (Broca 1867). Based on surface features of the bone surrounding the opening, Broca estimated that the patient had survived for approximately ten days. In the absence of visible skull fracture or other indication of why an opening might have been made in the skull, Broca hypothesized that the ancient surgeon might have been attempting to treat a subdural blood clot.

Not surprisingly, Broca's interpretation of Squier's skull was met with skepticism by some of his colleagues. Most physicians of the day were highly dubious of the idea that ancient peoples had ever performed surgery on the skull of a living patient. Even more controversial was the idea that such a procedure might have been done for medically appropriate reasons, and that a patient might have survived such an operation, if only briefly. In addition to the common belief among Western physicians that "primitive" cultures lacked the capacity for rational scientific thought, part of the skepticism arose from the practical experience of eighteenth- and nineteenth-century surgeons themselves. Until the introduction of aseptic techniques, mortality from infection following cranial surgery was very high, especially when performed in the disease-ridden hospitals of the day. Mortality rates following trepanations hovered around 75–90 percent in most hospitals (Aufderheide 1985; Martin 2003). For example, records from Glasgow Hospital in

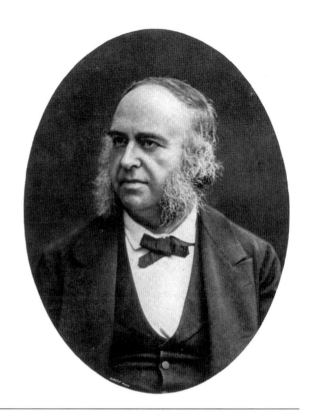

Figure 2.1
Paul Broca (1824–1880).
Courtesy of the National
Library of Medicine.

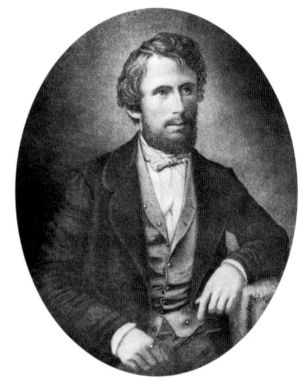

Figure 2.2
Ephraim George
Squier (1821–1888).
Courtesy of the National
Anthropological Archives,
Smithsonian Institution.

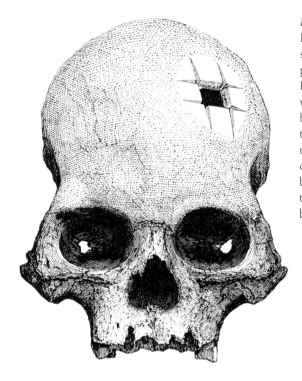

Figure 2.3
Illustration of a prehistoric skull found near Cuzco, first published in Squier (1877:457). In his book, the illustration was accidentally flipped horizontally, such that the trepanation appeared on the right instead of the left side of the frontal bone, and has been reproduced widely with this error. Here the image has been corrected.

Scotland from 1794 to 1839 report eight deaths in twenty-six patients (31 percent) with head injuries that were not surgically treated, while forty out of fifty-one (78 percent) who were trephined died (Bakay 1985:7). Some of the most distinguished and pioneering neurosurgeons of the day, such as Harvey Williams Cushing, had high mortality rates (Chapter 9). Given such a poor success rate, eighteenth- and nineteenth-century surgeons concerned with their reputations avoided drilling holes into their patients' skulls except as a last resort in intractable cases, such as a patient in a deep coma (Ruisinger 2003; Wehrli 1939). To them the idea that prehistoric people would be bold enough to attempt such a dangerous procedure seemed far-fetched.

Another reason for skepticism was that in the nineteenth century skulls had been discovered at Neolithic archaeological sites in Europe that had circular or oval pieces of bone cut from them. These discs were then perforated and apparently worn as amulets (Piggott 1940). Prior to Broca's presentation in 1867, any skull from a prehistoric site in Europe with a hole cut in it was assumed to reflect postmortem ritual practices, not surgery (Prunières 1874). But now, as surgeons were faced with a skull from Peru that Paul Broca was convinced showed evidence of surgery, the tide began to turn.

THE STORY OF SQUIER'S SKULL

In 1863, President Abraham Lincoln appointed Ephraim Squier to a legal claims commission charged with resolving a financial dispute between the governments of the United States and Peru. Squier happily accepted the appointment, as it would provide an opportunity for an extended visit to Peru and allow him to examine archaeological sites there. Squier already had an extensive background in the archaeology of North and Central America, and he was eager to expand his limited knowledge of Andean South America, which at the time was based primarily on his reading of William Prescott's 1847 book *History of the Conquest of Peru* (Finger and Fernando 2001).

After completing his diplomatic mission, Squier spent an additional eighteen months traveling throughout the country, visiting, photographing, and mapping some of its most important archaeological sites, including Pachacamac, the Pyramids of Moche, Chan Chan, and the Cuzco region, with a brief visit to the ruins of Tiwanaku in highland Bolivia. In 1877, he published a richly illustrated account of his travels and observations, *Peru: Incidents of Travel and Exploration in the Land of the Incas* (Squier 1877). In addition to maps, photographs, and drawings, Squier collected nearly sixty human crania from looted cemeteries on the north and central coast of Peru and from *chullpas* (burial towers) near Lake Titicaca, which he later donated to the Peabody Museum of American Archaeology and Ethnology of Harvard University. These crania were primarily of interest because they showed evidence of cranial deformation of various forms (Squier 1877:appendix B). One partial cranium that was shown to Squier in Cuzco, however, was most unusual.

While in Cuzco in 1865, Squier visited a private archaeology museum belonging to a prominent Cuzco woman, María Ana Centeno de Romainville (Lastres 1951), where he was shown the frontal portion of a skull with a square section of bone cut out (Figures 2.4 and 2.5). It had reportedly been found in an Inca cemetery in the town of Yucay, located in the Urubamba Valley about sixty-eight kilometers from Cuzco. Squier became fascinated by the idea that this opening might be evidence of Inca surgery on a living patient. He asked if he could take it back with him to the United States to seek the opinion of surgeons who might be able to confirm that it was an example of ancient surgery. His request was granted, and upon his return to the United States he presented the specimen to Dr. August Gardner, who examined it and presented his findings to the New York Academy of Medicine at its December 6 meeting in 1865. An excerpt from the minutes of that meeting is quoted by Stanley Finger and Hiran Fernando (2001:370): "The skull showed that during the patient's life an operation for trephining had been performed, a square-shaped piece of bone having been removed from the frontal bone, by what would appear to have been a gouging instrument. At one portion of the opening there seemed to be evidence of the attempt on the part of nature to form new bone, to repair the injury done by the operation."

While some members of the audience were convinced by Gardner's diagnosis, others were skeptical, not seeing clear evidence of bone reaction and suggesting that the opening may have been made postmortem. Given the lack of agreement, and not willing to give up easily, Squier decided to seek the opinion of one of the most prominent neurosurgeons and anthropologists of the day, Paul Broca. As the founder of the Société d'Anthropologie de Paris, Broca was one of the most influential and respected experts on the human skull and brain. Squier was certain that if Broca were to conclude that the opening was made in a living patient the issue would be settled.

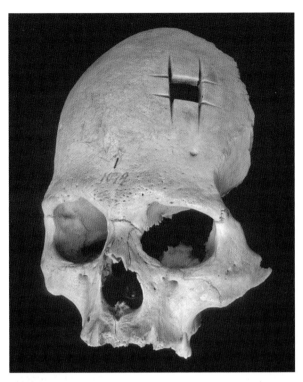

Figure 2.4
Squier's skull, front oblique view. American Museum of Natural History, catalog number 1/1079 © 2015, Division of Anthropology, American Museum of Natural History.

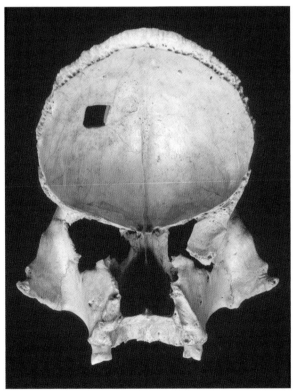

Figure 2.5
Squier's skull, posterior view. American Museum of Natural History, catalog number 1/1079 © 2015, Division of Anthropology, American Museum of Natural History.

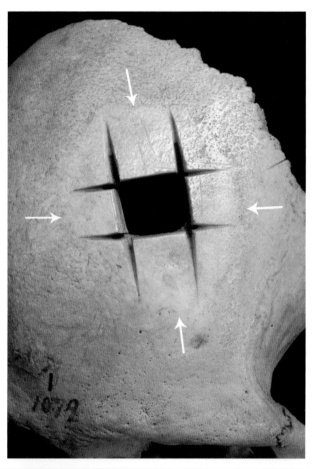

Figure 2.6
Close-up external view
of trepanation and
surrounding area of
bone reaction (arrows).
American Museum of
Natural History, catalog
number 1/1079 © 2015,
Division of Anthropology,
American Museum of
Natural History.

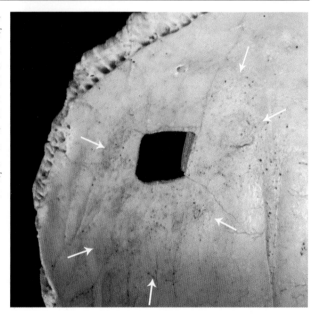

Figure 2.7
Close-up internal view of
trepanation, with arrows
indicating the patches
of porosities described
by Broca. American
Museum of Natural
History, catalog number
1/1079 © 2015, Division
of Anthropology,
American Museum of
Natural History.

Broca carefully examined the cranium and presented his conclusions at a meeting of the Société on July 4, 1867 (Broca 1867). Fernando and Finger (2003) have published a complete English translation of Broca's presentation, to which the interested reader is directed. Here I quote a few passages from Broca's introduction and conclusion, as translated by Fernando and Finger (2003:10–11). Broca begins boldly: "I have the honor to present to the Academy an ancient Peruvian skull on which trepanning was performed during the lifetime of the subject, following a procedure entirely different from that which is used in European surgery." After noting that the trepanation on the skull was made by four rectilinear incisions, he explains in detail the evidence of bone reaction surrounding the square opening that led him to conclude that the operation was done in a living patient:

> I shall now proceed to show that the trepanning was practiced during life. On the lateral portion of the right frontal bone there is a large white spot, quite regular, almost round, or rather slightly elliptical, forty-two millimeters wide and forty-seven long. . . . The surface is smooth and presents the appearance of entirely normal bone. Around this, to the edges, the coloration of the bone is notably darker; it is riddled with a great number of small holes caused by dilations of the small osseous canals. The line of demarcation between the smooth and the cribriform surfaces is abrupt; it is quite certain that the smooth surface had been denuded of its periosteum several days before death. . . . After considering the development of these perforations of the outer table . . . it seems to me impossible that the subject could have survived the denudations less than seven or eight days. Monsieur Nélaton, who carefully examined the specimen, thinks he may have survived fifteen days.

Figure 2.6 shows a close-up view of the trepanation, in which the area of color and texture changes noted by Broca can be clearly seen (indicated by arrows). Importantly, Broca's description of the bone changes is substantially more detailed than Gardner's reference to one portion of the opening showing what appeared to be an attempt at healing (see above). Broca then describes the appearance of the inner (endocranial) surface of the frontal bone, which he found quite distinct:

> The internal table around the opening is the seat of a very different alteration from that which existed on the external table around the denudation. It is the seat of little porosities in patches, which attest to the existence of osteitis [bone inflammation]. But this does not seem to have been the result of the trepanning, because it is not at all regularly distributed around the opening. It is entirely missing above the opening, it is minimal below, a little better marked on the outside, and is only really well pronounced about a centimeter and a half on the inner side of the internal border of the opening. These peculiarities and several others, which would take too long to detail, are well explained, if we suppose that there had been for some days before the operation an effusion of blood under the dura mater.

Figure 2.7 shows the approximate extent of the porosities Broca describes. As he notes, the appearance is distinctive from the changes seen on the outer table. Broca uses these observations to hypothesize why the skull might have been trepanned:

> In concluding, I call attention to one last question. For what motive was the trepanning performed? There is no fracture or fissure of either external or internal table. We notice, it is true, on the internal table several very delicate linear cracks [visible in Figure 2.7]. But these present all the ordinary characters of those produced by time, which are found in the majority of old crania. There was, then, no fracture; and the surgeon who performed the operation could consequently only be governed by functional troubles when diagnosing the existence of an intracranial lesion. Was this diagnosis correct? Did the operation succeed in evacuating a fluid poured into the cranium? . . . What astonishes me is not the boldness of the operation, as ignorance is often the mother of boldness. To trepan on an apparent fracture at the bottom of a wound is a sufficiently simple conception and does not necessitate the existence of advanced surgical arts. But here the trepanning was performed on a point where there was no fracture, and probably not even a wound, so that the surgical act was preceded by a diagnosis. Whether this diagnosis was correct, as is probable, or false, *we are in either case authorized to conclude that there was in Peru, before the European era, a surgery already very advanced—and this entirely new notion is not without interest for American anthropology* [italics mine].

Broca's detailed description of Squier's skull and his reputation in the scientific community were fundamental in convincing his audience and the wider academic world of the existence of prehistoric trepanation in Peru. It would inspire other anthropologists to explore the cemeteries and burial caves of Peru to collect more examples (Chapters 4–7). Broca's paper also led to the reexamination of defects in Neolithic European crania, many of which were revealed to be trepanations (Clower and Finger 2001; Piggott 1940). The question of why Squier's skull was trepanned continued to be a subject of debate, however. Some suggested that a small penetrating wound might have been the reason for the operation, the evidence of which was removed by the operation itself (Josiah Clark Nott and E. G. Squier in Squier 1877:579–80). In fact, later discoveries were made in Peru of small depressed and penetrating wounds surrounded by incomplete trepanations (Chapter 4). But in the case of Squier's skull, there remained no evidence of such a wound, leaving the question open.

TREPANATION IN ANDEAN SOUTH AMERICA

Paul Broca went on to publish various papers on ancient trepanation. The enthusiasm generated by this new research topic inspired museums and universities to send scientific expeditions to highland Peru and Bolivia to search for additional examples of trepanned skulls (Hrdlička 1914; MacCurdy 1923; Tello 1913). Hundreds would be discovered, eventually revealing that trepanation had been practiced not only by the Inca, but by a number of ancient Andean societies that predated the Inca Empire (Tello and Mejía Xesspe 1979; Yacovleff and Muelle 1932). We now know that trepanation was practiced in the Andean region for some two thousand years, from roughly the time of classical Greece (ca. 400 BC) until Spanish contact in the early sixteenth century (Verano 2003a). Isolated reports of trepanations performed by traditional healers continue well into the twentieth century, suggesting an even longer tradition in some isolated areas of the Andean highlands (Chapter 9; Bandelier 1904; Bastien 1987).

Before beginning a geographic and temporal survey of trepanation in ancient Peru, some basic issues need to be addressed regarding what is and what is not a trepanation, and how to tell the two apart. The following chapter reviews this issue, and describes the methods used in this study to record data on Peruvian trepanned skulls.

3 DIFFERENTIAL DIAGNOSIS OF HOLES IN THE HEAD

It is important to note that if only one or two skulls in a large amount of skeletal material have possible trephine holes, the diagnosis must remain tentative. Where practiced, trephination was usually performed on significant numbers of people—and the very nature of this operation must have required constant practice!

—(Steinbock 1976:35)

NOT ALL HOLES IN SKULLS ARE TREPANATIONS. IN FACT, THERE ARE MANY processes that can produce skull defects both in the living and in the dead (Bennike 2003; Campillo 2007; Merbs 1989). While distinguishing trepanations from other cranial defects can be relatively straightforward, in some cases it is more challenging. Particularly when faced with a healed defect in an isolated skull without medical history or archaeological context, one must be cautious, as R. Ted Steinbock recommends.

Differential diagnosis is a basic tool that paleopathologists use to distinguish the various causes of cranial defects. The process involves considering all possible causes, ruling out the most unlikely candidates, and reducing one's options until left with one or a few most likely diagnoses. In the case of trepanations, the easiest cases to diagnose are those with little or no healing, where visible tool marks provide direct evidence of the work of human hands. Although even in such clear samples one must be careful to rule out injuries produced by cutting weapons such as swords and axes or penetrating wounds from projectiles. Correct diagnosis is more difficult in healed defects of the skull, where the specific mechanism that caused a hole may be obscured by bone remodeling. Finally, postmortem damage to skulls (breakage, erosion of bone, carnivore or rodent damage) is common in archaeological material, and may produce defects that mimic trepanations.

DEFECTS REFLECTING NORMAL CRANIAL ANATOMY

In infants and children, gaps are normally present between developing vault bones. Fontanelles (fibrous tissue found between developing vault bones in infants) might be confused in archaeological material for a trepanation, in particular the large anterior fontanelle,

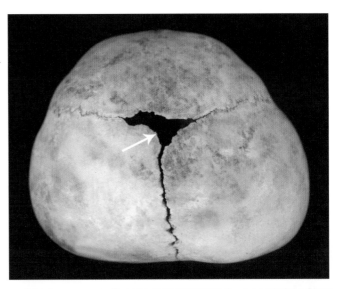

Figure 3.1
Superior view of the cranium of a 2.5- to 3.5-year-old child that shows delayed closure of the anterior fontanelle (arrow). Pacatnamú, Peru, Cemetery S1.

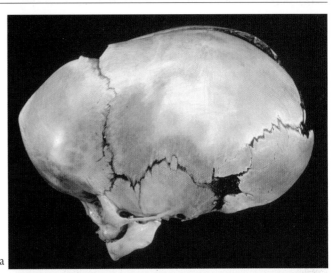

Figure 3.2
Lateral (a) and superior (b) views of the skull of an infant with hydrocephalus. This specimen shows great expansion of the cranial vault with forward projection of the frontal bones and an enlarged anterior fontanelle (see 3.2b). University of Nebraska, Lincoln, Anthropology Department, with permission of Karl Reinhard.

a

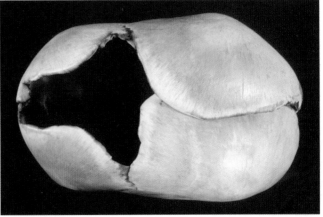

b

located between the developing halves of the left and right frontal bones and the parietals (Figure 3.1). But given that fontanelles are well-known anatomical features of the developing cranium, confusion with trepanations is unlikely, unless they are unusually large or remain open longer than normal. Some congenital and developmental defects of the cranium *have* been misdiagnosed as healed trepanations, so they must be considered here.

CONGENITAL AND DEVELOPMENTAL DEFECTS

Failure of Normal Ossification

Defects in the cranium may result from failure to ossify normally during growth and development. An example is partial or complete dysostosis, where cranial bones do not properly unite at the sutures, as in cleidocranial dysostosis or hydrocephalus (Figure 3.2). Small defects may also be produced by an outward bulging of the meninges (meningocoele), creating a smooth, round depression between sutures (Kaufman et al. 1997:fig. 1a–b; Stewart 1975). A common location for such defects is along the sagittal suture at or just posterior to the bregma, where the coronal and sagittal sutures meet (Figure 3.3). One case where meningocoele was not considered as a possible differential diagnosis is a cranium claimed to show one of the earliest trepanations known from Europe (Lillie 1998:fig. 2). Given its location and shape, and the fact that the cranium is a single isolated specimen in a region and time period without other convincing evidence of cranial surgery, meningocoele should be considered a more likely diagnosis. Cranial inclusion (dermoid) and epidermal cysts also

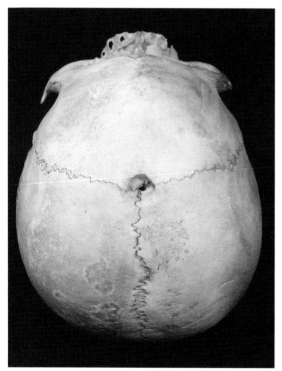

a

Figure 3.3 Superior (a) and oblique (b) views of a meningocoele. National Museum of Natural History 264629. Chicama Valley, Peru. Courtesy of David Hunt, Department of Anthropology, National Museum of Natural History, Smithsonian Institution.

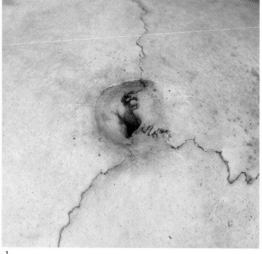

b

produce smooth-walled depressions and defects of the cranial vault that might be confused with healed trepanations (Barnes 2012; Klaus and Byrnes 2013; Ortner 2003).

Parietal Fenestrae (Enlarged Parietal Foramina)

Although not all authors distinguish between the parietal fenestrae and enlarged parietal foramina (e.g., Barnes 1994, 2012), M. H. Kaufman, D. Whitaker, and J. McTavish (1997:197) argue that the former term is the correct one, since parietal fenestrae are sometimes found near normal parietal foramina. Parietal fenestrae are typically oval in shape, although in some cases they are only narrow slits (Figure 3.4), and they are usually bilateral. Large fenestrae have been mistaken for healed trepanations (Goldsmith 1945), although their bilateral symmetry and the fact that they are usually found near the location of the parietal foramina should make one suspicious. The specific cause of parietal fenestrae is unknown, although they have been demonstrated to run in families, as in the case of "Catlin Marks" (Goldsmith 1945). I am unaware of any examples of parietal fenestrae in ancient Peruvian skeletal material, but examples probably exist, as they have been found in both Old and New World populations. One interesting Peruvian case that mimics parietal fenestrae is a cranium from Ollantaytambo, near Cuzco (Figure 3.5). It has two unhealed trepanation openings, one on each parietal bone. In this case, the openings are circular (not oval), show exposed spongy bone and clear evidence of cuts and scrape marks on and around their margins, and are located slightly anterior to where parietal foramina and fenestrae would normally be found. Had the trepanations healed, however, they might have presented a challenge to differential diagnosis.

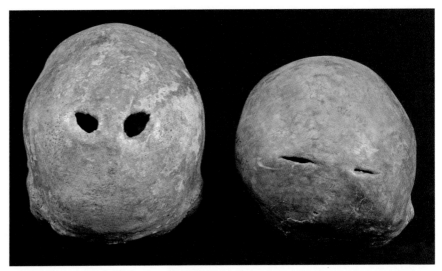

Figure 3.4 Parietal fenestrae. The cranium on the left shows the more typical oval defects. The cranium on the right shows the slit-like variant. National Museum of Natural History 276981, Ponce Mound, Santa Clara County, California (left); and National Museum of Natural History 276982, near Palo Alto, California (right). Courtesy of David Hunt, Department of Anthropology, National Museum of Natural History, Smithsonian Institution.

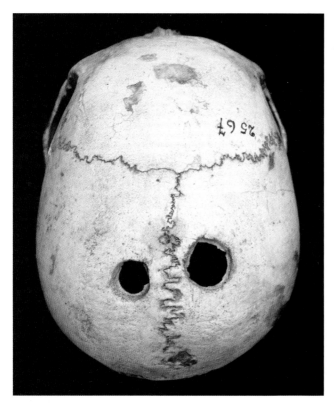

Figure 3.5
Double trepanation
with no evidence
of healing. Museo
Inka 2567.

Biparietal Thinning

Biparietal thinning is condition characterized by gradual thinning of the posterior-superior region of the parietal bones and loss of diploic bone, creating depressions (Figure 3.6). Pronounced cases may show small openings through the inner table, although these openings are most commonly the result of postmortem breakage. Biparietal thinning is most frequently seen in older adults (Cederlund et al. 1982; Wilms et al. 1983), although some cases have been reported in children as well (Barnes 1994, 2012). Examples of parietal thinning have sometimes been misdiagnosed as healed trepanations (Lisowski 1967:fig. 2). As in the case of parietal fenestrae, the location, symmetry, and characteristic shape of these depressions should distinguish them from healed trepanations, particularly in the case of a single isolated cranium found in a skeletal sample that shows no other examples of trepanation.

DEFECTS OF DIVERSE ORIGIN

Infection

Infection (osteomyelitis) of the vault bones of the skull caused by pyogenic bacteria, tuberculosis, or treponemal disease can produce defects that may be misdiagnosed as trepanations (Kaufman et al. 1997; Ortner 2003). If the infection was active at the time of death, then the margins of these defects will be porous and ragged, but if the infection healed,

Figure 3.6
Left (a) and right (b)
oblique lateral views of
an elderly adult cranium
with biparietal thinning.
The paper-thin bone
can be seen in areas of
breakage, particularly
on the left side, and the
parietal foramina rise above
the level of surrounding
bone. Modern anatomical
specimen, Department
of Anthropology,
Tulane University.

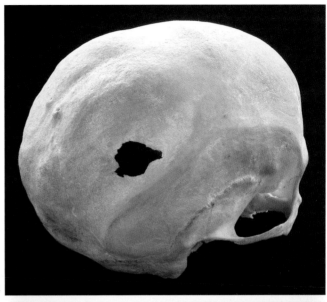

a

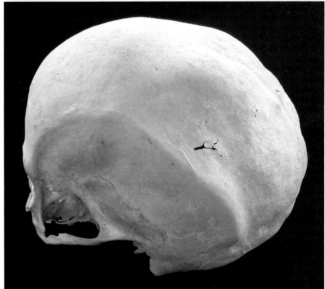

b

then the defects will be remodeled and could be confused with healed trepanations. Of course, both trepanation and osteomyelitis can appear in a single skull. Infection following a skull fracture or an open scalp wound might have been the motivation for trepanning, or the infection might have been a complication of the surgery itself. Many examples of trepanations surrounded by areas of inflammation are known (a number are illustrated in the chapters that follow), and it is not always clear which came first, the infection or the trepanation. Bone infection alone can result in cranial defects, however, so this must be considered when interpreting cases in which there is no clear evidence of cut or drill marks.

Neoplasm

Metastatic carcinoma and multiple myeloma can produce destructive lesions in the skull vault (Figures 3.7 and 3.8). These are primarily lytic (destructive) lesions produced by rapidly growing tumor cells that have metastasized from other parts of the body (metastatic carcinoma) or proliferate within the bone marrow (multiple myeloma). These defects show characteristic features, including ragged, "punched out" margins with little or no new bone formation. As they are the result of malignant tumors, healing is not expected in these cases. Thus, it is unlikely that these defects would be misdiagnosed as trepanations. Although some have speculated that trepanations may have been done to remove brain tumors, there is no evidence of this in prehistoric material from Peru or elsewhere in the world, as far as I know.

Trauma

Healed depressed fractures of the skull have frequently been misdiagnosed as trepanations (Figure 3.9). This is often due to the mistaken belief that trepanation defects heal by closing up the defect with new bone. In fact, this rarely occurs because bone remodeling in the cranium is very limited. More typically the margins of a trepanation close and actually retract slightly, rather than growing inward. Neurosurgeons know this well, as they frequently reattach plates of bone that are removed during surgery, or replace them with implants to protect the brain and maintain the normal contour of the skull vault (Verano and Andrushko 2008). Even in cases where bone plates are reinserted and wired in place by modern surgeons, they tend to show little or no union with the surrounding bone. In a study of eleven modern surgical specimens, Nerlich and colleagues made the following observation: "Despite very long periods of time (up to thirty-four years in our series), the trepanation defects do not show complete obliteration, even when the trepanned fragment is replaced properly. Additionally, there is no evidence that the defects show any tendency to decrease by marginal bone proliferation, as we did not see any significant new bone formation at the defect margins" (Nehrlich et al. 2003:49).

To my knowledge, only one example has been reported in which two surgical burr holes made during the same procedure show significant differences in healing. In this case, two small burr holes, each seven to eight millimeters in diameter, were drilled into the left and right side of the frontal bone. Approximately six years after the surgery, one hole had closed and was largely obliterated, while the other remained an open defect approximately seven millimeters in diameter. This example of differential healing was unusual enough to merit a case report in a major forensic science journal (Sauer and Dunlap 1985).

In comminuted fractures, where the cranial bone is broken into multiple fragments, isolated pieces of bone lose their blood supply, die, and are resorbed or sloughed off from the wound, or may be intentionally removed when a wound is cleaned. If the individual survives, there will be defects of variable size and form marking where bone fragments were lost. If there is extensive healing, it can be difficult to tell if any intervention was done to treat the fracture. A good example is the cranium of a child with comminuted and radiating fractures of the posterior portion of the left parietal bone (Figure 3.10). The fractured area shows extensive healing, as indicated by the rounded margins of the large defect and

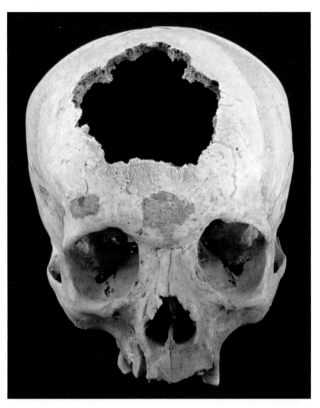

Figure 3.7
Large erosive lesion
on frontal bone.
Metastatic carcinoma?
Museo Nacional
de Antropología,
Arqueología, y Historia
del Perú, AF:7075.

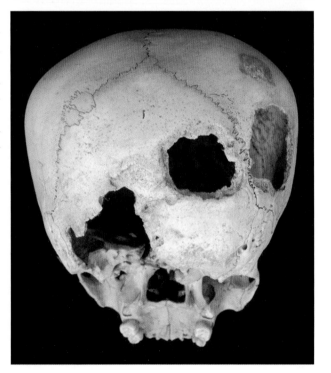

Figure 3.8
Multiple erosive
defects of the cranium
in a child. Neoplasm?
Museo Nacional
de Antropología,
Arqueología,
y Historia del
Perú, AF:6110.

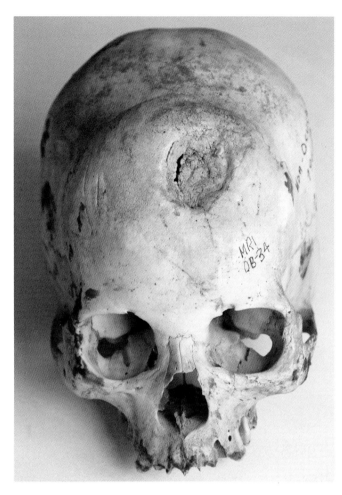

Figure 3.9
Healed depressed fracture on the frontal bone (mistakenly identified as trepanation in a museum catalog). Hacienda Ocucaje, Ica Valley, south coast of Peru. Museo Regional de Ica, 00292-12, MRI-DB-34.

the partial union of several of the fracture lines. Was the child trepanned as well? A semi-circular missing portion on the anterior margin of the large defect (marked with an arrow in the photograph) looks like a healed cut or drill mark, but it could also mark a punched out fracture from a star-headed club. Given the extensive healing, it is unclear if the child's wound was treated surgically.

Penetrating wounds to the skull have also been misdiagnosed as trepanations. If the wounds show no healing, their size and shape may allow matching them to particular weapons, such as spear points or star-headed maces, and to rule out the defect as a trepanation (Figure 3.11). If healed, it is more difficult to distinguish a penetrating wound from a small trepanation, although healed penetrating wounds are rare, due to their risk of infection and brain injury.

Skull Defects Made by Edged Weapons

In Europe and other parts of the Old World, sword and axe wounds are common during certain time periods (Campillo 2007), and some of these have been mistaken for

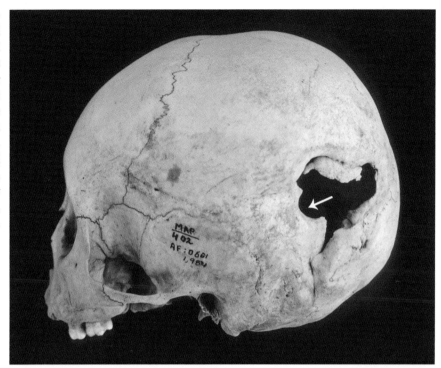

Figure 3.10
Cranium of a child with comminuted and radiating fractures of the posterior portion of the left parietal bone. The arrow points to a semicircular defect. Museo Nacional de Antropología, Arqueología, y Historia del Perú, AF:0561, MAP/402.

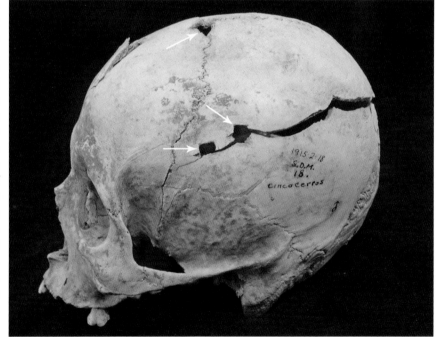

Figure 3.11
Cranium of an adult male with multiple small, rectangular, penetrating wounds (three are indicated by arrows) with a large radiating fracture extending posteriorly from two of them. The nature of the wounds and the lack of associated cut marks indicates that these are not trepanations. Cinco Cerros, central highland Peru. Hrdlička collection, San Diego Museum of Man, 1915-2-18.

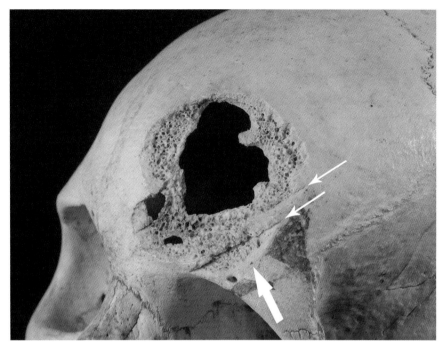

Figure 3.12
Cranium from West
Africa with a saber
wound on the frontal
bone. The large arrow
indicates the direction
of a glancing blow that
left several chatter marks
(small arrows) where the
blade cut into bone and
then bounced off, and
continued to cut through
bone, removing a large
fragment. The wound
shows no sign of healing.
National Museum
of Natural History,
Smithsonian Institution,
209434.

trepanations (Bennike 2003). Steel swords were unknown in the New World until after European contact, so wounds produced by these weapons are not expected to be found in prehistoric Peruvian skeletal remains. However, a few cases of possible wounds from Spanish weapons have been reported from early contact- and colonial-period sites (Murphy et al. 2010), so sword wounds should be considered as a differential diagnosis in a cranium of uncertain antiquity. Unhealed sword injuries should be distinguishable from trepanations by the form of their cut marks, as can be seen in Figure 3.12, an example of a saber wound from West Africa.

Suprainion Lesions

Lesions on the occipital bone in the area above the anatomical landmark of inion (the external occipital protuberance) were first suggested by Peruvian neurosurgeon Fernando Cabieses to be evidence of an unusual form of prophylactic trepanation done on infants. Pathologist Pedro Weiss subsequently examined the question by studying collections of crania from the central coast of Peru, where these lesions are relatively common. Suprainion lesions are shallow depressions on the squamous portion of the occipital bone showing thinning and occasional perforation of the bone (Figure 3.13). Cabieses and Weiss hypothesized that these were scars from intentional scraping of the occipital bone, and they classified them as trepanations. This interpretation is considered problematic by other scholars who have studied similar lesions in prehistoric Peruvian, Mexican, and North American crania. T. Dale Stewart executed the first comprehensive study of these lesions (Stewart 1976), noting that they were found in various cultures (including those of the central coast of Peru) in which infants' heads were strapped to cradleboards

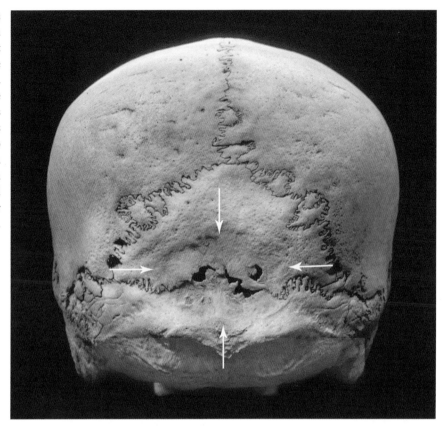

Figure 3.13
Healed suprainion lesion on an adult skull from the central coast of Peru. Arrows indicate the approximate margins of the lesion. Weiss collection, Museo de Arqueología y Antropología de la Universidad Nacional Mayor de San Marcos.

or other head-shaping devices. Stewart concludes that the lesions were the result of ischemia or inflammation caused by localized pressure on the back of the skull, not trepanation by scraping. In support of his argument he notes that no example is known of an unhealed trepanation showing tool marks from Peru or from anywhere else, and argues that unhealed cases would be expected, since a 100-percent survival rate for such procedures would be surprising, especially in infants. Unhealed suprainion lesions *have* been found in infants, but these are typically porous areas that do not show any evidence of cut marks or scraping (Figure 3.14). Stewart also notes that no other form of trepanation was practiced on the central coast of Peru, making it difficult to imagine that a procedure like this would evolve and become common in an area with no prior experience with cranial surgery. Stewart is probably correct here. We are aware of only four trepanned skulls reported to have been found on the central coast of Peru. Two crania with healed trepanations were surface collected from looted cemeteries at Pachacamac. The first is Cranium 11 from the Muñiz collection (Muñiz and McGee 1897:36–37; Chapter 4), and the second is an isolated cranium in the Museo Nacional de Antropología, Arqueología, y Historia del Perú (AF:4130, MAP PACH 39). Neither has a specific provenance or cultural association. Max Uhle reported an individual with a trepanned skull from an Inca cemetery at La Centinela, a site near Pachacamac (Uhle 1903:71, figs. 22a, 23, 23b). It has both a healed

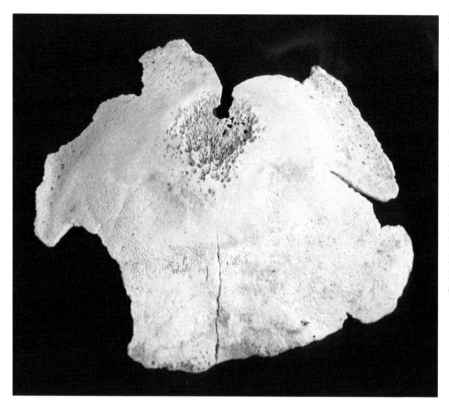

Figure 3.14
A suprainion lesion active at the time of death on the occipital bone of an infant less than six months old. It shows a focal area of osteoclastic activity (bone destruction) surrounded by a larger, smooth area of necrotic bone. L98-14, Huaca Cao Viejo Lambayeque Period burial, Chicama Valley, Peru. Courtesy of the Proyecto Arqueológico Complejo El Brujo.

trepanation and an incomplete opening made by the circular grooving method surrounding a penetrating wound to the left side of the skull. The fourth example is a cranium surface collected by Aleš Hrdlička from the site of Ancón, north of Lima, that has a series of drilled holes associated with a circular depressed fracture (NMNH 293877; Chapter 4). Although these four crania were found at central coast sites, it appears unlikely that trepanation was regularly practiced at Pachacamac or other nearby locations, as no other cases have been described from surface collections or from hundreds of scientifically excavated burials from these sites. Aleš Hrdlička collected some 2,200 crania from the surface of looted cemeteries at Pachacamac, none of which had trepanations (Hrdlička 1914). Were it a common practice there, one would expect to find other examples. And given that trepanation was widely practiced in the Inca heartland (Chapter 7), it would not be surprising to find a few trepanned skulls in coastal regions that were incorporated into the Inca empire.

A recent study of a Pueblo skeletal sample from southwestern New Mexico by Diane Holliday found a high frequency of suprainion lesions (both active and healed) associated with cradleboarding. Like Stewart, Holliday found no evidence of cutting or scrape marks that would identify trepanations. While most suprainion lesions heal and remain as simple depressions in adults, a recent case report concludes that, although rare, serious infection and death were potential risks of cradleboarding (Mendonça de Souza et al. 2008).

Debate continues on suprainion trepanation, despite evidence of a relationship between cranial deformation and suprainion lesions and a lack of unhealed suprainion lesions showing cut or scrape marks. This is particularly true in the case of the ancient Maya, among whom suprainion lesions have been reported, but there is no convincing evidence of trepanation (Tiesler 2012:45–47; Velasco-Suarez et al. 1992). From my own examination of many hundreds of deformed crania from the central and north coast of Peru, I have concluded that there is no evidence that suprainion lesions are the result of trepanation.

Postmortem Taphonomic Damage

Postmortem damage to crania can be produced by a variety of mechanisms, including breakage or erosion, surface weathering of exposed bone, and chewing by carnivores and rodents. Postmortem breakage or erosion of bone is normally fairly easy to recognize by the absence of bone reaction, such as inflammation or healing of the defect margins, or by the different coloration of broken edges indicating recent breakage (Figure 3.15). In coastal Peru, I saw two cases of sun-bleaching and abrasion by windblown sand that eroded away portions of the skull vault, mimicking large trepanations (Figures 3.16 and 3.17).

Carnivore gnawing is relatively easy to recognize by features such as puncture marks, deep grooves, and breakage of bone. Rodent gnawing is more subtle, and it has resulted in the misidentification of cranial defects as trepanations (Figure 3.18). Careful examination of the margins of a defect reveal the characteristic paired chisel marks of the rodent's central incisors, which leave small furrows along the margins of holes that are perpendicular to the edge of the hole. This pattern is unlike those created by a human cutting or scraping bone.

DIAGNOSTIC CHALLENGES AND PROTOCOLS FOR RECORDING TREPANATIONS

Without access to a subject's medical history or firm archaeological context and dating, diagnosing defects in skulls can be challenging. This is particularly true in the case of healed defects of the cranium, since bone remodeling normally erases the tool marks that identify surgical intervention. Unhealed holes in skulls, even if clearly made by human hands, also raise the question of whether trepanation was done on a living patient or as a postmortem experiment or ritual, such as the removal of bone discs in Neolithic Europe (Piggott 1940; Prunières 1874). Particularly challenging are isolated cases of crania found in regions where trepanation has not previously been identified. In discussing these, paleopathologist Donald Ortner made the following observation: "In such situations . . . the demonstration of unambiguous trephination in the same geographical area would certainly be significant in interpreting the equivocal cases" (Ortner 2003:171). Fortunately, in the case of Peru we have abundant evidence that trepanation was practiced in many geographic regions over more than two thousand years. Nevertheless, even in a region where skull surgery was common, differential diagnosis is important for confidently identifying trepanations.

During the initial stages of planning our study, we developed a laboratory form to record crania in a standardized fashion. The form was designed to simplify data entry, and includes standardized codes for bones present, estimated age and sex, and presence and form of cranial deformation. The final page of the form has space to draw standardized

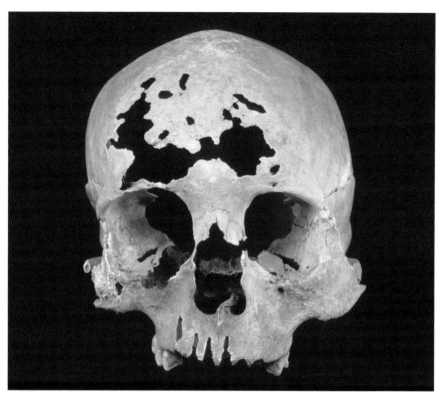

Figure 3.15
A cranium from Machu Picchu, showing postmortem erosion of the frontal bone and defects that mimic infection or scraping of the bone. The lack of bone reaction or cutting or scraping marks indicates that the damage was caused by humidity and soil conditions of the burial cave in which it was found. Machu Picchu Grave 77, 3219. Courtesy of the Yale Peabody Museum of Natural History.

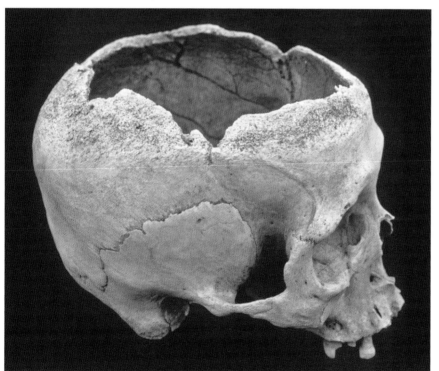

Figure 3.16
Cranium from coastal Peru with weathering and sand erosion of the top of the skull vault. Although superficially resembling a large trepanation, the margins of the defect show sun-bleaching and homogenous erosion, indicating that the top of the skull was exposed to the elements.

Figure 3.17
Cranium showing
sun-bleaching
and sand erosion.
Hacienda Ocucaje,
Ica, Peru. Museo
Regional de
Ica, 00868-12,
MRI-DB-4329.

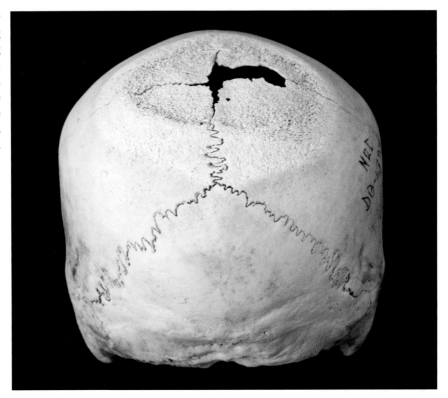

views of a cranium illustrating trepanations, cut marks, fractures, and other observations. Each cranium is divided into twenty-two numerically coded regions so that database searches can be made by side (left, right, or midline) or by particular bone (occipital, parietal, frontal, temporal, or sphenoid). Each of the parietal bones is further subdivided into four portions corresponding to functional areas of the cortex. We wanted to see if trepanations not obviously related to fractures might demonstrate patterning that would suggest that ancient surgeons had some understanding of specific functional areas of the brain, choosing to do "elective" trepanations in particular locations. We soon realized that there is no evidence to support this hypothesis, but nevertheless retained the numerical codes for consistency in data recording. We have also assigned numerical codes to cranial bones that were never trepanned (nasals, maxillae, malars) but that frequently have fractures, so that we can record trauma to the bones of the face as well as those of the skull vault.

For each trepanation opening, we recorded size (maximum length and width), method (scraping, linear cutting, circular grooving, drilling and cutting, or simple drilling), degree of healing (none, short-term, or long-term), evidence of cut marks and inflammation around the opening, and whether the trepanation was associated with a visible skull fracture. We also recorded whether trepanations cut through major muscles (temporalis or nuchal musculature) or cranial sutures. We predicted that trepanners would avoid, if possible, cutting through major muscles of the temporal and neck regions because of the risk of bleeding and nerve damage. We also predicted that cranial sutures (particularly the

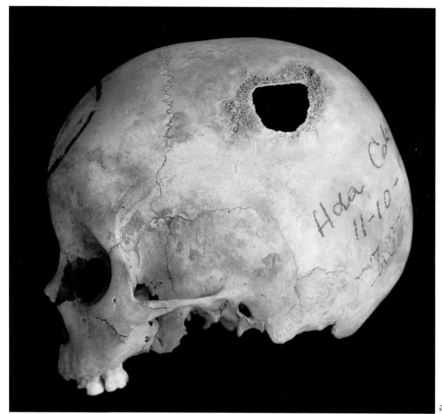

a

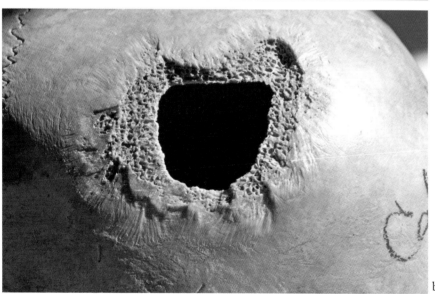

b

Figure 3.18
Overall (a) and
detail (b) views of a
cranium cataloged as
"trepanned," but which is
more likely an example
of postmortem breakage
and rodent gnawing.
Hacienda Cabildo, Peru.
Museo Regional de Ica,
00863-12, 11-10-1969.

sagittal suture, which lies over a major venous sinus) might have been avoided as well. Hippocrates advised against trepanning over the sutures, and nineteenth-century Berber surgeons of Algeria reportedly avoided them as well (see Chapters 1 and 8). Even modern neurosurgeons prefer not to do craniotomies over the sagittal suture, to avoid the risk of tearing the sagittal sinus.

All trepanned crania were photographed, as were non-trepanned crania with fractures. In the early stages of this study, we did some experimentation with radiography and computed tomography (CT) scanning of crania at the National Museum of Natural History (NMNH), but x-ray and tomography equipment was not available at most museums we visited, so we limited our study to macroscopic observations. We also decided to leave microscopic studies of cut marks and trepanation openings for a future project.

DRIVING INLAND FROM THE CITY OF LIMA UP THE CARRETERA CENTRAL, one leaves the frequently overcast and gray coast to emerge in the sunny foothills of Chosica, today a popular lunch spot and escape from the capital city. Continuing inland one follows curving roads higher into the western chain of the Andean *cordillera* and enters the province of Huarochirí (Figure 4.1). Here in remote areas adjacent to modern towns are ruins of habitation sites, burial houses (*chullpas*), and burial caves (*machays*) dating to Inca times and earlier. The burial houses and caves once were filled with mummies and skeletal remains of the ancestors of the modern Huarochirí population. Centuries of abandonment, intentional destruction by colonial authorities, and depredation by explorers and artifact hunters have emptied most of these structures of all but a few scattered bones and pottery fragments. At one time, however, they contained a wealth of physical evidence of trepanation.

The central highlands of Peru are important to the trepanation story for several reasons. The largest number of trepanned skulls in the New World come from two provinces in this region: Huarochirí and Yauyos. More than five hundred of these skulls are in the collections of major anthropology museums, and many others are in regional museums and private collections. The central highlands skulls are important because they are the principal data source for the great majority of publications on trepanation in ancient South America. They form the basis for most published statistics on success rates, surgical techniques, and possible motivations for trepanning.

Unfortunately, most skeletal collections from the central highlands lack detailed information on provenance, context, and dating. Most were collected in the late nineteenth and early twentieth centuries from the floors of caves, rock shelters, and above-ground burial structures (Figures 4.2 and 4.3). Human remains in these tombs were mixed and scattered, and most collectors had little interest in determining the antiquity or cultural affiliation of the material. The problem of dating these burial structures continues, as William Isbell notes in his book *Mummies and Mortuary Monuments*: "Much like adjacent Junín, above-ground tombs of the chullpa variety are very common in the western Andes, but they have not been investigated enough to date them definitively. Popular knowledge associates

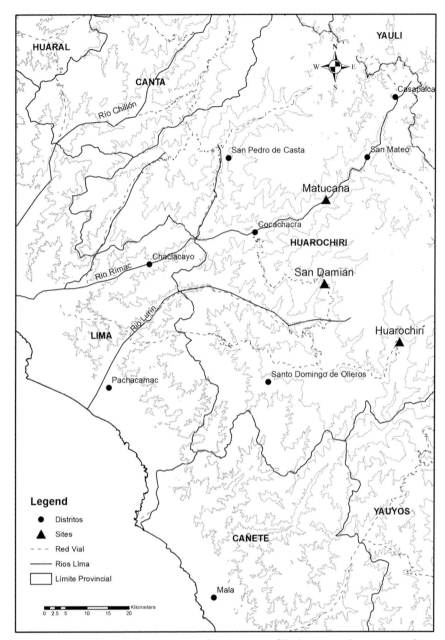

Figure 4.1 Map of Huarochirí Province, indicating some of the locations where trepanned skulls were collected by Julio Tello and Aleš Hrdlička. Map by Bebel Ibarra Asencios.

HOLES IN THE HEAD

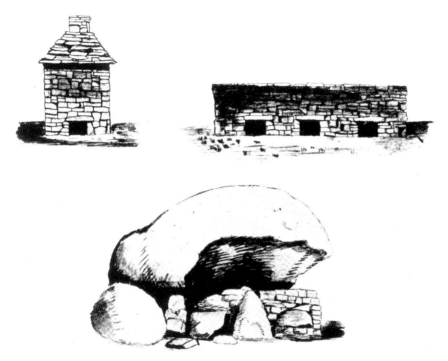

Figure 4.2
Two forms of chullpas and a machay from the sierra de Huachupampa, north of Matucana, Huarochirí Province. From a drawing by C. Palma, given to Aleš Hrdlička by Julio Tello (Hrdlička 1914:pl. 4).

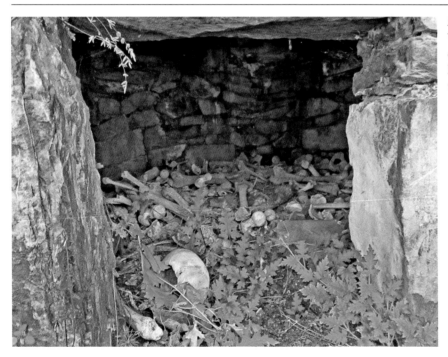

Figure 4.3
View of the interior of a chullpa with human bones littering the surface.

them with the people who occupied the area before the arrival of the Incas, implying a Late Intermediate Period date [ca. AD 1000–1400], with a continuation of the tradition into the Late Horizon and early colonial era" (Isbell 1997:192).

The best documented central highlands collections have information on the collection site, but many lack specific details even on their collections' places of origin or antiquity. Nevertheless, some skulls can be provisionally assigned a probable central highlands origin based on trepanation technique or the collection history of a particular museum.

THE COLLECTORS

Two anthropologists are responsible for amassing the largest collections of trepanned skulls from the central highlands: Julio C. Tello and Aleš Hrdlička (Figures 4.4 and 4.5). Both made systematic collections of human skulls and other skeletal material in the first decades of the twentieth century. While Tello's collecting focused primarily on trepanned skulls and examples of skeletal pathology, Hrdlička's was more broad. In addition to pathological specimens, Hrdlička set out to collect all the skulls he could find for the purpose of defining the "physical type" of ancient Peruvians, as well as to assist in building the

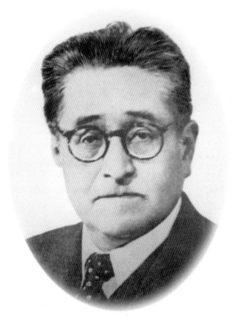

Figure 4.4 Julio César Tello. Courtesy of the Universidad Nacional Mayor de San Marcos, Lima.

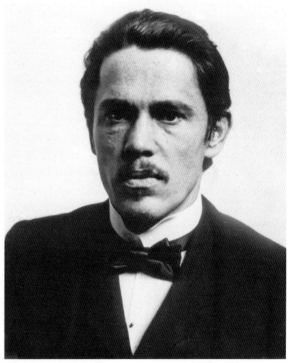

Figure 4.5 Aleš Hrdlička. Courtesy of the National Anthropological Archives, Smithsonian Institution.

skeletal collections of the United States National Museum, where he had been invited to direct the new division of physical anthropology in 1903 (Ubelaker 1999). Hrdlička's systematic collection of all complete crania makes his collections more useful for examining the frequency of head injuries, as will be described below. Tello's focus on trepanation and skeletal pathology resulted in collections that are more selective, although for the study of trepanation they remain unique and important resources.

EARLY DISCOVERIES OF CENTRAL HIGHLAND TREPANNED SKULLS

Tello and Hrdlička were not the first to explore central highland tombs in search of trepanned skulls. Some travelers and artifact collectors, like Manuel Antonio Muñiz, preceded them. Muñiz first called attention to this region and drew Tello's and Hrdlička's interest to the tombs of the Peruvian central highlands and their potential to shed light on ancient trepanation. During his travels throughout Peru in the early 1890s, Muñiz, who was then surgeon general of the Peruvian army, collected archaeological material. His particular interest, as a medical doctor, was in human remains, but as a military man he was also interested in weaponry, and he collected mace heads and other ancient weapons as well as skulls that showed injuries caused by them. With the assistance of local officials, he reportedly amassed a collection of more than a thousand crania, including nineteen with trepanations. The trepanned skulls came primarily from the Peruvian highlands in the Cuzco and Huarochirí regions, although two are recorded as coming from coastal sites: one from Pachacamac in the Lurín Valley and one from the Cañete Valley farther south. The Huarochirí skulls were collected from chullpas by the older brother of Julio Tello and presented to Dr. Muñiz by their father, then governor of Huarochirí.

In 1893, Muñiz brought his collection of trepanned skulls to the United States to be exhibited at the Columbian Exposition in Chicago, and he later donated them to the Bureau of American Ethnology in Washington, D.C. The collection was subsequently transferred to the National Museum of Natural History, Smithsonian Institution, where it can be found today. The fact that Dr. Muñiz brought the skulls to the United States turned out to be fortunate for their preservation, because while he was in the United States, political unrest broke out in Peru and his home was sacked and burned, resulting in the loss of his library and all of his archaeological collections.

In Chicago, Muñiz presented a paper describing his trepanned skull collection. This would later be included in an 1897 publication he coauthored with William McGee, then director of the Bureau of American Ethnology (Muñiz and McGee 1897). Muñiz begins his paper by noting that trepanation is generally recognized to have been practiced by prehistoric peoples in both the Old and New Worlds not only for religious purposes but also for practical surgical reasons, such as trauma and certain "cerebral diseases." In the case of Peru, he emphasizes that the types of weapons used in warfare (clubs, hatchets, and sling stones) produced a high frequency of depressed fractures of the skull. He argues that ancient Andean peoples developed advanced medical knowledge in the diagnosis and treatment of these fractures, as well as infections and other diseases, and that trepanation is a prime example of these medical advances. Muñiz further emphasizes that Peruvian trepanations were surgical procedures performed on living patients, not (as had been suggested for some Neolithic European skulls) postmortem operations for the collection of rondelles or amulets:

> The exaggerated veneration of the ancient Peruvians for their dead completely disproves the supposition, which as been advanced in regard to some other countries or peoples, that trephining was performed only for the purpose of procuring amulets from persons noted for valor, intelligence, or virtue. This profanation, if we may so call it, of the bodies of the dead was impossible in ancient Peru, and this fact is proved, since to this day there has never been found any fragment of human bone which could have been used as an amulet (Muñiz and McGee 1897:12).

Muñiz was probably correct, although Tello claimed to have found bone amulets in Huarochirí and in some Chanca burials. These were never published, however, and Pedro Weiss, who inquired about them, reported that "unfortunately, they have been lost" (Weiss 1958:521).

Later in the 1897 joint publication, William McGee describes the individual skulls and provides his own interpretation of their significance. It is here that a clear disconnect between the two authors appears, as McGee systematically discredits the notion that ancient trepanation demonstrates any real knowledge of anatomy or of skill in execution. McGee begins by presenting an evolutionary typology of trepanation, contrasting prehistoric and modern surgery by comparing their "methods," "motives," and "culture-grade." He concludes that modern surgical methods are "specialized" (using tools created for a specific purpose) and "refined" (skillfully performed), with a "therapeutic" motive that is "scientific" and "empiric"—all characteristics of a "civilized culture-grade." In contrast, prehistoric surgical methods are "primitive" (not using tools specifically created for surgery), with motives that are "thaumaturgic" (acting in an "occult or mystical way"), and reflect an "uncivilized" culture-grade. McGee concludes from his typology that "trephining was not originally a curative treatment; indeed, the early practitioners had no conception of real curative or restorative treatment, no glimmering of physiologic or etiologic knowledge, no idea of relation between health and disease, no definite notions concerning the conditions of life and the causes of death" (Muñiz and McGee 1897:20).

McGee saves his most brutal comments for the ancient Peruvian surgeons who performed the trepanations on the skulls in the Muñiz collection. Not only does he denigrate their medical and manual skills, but he goes further, even questioning their sense of geometric aesthetics: "There are many indications that the operators were (1) inexpert in manipulation, (2) ignorant of physiology, (3) skilless [sic] in diagnosis and treatment, and (4) regardless of the gravity of the operations performed. . . . and the apertures display an irregularity of form attesting unfamiliarity either with geometric proportion in general or with the production of geometric figures by means of the facilities and under the conditions represented by the work" (Muñiz and McGee 1897:61). McGee concedes that several trepanations in the Muñiz collection are associated with depressed skull fractures, and thus

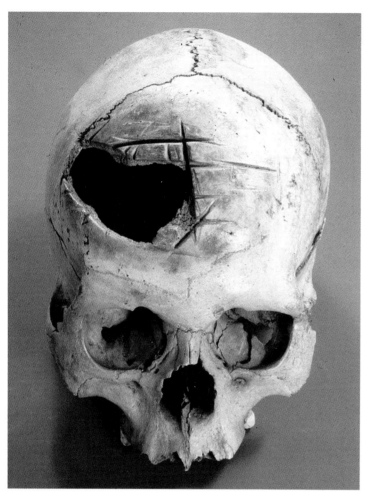

Figure 4.6
Trepanned cranium
from Huarochiri.
Muñiz collection.
National Museum
of Natural History,
Smithsonian
Institution, 178473.

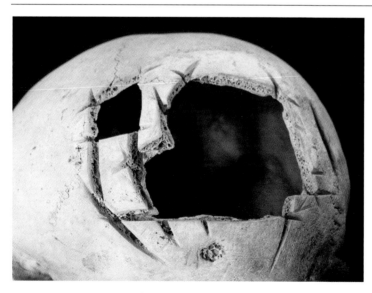

Figure 4.7
Trepanned cranium
collected by Hrdlička
from the site of Cinco
Cerros, near San
Damian. National
Museum of Natural
History, Smithsonian
Institution, 293785.

presumably were done for rational therapeutic purposes, although he characterizes them as poorly executed. He concludes: "In short, Peruvian trephining, as exemplified in the Muñiz collection, can only be regarded as crude in plan and bungling in procedure; and study of the procedure only occasions surprise that the results were not worse, and awakens admiration for the powerful vitality which enabled so large a proportion of victims to survive" (Muñiz and McGee 1897:63).

A "powerful vitality" seems to be the only positive thing McGee can say about ancient Peruvians. One can only imagine the disappointment Dr. Muñiz must have felt upon reading McGee's words. The two did not collaborate further, and although McGee notes in the prefatory note to the publication that "a more exhaustive discussion of primitive trephining in Peru by Dr. Muñiz may be looked for in the future" (Muñiz and McGee 1897:6), it appears that after this experience he lost interest in the subject. Given Dr. Muñiz's political problems back home, he also may have been preoccupied with other concerns.

William McGee's characterizations of "primitive" thinking and medical practices would disturb the sensibilities of any anthropologist today. To put this in perspective, however, it should be noted that Neolithic trepanners in Europe have been maligned by some authors as well. In 1929, paleopathologist Roy Moodie wrote: "Trephining arose among the ignorant, cave-dwelling, skin-clad hunters of the western part of Europe, who built no fine temples and palaces as did the ancient Egyptians and Greeks. They were crude and did not cultivate the love of the beautiful as did the ancient Peruvians" (Moodie 1919:495–496). At least Moodie gave some credit to ancient Peruvians for their sense of aesthetics.

Why was McGee so adamant about the lack of skill of ancient Peruvian surgeons? The answer may lie in some of the trepanations in the Muñiz collection. One skull from Huarochirí seems to have convinced McGee that ancient Peruvian trepanners were "bungling." The skull in question is one I sometimes refer to in my own lectures as an example of "surgery by committee." It appears that whoever was performing this procedure was uncertain how to approach the problem. The skull has a large, irregular opening in the frontal bone made by a series of cuts of varying orientation (Figure 4.6). McGee counted at least twenty cuts and grooves on the skull. Overall, their placement indeed suggests uncertainty and poor planning. The trepanation is surrounded by an area of dead bone, suggesting a prior head wound that led to necrosis. Alternatively, the periosteum may have been stripped from the skull during the trepanation procedure itself, causing subsequent death of the exposed bone. Whatever the case, the operation was unsuccessful, judging from the lack of any remodeling at the margins of the opening, and by the fresh appearance of the cuts and grooves around it.

Other skulls in the Muñiz collection do not show such apparent uncertainty. Most are relatively small single openings, and many show long-term healing, indicating a successful outcome. Of course, we cannot know why this particular skull proved so challenging to the operator or operators. Other examples of "indecisive" trepanations are known from the central highlands of Peru (e.g., Figure 4.7), and this has led some to suggest that ancient Peruvian trepanners may have experimented on cadavers (Moodie 1919; Ortner 2003). Personally, I agree with Muñiz that experimentation on cadavers is unlikely. Andean mortuary practices placed great emphasis on preserving the bodies of one's ancestors, and there was great fear associated with postmortem mutilation or lack of proper burial (Doyle 1988; Isbell 1997; Salomon 1995). Surgical training on cadavers seems unlikely in this cultural context, and hospitals and medical schools are not known to have existed in ancient Peru. Experimentation on dead or living enemies is conceivable, but trepanned skulls from the central and southern highlands are found in community mortuary structures and caves—an unlikely place to deposit the skulls of enemies. An alternative scenario for such poorly trepanned skulls might be a hurried operation on a gravely wounded and bloody patient. In such cases, as in modern-day trauma surgery, the need for quick intervention may have superseded concerns over aesthetics and geometric harmony. As will be seen, a significant number of central highlands trepanations treated skull fractures, some of which clearly were severe and life-threatening.

TELLO'S CENTRAL HIGHLANDS COLLECTIONS

Julio Tello was a native of Huarochirí and thus was intimately familiar with the abandoned ruins and chullpas in the region and the skeletal remains and mummies to be found therein. He was born in 1880, and would have been about eight to ten years old when his father presented Muñiz with twelve trepanned skulls from chullpas at the site of Chuicoto (Gonzáles and Daggett 2005; Lothrop 1948). Years later, as a college student, Tello came across Muñiz and McGee's 1897 publication while cataloguing books at the Biblioteca Nacional del Perú. He recognized some of the skulls he had seen and touched many years before. His childhood interest once again sparked, Tello spent his medical school breaks in 1905 and 1906 collecting skeletal material from tombs in Huarochirí and Yauyos. His collecting zeal reportedly led to some run-ins with local police (Astuhuamán Gonzáles and Daggett 2005) and made inhabitants of the region uncomfortable. Frank Salomon, who conducted ethnographic research in the Huarochirí area, wrote:

> Modern rural culture conserves a shadow of the conviction that in conducting the routines of production one is treading the domain of the dead, and that this warrants ritual caution. "The beautiful grandparents" (*los hermosos abuelos*) is a phrase by which modern Huarochiranos refer to the despoiled bones of ancestors, common in local ruins and caves. . . . In Huarochirí, this author repeatedly heard it said that the ancestors sent the pioneer archaeologist and Huarochirano Julio C. Tello a horrible disease to punish him for putting the mummies of his home into museums (Salomon 1995:336).

Despite some local resistance, Tello managed to gather an impressive collection of skeletal material from his home and neighboring provinces, a collection reported to have included more than ten thousand skulls (although this number is probably an exaggeration) and some four hundred trepanned skulls (Tello 1913). Tello gave lectures on this material while a medical student in Lima, and he originally considered writing his medical thesis on surgery in ancient Peru. Although he later decided to write his thesis on the skeletal evidence for syphilis in ancient Peru (Tello 1909), he did not lose interest in trepanation. In 1912, he presented the paper "Prehistoric Trephining among the Yauyos of Peru" at the Twenty-Eighth International Congress of Americanists in London. The paper was well received and published in the congress proceedings (Tello 1913). In this paper, Tello counters McGee's argument that trepanation in ancient Peru was practiced largely for religious or "thaumaturgic" reasons. He proposes instead that trepanation was inspired by four principal motives, all of which were therapeutic: (1) for antecedent fracture; (2) for scalp injuries that denuded the periosteum; (3) for circumscribed infection (periostitis or osteitis); and (4) for syphilitic lesions. Tello presents examples from his collection that highlight each of these, emphasizing the rational and appropriate surgical approach in each case. He concludes that the ancient trepanners of the Yauyos region were surprisingly successful, with approximately 250 out of 400 trepanned skulls (63 percent) showing some degree of healing.

Unfortunately, despite his plans to write more extensively on trepanation, Tello did not publish anything else on the subject. Before giving his paper in London, he had sold a portion of his trepanned skull collection to the Warren Museum of the Harvard Medical School (later transferred to the Peabody Museum of Archaeology and Ethnography). The remainder of his osteological material was divided between the Museo Nacional de Antropología, Arqueología, y Historia del Perú and the Museo de Arqueología y Antropología de la Universidad Nacional Mayor de San Marcos. Tello's collection at the Peabody Museum has been studied and described in part by T. Dale Stewart (1958), and it was the focus of a Harvard honors thesis (Meyer 1979), but it has not otherwise been published. The portion of Tello's collection donated to the MNAAHP has been examined, photographed, and included in publications by various Peruvian researchers (Graña et al. 1954; Lastres and Cabieses 1960; Weiss 1953, 1958), but these are general overviews of ancient trepanation that provide little information on the geographic origin or context of the crania.

After his early interest in trepanation in the central highlands, Tello became involved in numerous archaeological research projects on the coast and in the highlands of Peru. In 1925, he found trepanned skulls littering the surface around recently looted tombs at the early site of Paracas on the south coast of Peru. Tello made brief descriptions of these skulls in his report of the excavations (Tello and Mejía Xesspe 1979), but he apparently decided to leave detailed study of the collection to others (see Chapter 8).

ALEŠ HRDLIČKA

Among the attendees at Tello's presentation to the International Congress of Americanists in 1912 was Aleš Hrdlička. At the time, Hrdlička was actively building skeletal collections at the Smithsonian Institution in Washington, D.C., and he asked Tello for assistance in locating suitable collection sites in Peru. In 1913, Tello guided Hrdlička to sites around Huarochirí, where Hrdlička made substantial collections of skeletal material, including many trepanned skulls (Gonzáles and Daggett 2005).

Aleš Hrdlička was born in 1869 in Humpolec, Bohemia (now the Czech Republic) and immigrated with his father to the United States at age thirteen. After completing his secondary education, Hrdlička went on to study medicine at the Eclectic Medical College of the City of New York and the New York Homeopathic Medical College. After a brief stint in private practice, he accepted a position as a staff physician at the State Homeopathic Hospital for the Insane in Middletown, New York. At this post, Hrdlička developed an interest in applying anthropology to the study of mental illness, and he was invited to be an anthropology associate on a newly formed research team at the Pathological Insitute of the New York State Hospitals. To better prepare himself for this appointment, Hrdlička requested leave to attend classes at the École d'Anthropologie and to study anthropometric techniques at the École Pratique des Hautes Études in Paris. After completing these studies and visiting a number of medical and anthropological research centers in Europe, he returned to the Pathological Institute, where he recorded anthropometric data of patients and collected skeletons and autopsy specimens for further research. In 1899, he resigned from the Pathological Institute and became affiliated as a field anthropologist with the American Museum of Natural History, where he conducted anthropometric surveys of American Indians of the southwest United States and northern Mexico from 1899 to 1902 (Buikstra et al. 2012; Loring and Prokopec 1994; Spencer 1997).

In 1903, Hrdlička moved to Washington, D.C., to accept the post of assistant curator in charge of establishing a physical anthropology division in the United States National Museum. He was promoted to curator in 1910 and would spend the rest of his career at what is today the National Museum of Natural History (NMNH) at the Smithsonian Institution (Stewart 1981). Considered the founder of American physical anthropology, Hrdlička devoted a significant amount of his time to building the human osteology collection of the NMNH, which remains to this day the largest collection of its kind in the world. In 1910 and 1913, he made expeditions to Peru to collect material for the museum. Interested in the peopling of the New World and in the antiquity of human occupation of the Americas, he judged Peru a particularly important area of study. In the introduction to his short monograph on the results of his first expedition he writes:

> Peru may be regarded, even in its present territorial restriction, as the main key to the anthropology of South America. Due to the numbers of its ancient inhabitants, and to their far-reaching social differentiations, indicating long occupancy, a good knowledge of the people of Peru from the earliest times is highly desirable, and would constitute a solid basis from which it should be relatively easy to extend anthropological comparison to all the rest of the native peoples of the Southern Continent (Hrdlička 1911:1).

Peru also attracted Hrdlička because of the extensive looting of prehistoric cemeteries occurring at the time. Although the disturbance of tombs can be traced to ancient times in Peru, the large-scale destruction of cemeteries and monumental architecture began with commercial looting projects of the early colonial period that literally "mined" pyramids and tombs for precious metals (Zevallos Quiñones 1994). More informal looting of ancient cemeteries in search of ceramics, textiles, and other artifacts was ongoing in the late nineteenth and early twentieth centuries, when archaeologists and physical anthropologists began scientific fieldwork there. Hrdlička found cemeteries all along the coast of Peru being actively worked by *huaqueros* (grave robbers), who left objects deemed to be of little commercial value (undecorated ceramics, simple textiles, and mummies and bones) scattered on the surface (Hrdlička 1914:fig. 1).

Visiting the great pilgrimage center and burial ground of Pachacamac in 1910, Hrdlička was amazed by what he saw, although he admitted that at the same time he was excited by the opportunity presented to him: "On the writer's arrival, the place looked like a veritable Golgotha, or some great barbaric battlefield, with skulls and bones whitening the ground and ruins in every direction." But, he continues, "in one sense, of course, these conditions, however they may be regretted, proved of great service, giving an invaluable opportunity for investigation and collection of skeletal material" (1911:5). Hrdlička collected more than 2,200 skulls and thousands of postcranial bones from the surface of Pachacamac and shipped them back to the Smithsonian. He then traveled north to the Chicama Valley, a short drive north of the city of Trujillo, where he was a guest at the hacienda of Victor Larco, a prominent landowner. Larco generously offered Hrdlička transportation and manpower to visit and collect skeletal material from the surface of over thirty looted cemeteries in the Chicama Valley. During this expedition, Hrdlička collected more than 1,100 crania and thousands of postcranial bones. Hrdlička noted that skull fractures were common at Pachacamac, and he mentions finding one trepanned skull there, although he does not illustrate or describe it further (Hrdlička 1911:12). He found no trepanned skulls in any of the Chicama Valley cemeteries. This is consistent with later archaeological investigations; apparently trepanation was not practiced on the north coast of Peru.

In 1913, Hrdlička returned to Peru for a longer and more ambitious collecting mission. The directorate of the Panama-California Exposition, which would be held in 1915 in San Diego, California, requested his help in assembling an exhibit on physical anthropology. Ancient disease and surgery were to be the focus of one section of this exhibit, and Hrdlička was asked to assemble examples of skeletal pathology. He spent three months in Peru in early 1913 collecting more than one thousand pathological specimens from both coastal and highland sites. As in his 1910 expedition, he did not excavate, but instead took advantage of the ongoing looting of cemeteries on the coast and the accessibility of highland caves and above-ground mortuary structures, which provided large and easily collected samples. After personally supervising the installation of the exhibit in San Diego, he donated the pathology collection, including fifty-nine trepanned skulls, to the San Diego Museum of Man (SDMM). The remaining portion of the collections Hrdlička made on his 1913 expedition, including non-pathological specimens he gathered for population studies as well as seventy-five trepanned skulls, were accessioned into the collections of the National Museum of Natural History.

Reading Hrdlička's account of his 1913 expedition, it is clear that it was very successful, but not as pleasant as his first experience in Peru. Unlike what must have been first-class treatment as a distinguished guest at the Larco hacienda in the Chicama Valley in 1910, his second visit to Peru was more challenging, particularly in the remote highland areas he visited:

> Due to adverse climatic conditions, poor means of communication and transportation, the backward state of the people, and the prevalence of infectious diseases, the journey proved uncommonly difficult. . . . Serious obstacles were encountered

on the part of the natives, ignorant, superstitious, unwilling, and enfeebled by alcohol. Reliable information or help was out of the question; and due to the general poverty and the season, it was almost impossible to secure the necessary animals, or food for them when secured (Hrdlička 1914:1, 8).

Hrdlička's expedition coincided with the beginning of the rainy season in the highlands, and he traveled through areas where bartonellosis, a serious and potentially fatal disease, was endemic. In the highlands, he traveled by mule, and sometimes he had to climb steep mountain trails at night or in the rain, something he found most unpleasant. His characterization of natives as "superstitious" is in reference to guides and field assistants who did not share his eagerness to crawl into highland tombs and handle human remains.

Hrdlička was also disappointed that many of the tombs in the Huarochirí area had already been picked over for pathological skeletal material. He complained that "the exploration would have been prolonged had it not been found that the majority of the more approachable ruins had been visited by Tello or his native friends, who secured whatever seemed more valuable of the skeletal remains for the collection that was later sold to Harvard" (1914:8–9). One gets the impression that Hrdlička was cranky on this second trip. But he managed, despite obstacles, to achieve his objective. He returned to the United States with an exceptional paleopathological collection, as well as much additional skeletal material for the National Museum of Natural History.

Other than his 1911 and 1914 reports on his Peruvian expeditions and their preliminary findings, Hrdlička never published extensively on these skeletal collections, although he personally cataloged the material and wrote descriptions of each pathological specimen for the San Diego Museum of Man's accession records (Rogers 1938:322). He included a discussion of New World trepanation in a short article in the *Journal of the American Medical Association* in 1932, and he wrote a broader survey of trepanation for a 1939 *Ciba Symposia* publication (Hrdlička 1932, 1939). This second article briefly surveys ancient trepanation worldwide and then focuses on ancient Peru, illustrating his arguments with photographs and descriptions of some of the skulls he brought back from his 1913 expedition. Like Tello, Hrdlička argued against McGee's theory that ancient trepanation in Peru was done crudely, irrationally, and primarily for magical reasons. He also praised the high success rate of ancient New World trepanners: "The operation, present large collections show, was not in general of thaumaturgic nature, as had been supposed, but surgical and curative, partly for wounds of the skull, partly in all probability for painful and other affections of the head and brain." And: "With rare exceptions, the operation among the Indians, everywhere, was followed by normal healing, without the bones showing any signs of inflammation or suppuration" (Hrdlička 1939:177).

Hrdlička's observations on possible motivation and survival rates are sound, as they are based on his careful examination of specimens collected in Peru. One exception, however, is his belief, based on secondary accounts, in the use of "stoppers" to plug trepanation holes:

While most of the perforations were of moderate size, at times the wound was so extensive that it involved a large opening, with the consequent danger of extrusion (hernia) of the brain. In such cases the Andean primitive surgeons used various objects for "stoppers." In some cases these consisted of a gourd, or perhaps a bone; in others they used portions of shell; and in still others, though these were rare, they used beaten silver. (The writer heard of three such cases in Peru.) These stoppers were evidently effective, for the several skulls in the U.S. National Museum collection which indicate their use show that the subject survived the operation for a sufficient length of time to permit more or less cicatrisation (1939:174–175).

Hrdlička never directly observed examples of these "stoppers," but apparently believed accounts he had heard in Peru. Stories of gourds or other objects used to cover trepanations continue to be repeated (Marino and Gonzales-Portillo 2000; Verano and Andrushko 2010), although there have never been any convincing cases documented. The lack of decisive evidence, as well as the knowledge that foreign objects in wounds are not tolerated by the body, has led most to doubt such secondhand accounts (Cabieses 1974:2:281; Lastres and Cabieses 1960:156–157; Weiss 1958:620). While Tello did find a mummy at Paracas with a thin hammered sheet of gold placed over an unhealed trepanation, this was more likely a grave offering than a surgical implant (see Chapter 8).

Two other cases of trepanations covered with metal are exhibited in a private museum in Lima and have been illustrated in several publications (e.g., Marino and Gonzales-Portillo 2000:fig. 20). The skulls have rectangular trepanations with openings perfectly sealed with gold plates. The skulls have no documented provenance (although the form of the trepanations is typical of the central highlands), and their authenticity is questionable, as is the case with many of the Pre-Columbian metal objects in the museum (Verano and Andrushko 2010). It is more likely that these specimens were "accessorized" to make them more appealing to a private collector. Nothing like this was ever found in the hundreds of trepanned skulls collected by Tello, Hrdlička, and others.

RESEARCH ON HRDLIČKA'S TREPANNED SKULLS

Although Hrdlička did not publish much on his trepanation collection, other scholars have conducted studies of individual specimens (Burton 1920) or examined broader issues, such as trepanation techniques and healing (Moodie 1919; Rogers 1938). In 1980, the San Diego Museum of Man published a photographic catalog of the entire Hrdlička paleopathology collection, with detailed descriptions of each specimen by paleopathologist Charles Merbs (Tyson and Alcauskas 1980). This catalog, with its excellent photographs and descriptions, proved most useful for our own study.

T. Dale Stewart, who assumed Hrdlička's position upon his retirement, did not examine the SDMM collection, but he published several important articles based on his observations of Tello's collection at Harvard University and the trepanned crania that were brought back by Hrdlička to the Smithsonian Institution (Stewart 1950, 1956, 1958). Together, these two collections include 187 skulls with a total of 214 trepanations (Stewart 1958). Stewart's 1958 article is important because it is one of the few studies of a large collection of trepanned skulls that presents numeric data on survival rates and the locations where trepanations were placed. Most preceding publications, and many since, lack systematic observations, making it hard to evaluate their conclusions.

In the Tello collection skulls (112 operations), Stewart found that most trepanations were located on the frontal (53.6 percent) and parietal bones (33.0 percent), with fewer on the occipital area (15.4 percent). He noted that 48.2 percent of trepanations were placed on the left side of the skull, 29.5 percent on the right side, and 22.3 percent on the midline. According to Stewart, these differences make sense if trepanations were done to treat skull injuries resulting from face-to-face violent encounters. The front of the skull would be most vulnerable to such injuries, and the left side more prone to injury from a right-handed assailant wielding a club. He found no evidence that specific areas of the skull (such as over the sagittal and transverse venous sinuses or over the frontal sinuses) were avoided in surgery. Stewart also noted that children were trepanned as well, and that more than half of these children had skull fractures that appear to have been the motivation for trepanning.

To generate an estimate of survival rates, Stewart combined the Tello and NMNH collections with his observations on a collection of twenty-seven trepanned skulls from the southern highlands of Peru and Bolivia at the American Museum of Natural History. He produced the following statistics, based on a total of 214 trepanations:

Complete healing:	55.6 percent
Beginning healing:	16.4 percent
No healing:	28.0 percent

Keep in mind that these numbers are based almost exclusively on trepanations from the central highlands. Stewart's sample does not include Paracas skulls, which show lower success rates (see Chapter 5), and it contains only a few southern highland trepanations, a region in which substantially higher success rates are found (see Chapter 7).

THE CENTRAL HIGHLANDS SAMPLE

For this study, we recorded data on central highland trepanned skulls from the following museum collections: the National Museum of Natural History, Smithsonian Institution; the Peabody Museum of Natural History, Harvard University; the San Diego Museum of Man; and the Museo Nacional de Antropología, Arqueología, y Historia del Perú in Lima, Peru. In total, our database contains 421 trepanned skulls from this region. We also examined all non-trepanned central highland skulls in these collections in order to record the frequency and location of skull fractures. We suspected that head injury was common in ancient inhabitants of this area based on a cursory review of the Hrdlička paleopathology collection, which contains some spectacular examples of skull fracture. Our examination of the other collections confirmed our suspicions: skull fractures were indeed very common. As will be discussed below, central highlands trepanned skulls show the most frequent association with skull fractures of any regional sample from Peru, suggesting that trepanation flourished here as a practical treatment for head injury.

Sample Size and Demographic Characteristics

The age and sex distribution of the central highlands sample is presented in Table 4.1. Among adults, males clearly outnumber females, and this is a highly significant difference ($\chi^2 = 18.4$, $df = 1$, $p < 0.001$). This may reflect the fact that males have a higher frequency of skull fractures than do females, and thus they were more likely to receive trepanations to treat these injuries (see Motives for Trepanning, below). Unlike some other regions of Peru and Bolivia, intentional cranial deformation is rare in the central highlands, and only a few trepanned skulls in our sample show cultural modification of skull shape. This is important, because the data dispel the notion that trepanation was done to treat headaches or other neurological side effects of skull shaping, at least in the central highlands (Figure 4.8).

What most distinguishes this sample from other Andean regional collections, however, is the number of trepanations performed on children. Other than three crania from the Chachapoyas region of northern highland Peru (see Chapter 6) and two from the Cuzco region (see Chapter 7), we have not found trepanned children in any of the other South American samples. Apparently this was a practice limited primarily to the central highlands. The Tello and Hrdlička collections contain a total of nineteen trepanned children (Table 4.2). Based on dental development, the youngest was a toddler, approximately three years of age (Figure 4.9). The cranium has some preserved soft tissue and three cervical vertebrae still attached to the base. In the superior view (Figure 4.9a), the parietal bones show an unusual degree of lateral expansion, and bone reaction (both lytic and blastic) is visible around the margins of a large defect on the top of the cranium. While there is some postmortem breakage, most of the defect's margins seem to be intact, suggesting that the cranium had an unusually large anterior fontanelle. The expanded vault and large defect in the parietal bones suggests that the infant may have suffered from hydrocephaly, and that the trepanation was done in an attempt to relieve intracranial pressure. The only indication of surgical intervention is a linear grooved cut on the right parietal bone parallel to the sagittal suture. The cut shows no evidence of bone remodeling, indicating that the infant died during or shortly after the operation.

The other children in the central highlands sample range in age from about five to twelve years, with most falling in the seven- to ten-year age range. The motivation for trepanning many of these children was to treat acute head injury. Fifteen of nineteen, or 80 percent, are associated with visible skull fractures or penetrating wounds (Figures 4.10 and 4.11). Two crania show trepanations associated with fractures and areas of necrotic bone that were in the early stages of healing, but they apparently became infected (Figures 4.12 and 4.13). Of the children who had skull fractures treated by trepanation, only one case shows long-term healing (Figure 4.14).

Table 4.1 Age and sex distribution of the central highlands sample (n=421).

ADULT MALES	ADULT FEMALES	ADULTS OF UNCERTAIN SEX	CHILDREN AND ADOLESCENTS
238 (65.7%*)	124 (34.3%*)	22	37

*percentage of adult males and females that could be sexed.

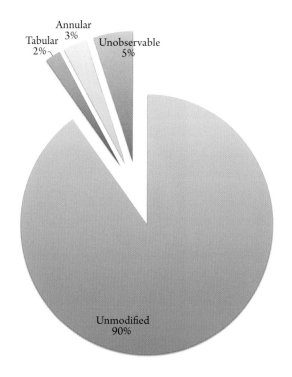

Figure 4.8
Cranial deformation
in central highlands
trepanned skulls (n=421).

Annular
3%
Tabular
2%
Unobservable
5%

Unmodified
90%

Table 4.2 Trepanned children and association with skull fractures in the central highlands sample.

DATABASE REFERENCE NUMBER	AGE	ASSOCIATED WITH VISIBLE INJURY?
NMNH 006	9–11 years	yes
NMNH 035	10–11 years	yes
NMNH 068	7–8 years	no
NMNH 077	8–10 years	yes
NMNH 079	child, uncertain age	yes
NMNH 082	child, uncertain age	yes
MNAA 020	10–12 years	no
MNAA 021	7–10 years	yes
MNAA 043	4–6 years	no
MNAA 106	child, uncertain age	yes
MNAA 164	7–9 years	yes
MNAA 173	5–6 years	yes
PEA 023	2–3 years	no
PEA 082	6–7 years	yes
PEA 119	6–7 years	yes
PEA 150	5–6 years	yes
PEA 172	10–11 years	yes
PEA 211	11–12 years	yes
PEA 246	6–7 years	yes

Figure 4.9

(a) Superior view (anterior is up) of the cranium of a three-year-old child with a linear cut visible on the right parietal bone (white arrow); and (b) inferior view of the same cranium, showing erupted deciduous teeth, preserved soft tissue, and several cervical vertebrae still attached by mummified tissue. Collected by Tello from Sacsa. Peabody Museum of Archaeology and Ethnology 56-42-30/ N8378.0 © 2016 President and Fellows of Harvard College.

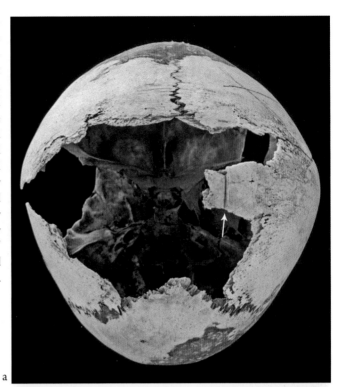

a

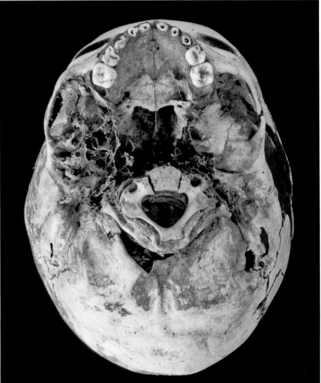

b

HOLES IN THE HEAD

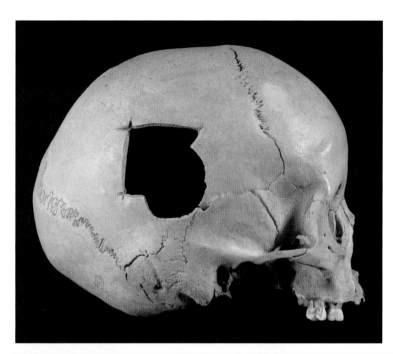

Figure 4.10
Cranium of an eight-
to ten-year-old child
collected by Hrdlička
from Cinco Cerros. It
shows a semicircular
broken area (possible
sling stone injury)
with a triangular area
cut out of its superior-
posterior margin.
There is no evidence
of healing. National
Museum of Natural
History, Smithsonian
Institution, 293315.

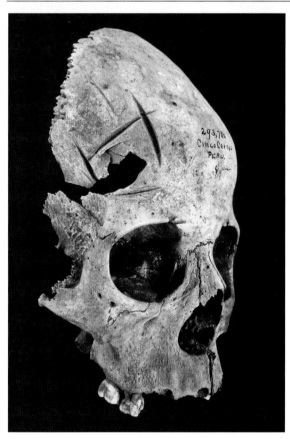

Figure 4.11
Partial cranium of a
ten- to eleven-year-old
child with a depressed
fracture or penetrating
wound of the right frontal
bone, with an attempted
trepanation by linear
cutting. The trepanation
was not completed, and
there is no evidence of
bone reaction. Collected
by Hrdlička from
Cinco Cerros. National
Museum of Natural
History, Smithsonian
Institution, 293780.

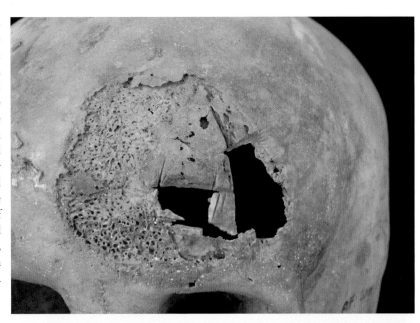

Figure 4.12
Cranium of a seven- to nine-year-old child with apparent skull fracture, necrotic bone, and inflammation of the frontal bone. Multiple linear cuts through the necrotic bone and fractured areas appear to mark an unsuccessful attempt to treat the wound. From the site of Tuna. Museo Nacional de Antropología, Arqueología, y Historia del Perú, AF:9993.

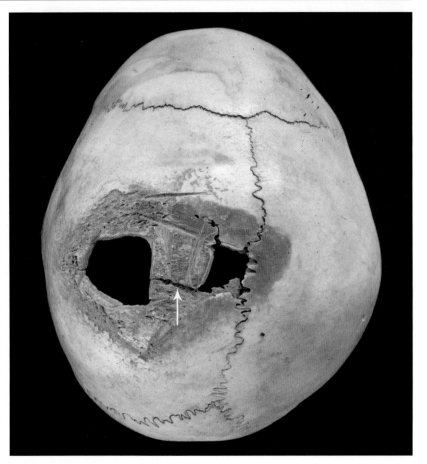

Figure 4.13
Cranium of a five- to six-year-old child with a large patch of necrotic bone and a linear fracture extending laterally from the sagittal suture (arrow). Two trepanations are located in the area of necrotic bone. The one on the left shows smoothing of its margins, indicating partial healing; the smaller opening to the right appears to show some healing as well. The openings may have been made to treat the fracture, but without success. From the Tello collection (no provenance), Museo Nacional de Antropología, Arqueología, y Historia del Perú, AF:10003.

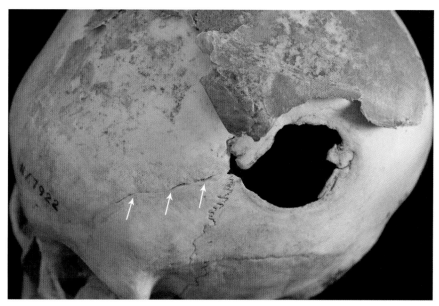

Figure 4.14 Cranium of a five- to six-year-old child collected by Tello from Auguipa. It shows a healed trepanation on the left parietal bone associated with skull fracture, marked by adherent bone fragments on the margins of the defect and a linear fracture extending along the frontal bone from the anterior margin of the defect (arrows). Smoothing of the margins of the defect and partial union of the edges of the linear fracture indicate survival for some period of time. Peabody Museum of Archaeology and Ethnology 56-42-30/N7922.0 © 2016 President and Fellows of Harvard College.

Trepanation Locations

Central highlands trepanations are most frequently located on the frontal bone (43.1 percent), followed by the left side of the vault (22.9 percent), right vault (14.7 percent), occipital (13.5 percent), and along the midline (6 percent) (Figure 4.15). Areas of the cranium covered with heavy musculature, such as the nuchal region of the occipital and the temporal fossa, appear to have been avoided. Only one trepanation was found in the nuchal area and only 7.5 percent of trepanations in the temporal fossa. We predicted that these areas would be avoided due to the risk of heavy bleeding and damage to important neck and chewing muscles, and the low frequencies support this. Apparently no attempt was made to avoid cranial sutures, however, since 38 percent of central highland trepanations cut through them.

Trepanation Number

Unlike in the southern highlands (Chapter 7), individuals with multiple trepanations are relatively rare in the central highlands collections. Of the 421 skulls in our sample, 363 have single trepanations, 55 have two, and only 2 individuals have three trepanations done at different times. These numbers do not include skulls in which multiple openings were made during a single operation. Most examples of these are trepanations using the drilling or drilling and cutting method, in which multiple holes were drilled into the skull (see

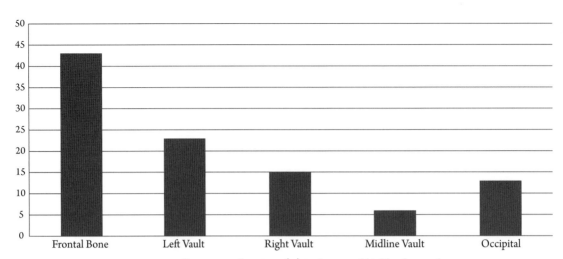

Figure 4.15 Trepanation locations (%) in the central highlands sample.

Techniques and Tools, below). In other cases, multiple openings—typically linear cuts, but also circular openings—appear to mark exploratory openings placed around the site of a depressed fracture (Figures 4.16 and 4.17). I recall discussing cases such as these with an emergency physician some years ago. He noted that these exploratory openings were precisely what he might do if he were presented with a skull fracture and possible blood clot and did not have access to x-ray or CT equipment. Clearly, ancient trepanners had to rely on experience and simple diagnostic techniques; these isolated cuts may have been attempts to identify sites of intracranial bleeding.

In contrast to the southern highlands of Peru (Chapter 7), relatively few central highlanders with a successfully healed trepanation returned for another. Identifying such cases is straightforward if the degree of healing differs markedly between one opening and another, as in a cranium from the Tello collection (Figure 4.18). Likewise, where healed trepanations are located on different areas of the skull and do not have margins that overlap one another, they may be assumed to have been done at different times (Figure 4.19). In cases where multiple openings are located adjacent to one another and are linked by areas of remodeled bone, such as in Figure 4.20, it is difficult to know if all of the holes were made at once or at different times.

Success Rates

Survival following a trepanation procedure is determined by evaluating bone reaction around the margins of each defect. Of a total of 497 trepanations, 161 (32.4 percent) show no sign of bone reaction. In these examples, scraped or cut bone still shows the striations left by the instrument used to make the holes, and there is no smoothing of edges or porosity surrounding the opening that would indicate a vital response. In these cases, the patient would have died during the procedure or within about a week following it. A total of seventy-four trepanations (14.9 percent) show porous areas and necrotic bone around the margins of the defects, marking hyperemia and the initial phases of bone remodeling,

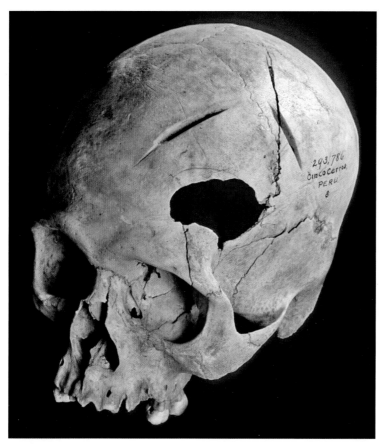

Figure 4.16
Cranium of an adult male with a skull fracture marked by a jagged-edged defect with radiating and concentric fractures. Two linear cuts were placed above and posterior to the defect, one crossing a linear fracture extending out from its posterior margin. No evidence of bone reaction. Collected by Hrdlička from Cinco Cerros. National Museum of Natural History, Smithsonian Institution, 293786.

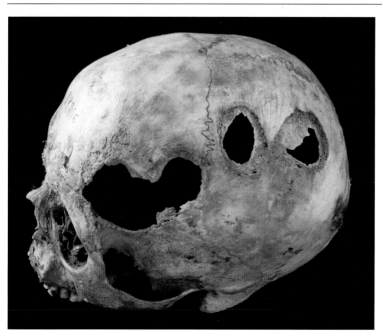

Figure 4.17
Cranium with a fracture to the left frontal bone showing short-term healing (porous areas and osteoclastic activity around the anterior margins of the defect) and three trepanations. The most anterior trepanation intersects the area of skull fracture, while the other two are located posterior on the left parietal bone. The trepanations appear fresh, with no signs of healing. Collected by Tello from Paukaruri. Peabody Museum of Archaeology and Ethnology 56-42-30/N8206.0 © 2016 President and Fellows of Harvard College.

Figure 4.18
Adult male with two trepanations done at different times, as indicated by degrees of healing. The first (above) shows extensive remodeling of the edges of the opening and what was probably necrotic bone surrounding it. The second trepanation, which is associated with a depressed skull fracture and an area of necrotic bone in the early stages of remodeling, shows no evidence of bone reaction. Collected by Tello from Cushula. Peabody Museum of Archaeology and Ethnology 56-42-30/N7936.0 © 2016 President and Fellows of Harvard College.

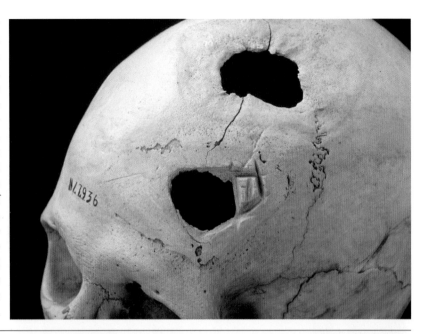

Figure 4.19
Adult male with three well-healed trepanations. Collected by Hrdlička at Cinco Cerros, near Matucana. San Diego Museum of Man, 1915-2-310.

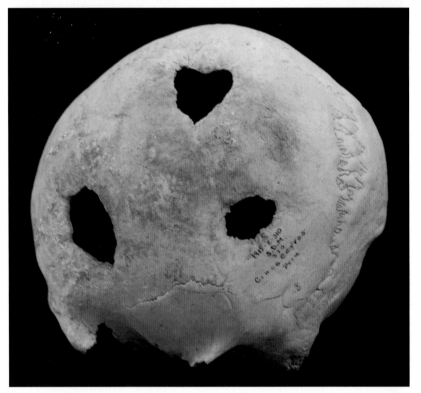

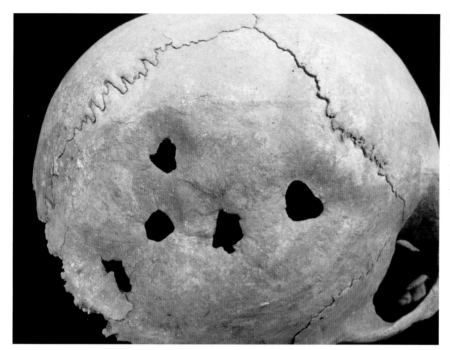

Figure 4.20
Adult cranium with a large oval area of remodeled bone with five small openings that appear to have been made at the same time. Museo Nacional de Antropología, Arqueología, y Historia del Perú, AF:4912, Wambu Chaka.

indicating survival of perhaps several weeks. A further 262 trepanations (52.7 percent) show extensive remodeling of their margins, marking long-term survival (Figure 4.21). These statistics are quite similar to Stewart's data, referenced above, and indicate that more than half of the central highlands trepanations were successful. By today's standards this might not seem impressive, but it is far superior to the 75–90 percent mortality rates reported by nineteenth-century surgeons in Europe and North America (Chapter 9; Aufderheide 1985).

While healed trepanations are easily distinguished from unhealed trepanations, interpreting the sequence of events in cases of trepanations surrounded by necrotic or inflamed bone is more complicated. Areas of dead bone and osteoclastic activity surrounding a trepanation may represent postoperative infection or bone necrosis from loss of blood supply when the scalp and periosteum were cut or removed. Stewart has conducted the most detailed study of these cases (Stewart 1956). He notes that roughened areas around healed trepanations from the central highlands are often angular in shape, and suggests that they mark where the scalp and periosteum were removed during surgery. Stewart identifies a number of healed trepanations in the Hrdlička collection that clearly demonstrate his hypothesis (Figures 4.22 and 4.23). Given the regular shape and clearly defined borders of many of these roughened areas, Stewart rules out infection, since there is no anatomical basis for infection spreading and stopping so regularly without natural barriers to proliferation, such as muscle attachments or sutures. Stewart concludes that the roughened areas indicate that instead of cutting a scalp flap and retracting it, a rectangular section of scalp was simply cut away. He theorizes that the bone reaction seen on the outer table was caused not by infection but perhaps by the application of some caustic substance to the

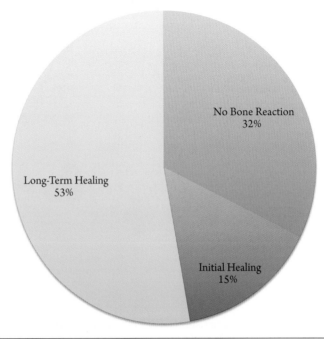

Figure 4.21
Success rates of
central highlands
trepanations (%).

No Bone Reaction
32%

Initial Healing
15%

Long-Term Healing
53%

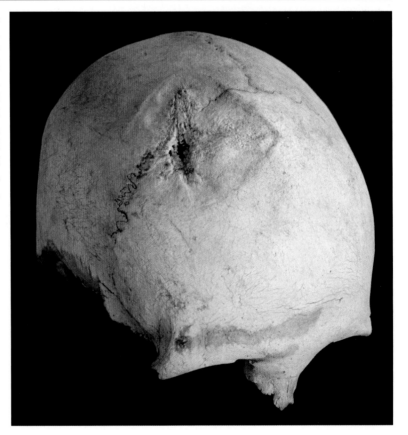

Figure 4.22
Partial adult cranium
with a healed irregular
opening surrounded
by a square area
of remodeled
bone. Collected
by Hrdlička at San
Damian. National
Museum of Natural
History, Smithsonian
Institution, 293384.

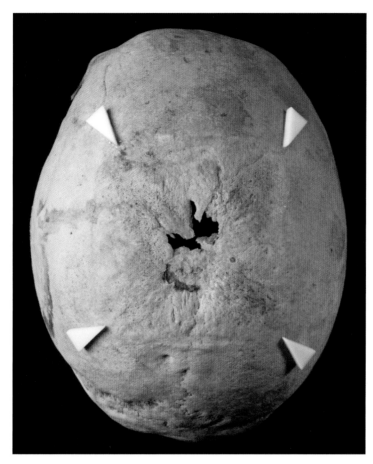

Figure 4.23
Adult female with a healed irregular opening surrounded by a square area of remodeled bone. The white triangular markers indicating the four corners of the remodeled area were attached when the skull was put on display at the National Museum of Natural History. Collected by Hrdlička at Cinco Cerros, near San Damian. National Museum of Natural History, Smithsonian Institution, 293790.

wound following surgery. Stewart's argument for cutting away rectangular pieces of scalp would be strengthened if cuts marking the outline of these areas could be identified in skulls with unhealed trepanations. In our study, we looked carefully for these, but to date have observed only scattered and isolated cuts, none of which clearly mark the margins of such a rectangular area.

In some skulls, prior infection or bone necrosis from a blow to the head may, in fact, have been the reason for trepanning. Lastres and Cabieses, following an argument originally made by Tello (1913:78–79), suggest that in many cases the porous and necrotic bone surrounding trepanation openings predates the surgery (Lastres and Cabieses 1960:fig. 132). In other cases, however, they conclude that necrotic bone marks postoperative osteomyelitis (Lastres and Cabieses 1960:figs. 125, 128, 129). More recently, Donald Ortner discussed the problem of determining the sequence of events in trepanations associated with infection and bone necrosis. He used as an example a cranium from the Hrdlička collection that he interpreted as an aborted trepanation of a necrotic bone fragment surrounded by an inflammatory reaction (Ortner 2003:173–174). In his 1956 article, Stewart describes the same cranium and interprets it as infection following the trepanation. In the absence of clinical data on these skulls, the issue remains a mystery.

Techniques and Tools

Central highlands trepanners experimented with a variety of techniques. These include scraping, drilling, drilling and cutting, circular grooving, linear cutting, or some combination of the above (Figures 4.24 and 4.25). The method most distinctive to the central highlands is that of rectangular or polygonal openings made by intersecting linear cuts (Figure 4.26). It is rare elsewhere in the Andes. Only three trepanations using this method have been reported from the Cuzco region of the southern highlands (Squier's skull and two other examples described in Chapter 7). This is also the least common trepanation technique worldwide. Only two prehistoric examples of rectangular trepanations have been reported from the Old World. Both were found at the site of Lachish (Tell Dueir) in Israel (former Palestine) and have trepanations made by intersecting linear incisions. They could easily be confused with central highland Peruvian examples (Parry 1936; Risdon 1939; Starkey 1936).

Various researchers have argued that the linear cutting method was a particularly dangerous one. Stewart considered it "technically unsound" because the linear cuts (which usually extend considerably outward from the trepanation opening) would require a larger area of skull to be exposed than trepanations by scraping or circular grooving. This made more of the skull surface vulnerable to infection and loss of blood supply (Stewart 1958:482). Others have noted that the cuts made by this method produce "canoe-shaped" (Muñiz and McGee 1897) grooves that, given the convex curvature of the skull, are deepest at their central point, increasing the risk that the dura mater might be cut accidently, leading to infection and death. Some have even suggested that the technique was never successful, since examples of well-healed trepanations by this method have not been identified.

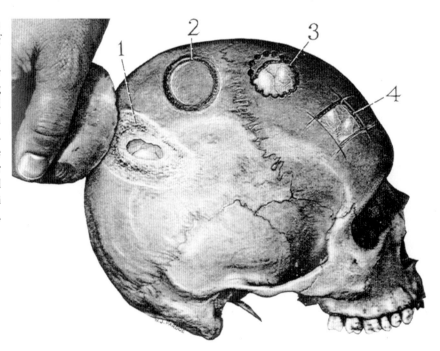

Figure 4.24
Illustration of trepanation methods: (1) scraping, (2) circular grooving, (3) drilling and cutting, and (4) linear cutting with angular intersections. Not shown: simple drilling and linear cutting with curved margins (Lisowski 1967:fig. 1).

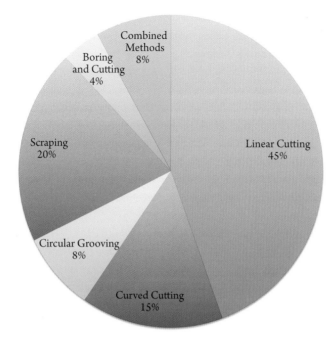

Figure 4.25
Trepanation techniques in the central highlands (n=226 unhealed or partially healed trepanations).

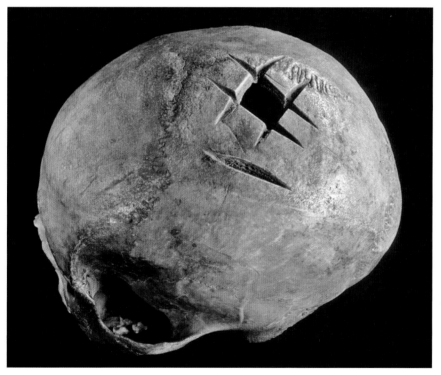

Figure 4.26
Adult male from Huarochirí with a rectangular trepanation and an isolated linear cut lateral to it. Fine cut marks, presumably from cutting the scalp, can be seen below the isolated cut and both anterior and posterior to the rectangular opening. There is no indication of bone reaction. From the Muñiz collection, National Museum of Natural History, Smithsonian Institution, 178469.

Fernando Cabieses, a Peruvian neurosurgeon who has long had an interest in ancient trepanation, disagrees with the suggestion that no healed rectangular trepanations exist. In a publication with medical historian Juan Lastres (Lastres and Cabieses 1960), he includes an extensive discussion of the healing of trepanations, arguing that contrary to common belief, the margins of trepanned openings do not grow inward during healing, but retract as a result of inflammation and the resorption of dead bone, creating an enlarged defect with beveled edges. He argues further that the healing process itself obliterates any evidence of the original cut or saw marks around the trepanation, producing an opening that is roughly oval or circular in form. Cabieses suggests that well-healed rectangular trepanations would have a final shape indistinguishable from a scraped trepanation of similar size. He made a similar argument for trepanations made by the drilling and cutting method.

Cabieses's argument has merit. It is hard to imagine that a trepanation technique almost invariably fatal to the patient would be practiced so frequently in the central highlands of Peru. Although it is true that many trepanations by linear cutting were not successful, a significant proportion of these are associated with skull fractures, often severe (see below), and a number of cases document an attempt to save the life of a severely injured patient. It is indeed hard to find healed trepanations that preserve any evidence of linear cutting around their margins. In my own examination of more than four hundred central highlands crania with trepanations, I have found only one with a healed opening that may show the trace of a linear cut. It was collected by Tello from the locality of Hushana (Yauyos) and has a well-healed trepanation on the left parietal. On the anterior border of the opening is a linear depression that may mark a healed cut (Figure 4.27). Given its irregular and remodeled surface, one has to use one's imagination to see a linear defect crossing the anterior margin. This is as close as I have come to finding what may be a well-healed rectangular trepanation.

Given the uncertainty of identifying trepanation technique in healed cases, only cases where the technique is unambiguous (unhealed or short-term healing only) are considered here. As can be seen in Figure 4.25, trepanation executed by cutting, whether linear, curved, or circular, was the most common technique used in the central highlands. Here, I classify linear cutting as trepanations in which straight lines intersect to create openings in the form of squares, rectangles, or polygons (see, for example, Figures 4.11 and 4.26). "Curved" cutting refers to trepanations in which oval or other curved-edge openings were cut out (Figure 4.28). Circular grooving is a method in which a circular piece of bone is cut out, leaving a distinctively beveled hole (Figure 4.29). Unhealed scraping trepanations typically show broad areas with striations marking where the bone was gradually scraped away. The scraping may be limited to the outer table and diploe, or may continue through the inner table (Figure 4.30). The drilling and cutting method involves drilling a series of holes and cutting from one to the next to allow the removal of a disk of bone (Figure 4.31 and 4.32). "Combined methods" are those in which two or more techniques were used in a single trepanation procedure. The most frequent combination in the central highlands sample is linear cutting combined with scraping (Figure 4.33), but others, such as drilling and linear cutting, are found as well (Figure 4.34).

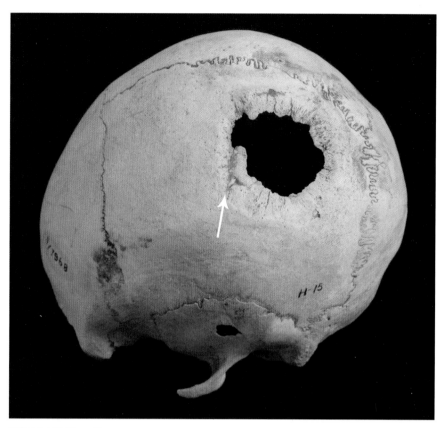

Figure 4.27
Adult female with a healed trepanation that preserves what may be evidence of a linear cut on its anterior margin (arrow). Collected by Tello from Hushana. Peabody Museum of Archaeology and Ethnology 56-42-30/N7968.0 © 2016 President and Fellows of Harvard College.

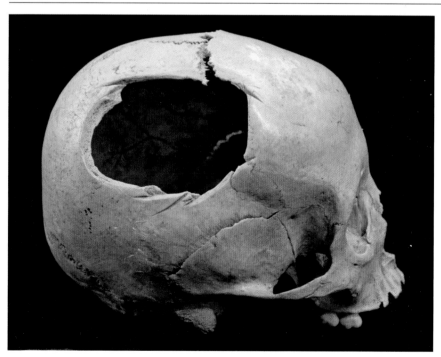

Figure 4.28
Adolescent female with an unhealed trepanation made by a series of curved cuts. Possibly associated with a skull fracture that separated the coronal suture and fractured the right parietal. Collected by Hrdlička at Cinco Cerros, near San Damian. San Diego Museum of Man, 1915-2-257.

Figure 4.29
Adult male with an
unhealed trepanation
created with the circular
grooving method.
This skull also has a
healed trepanation
or depressed fracture
(or both) above the
forehead. Collected
by Hrdlička at Cinco
Cerros. National
Museum of Natural
History, Smithsonian
Institution, 293792.

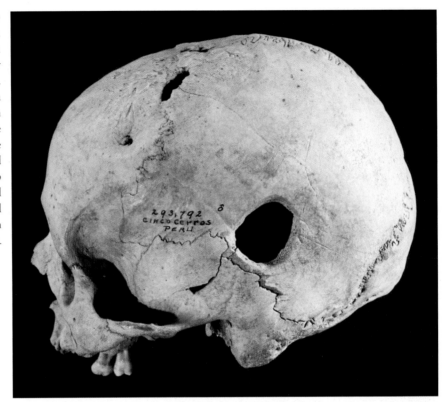

In some cases, classifying trepanation methods into discrete categories is more challenging. An example is a skull in the Tello collection from the site of Paukaruri (Figure
4.35). Two unhealed trepanations are present along the sagittal suture. One is complete
and shows the classic features of the circular grooving method. The other trepanation is
only partially complete. Although it shows a circular groove around its outer margin, the
center of the circular area was also scraped away, revealing the spongy bone beneath. Had
the scraping continued through the spongy bone and inner table, no circular bone plug
would have been removed, as is normally assumed in trepanations by circular grooving. In
this case, bone was removed through the action of both scraping and grooving, but only
the former is visible because one of the trepanations was not completed. A similar case
from the Tello collection is a skull from the site of Pukutay (Figure 4.36). Here, an area of
scraping is overlaid by a series of intersecting linear cuts. It appears that the area was first
scraped, and then a rectangular area was traced out by four perimeter cuts. Two deeper
oblique cuts connect with the former. Had the rectangular portion been removed, the
evidence of surface scraping would have been lost. Why were these two methods used?
Perhaps the initial scraping was done to examine a superficial contusion, and then it was
decided to remove a portion of bone. Whatever the motivation, the result was not successful, as there is no indication of bone healing.

A number of skulls from the central highlands show isolated linear cuts or clusters of
cuts that do not intersect to define a portion of bone to be removed. These enigmatic cuts

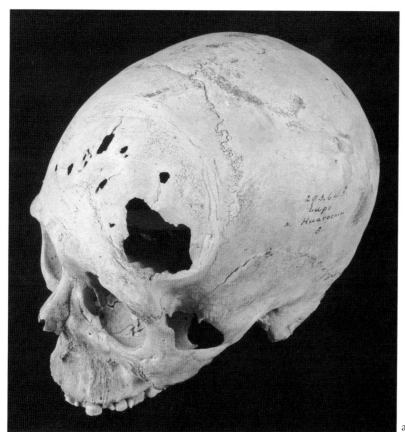

a

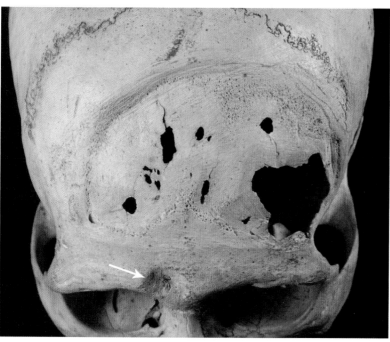

b

Figure 4.30
(a) Adult male with a
large trepanation created
with the scraping method,
apparently associated with
a fracture above the left
eye; and (b) a healed injury
over the right eye (arrow).
Collected by Hrdlička at
Lupo, near Huarochirí.
National Museum of Natural
History, Smithsonian
Institution, 293643.

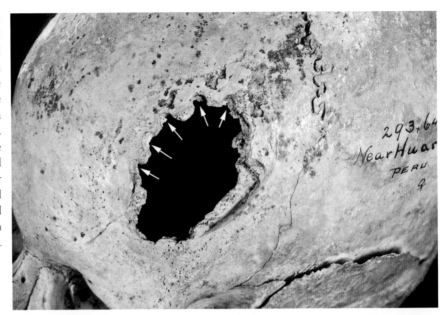

Figure 4.31
Trepanation created using the drilling and cutting method, with holes drilled around the margins of a fracture and through an area of necrotic bone. There is no evidence of healing. Collected by Hrdlička near Huarochirí. National Museum of Natural History, Smithsonian Institution, 293642.

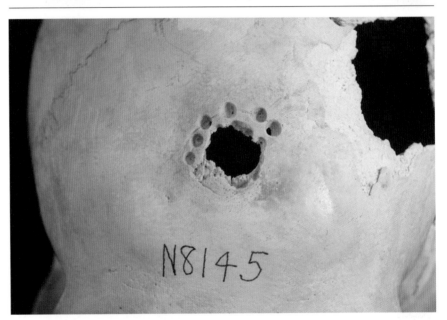

Figure 4.32 Cranium of an adult male from Llactashica, showing incomplete trepanation using the drilling and cutting method placed around the margins of a depressed fracture or penetrating wound. Tello hypothesized that these holes were made by percussion with a copper rod (Tello 1913:82–83). Peabody Museum of Archaeology and Ethnology 56-42-30/ N8145.0 © 2016 President and Fellows of Harvard College.

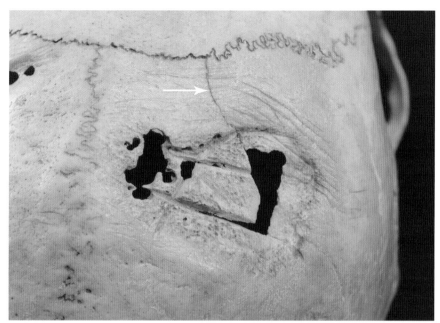

Figure 4.33
Combined trepanation using both the scraping and linear cutting techniques, apparently to treat a fracture (arrow). Cranium collected by Hrdlička at Lupo, near Huarochirí. San Diego Museum of Man, 1915-2-284.

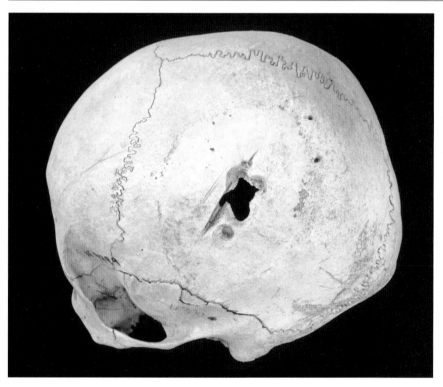

Figure 4.34
Combined trepanation involving both the drilling and linear cutting techniques. Cranium from Tuna. Museo Nacional de Antropología, Arqueología, y Historia del Perú, AF:9999.

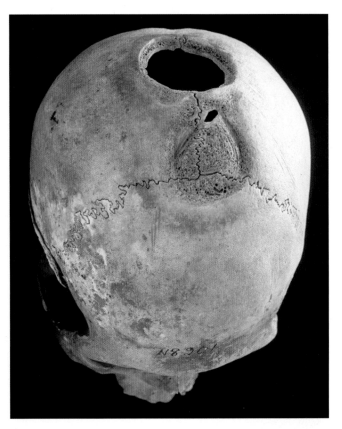

have been noted by various observers and interpreted as either incomplete operations, in
which the patient died before they were completed, or as openings made to allow for drainage or release of intracranial pressure (Lastres and Cabieses 1960:129; Weiss 1958). Indeed,
some cases appear to be trepanations that were begun but not completed for some reason,
such as in skulls from the sites of Tuna (Figure 4.37) and Cinco Cerros (Figure 4.38). In
other cases, the cuts appear to be exploratory, such as the cranium in Figure 4.16 and in
one Muñiz collection cranium from Huarochirí (see Figure 4.26). The latter example has a
classic square trepanation of intersecting cuts with a single isolated cut nearby. The isolated
cut is just as deep and carefully made as the others, indicating that it was not a false start
or slip of the knife. Perhaps it was an exploratory cut made prior to or after the cutting and
removal of the rectangular piece of bone.

Since the 1897 publication by Muñiz and McGee there has been continued specula-
tion about what tools were used to trepan skulls in the central highlands. McGee ruled
out metal tools, arguing that repeated grooving with stone tools were used to make linear
cuts. In a detailed description of an unhealed trepanned skull from Huarochirí, he writes:

> The preservation of the specimen is so perfect as to reveal even the faintest scratches
> produced in connection with the operation, and thus to indicate the character of
> the instrument and the mode of its use. The scratches, both random and at the

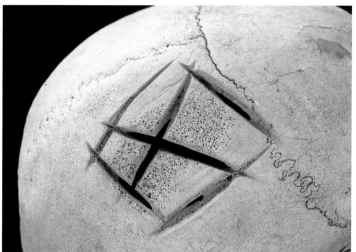

Figure 4.36
Combined
trepanation method
of linear cuts
superimposed on
a scraped area.
Cranium collected by
Tello from Pukutay.
Peabody Museum
of Archaeology and
Ethnology 56-42-30/
N8237.0 © 2016
President and Fellows
of Harvard College.

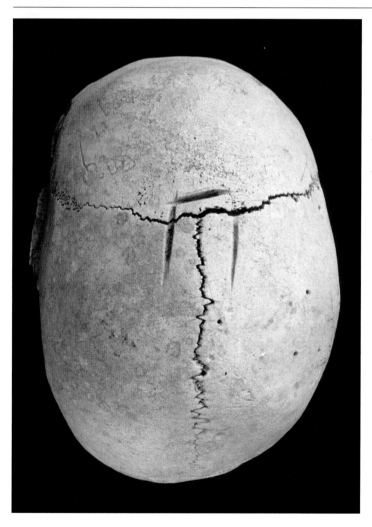

Figure 4.37
Incomplete
trepanation consisting
of three linear cuts.
Cranium from Tuna.
Museo Nacional
de Antropología,
Arqueología, y
Historia del Perú,
AF:9998.

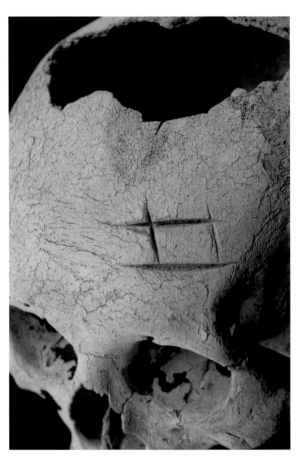

Figure 4.38
Incomplete trepanation
made by four intersecting
cuts. Collected by Hrdlička
at Cinco Cerros, near
San Damian. San Diego
Museum of Man, 1915-2-271.

ends of some of the incisions, show that the instrument had a single moderately
sharp point, thickening rapidly to three or four millimeters within six or seven
millimeters from the tip; that not only the point but the sides bit into and ground
away the bone as it was manipulated; and that the manipulation could only have
been a reciprocal motion back and forth from end to end of the incision, accompanied by considerable pressure. It is noteworthy that no known metal instrument
or implement would produce the general and special features of the incisions in
this cranium, while all the features of incisions and scratches are precisely such as
would be produced by a sharpened stone in the form of a spearhead, arrowpoint,
or knife (Muñiz and McGee 1897:27).

Most subsequent writers agree that a stone tool is the most likely candidate for both linear
cutting and scraping trepanations in the central highlands (Lastres and Cabieses 1960:137–
140; Tello 1913). Although no tools specifically identified as trepanation "kit" have ever
been found in the central highlands, obsidian was available from highland sources and
was exchanged widely (Burger et al. 2000). Experiments performed by several Peruvian
surgical teams using actual Inca metal tools found that *tumis* (knives with crescent-shaped

HOLES IN THE HEAD

blades) were suitable for cutting the scalp and periosteum, but not of any use in cutting through bone. In two experiments done on living patients, success in removing a portion of cranial bone was achieved only by using a chisel-shaped metal tool and a hammer (Chapter 8; Graña et al. 1954; Lastres 1951).

With regard to trepanations by drilling and cutting, Tello suggested that the small, pointed, copper rods that he found in some Huarochirí tombs may have been used to punch out, rather than drill, the holes. With reference to a cranium he collected from the site of Llactashica (Figure 4.32), he wrote:

> The regularity of the markings of the hollows and the absence of any scratch round them make it probable that one of these rods acted perpendicularly by percussion . . . causing only the breaking of the outer layer. A stone instrument acting as a drill could not leave a trace of this nature. . . . This induced the writer to repeat the operation, by way of experiment, with one of the copper rods on a fresh cranium. The result obtained by percussion was an incision identical to that presented by the cranium now before us (Tello 1913:82–83).

Percussion would seem to be a particularly dangerous way to perforate the skull of a living patient. Drilling, while certainly a more time-consuming process, benefits from its gradual nature. But if a drill was used, what was it made of? Peruvian neurosurgeons Francisco Graña, Esteban Rocca, and Luis Graña sought to determine if bifacially flaked knives made of obsidian could have produced these holes. They found that the brittle volcanic glass fractured into small pieces and concluded that obsidian tools would not have worked as cranial drills (Graña et al. 1954). A skull that Hrdlička found at the site of Matucana may indicate otherwise. It has an incomplete trepanation in the form of eight holes drilled through the outer table. Embedded in the external wall of one of the holes is a fragment of dark material that appears to be stone or volcanic glass (Figure 4.39). No laboratory tests have been done to identify the composition of the fragment, so this awaits confirmation (Rose Tyson, personal communication 2007). The only other similar case I am familiar with is a prehistoric California skull with scraping and drilling marks on its frontal bone that have small fragments of obsidian embedded in them (Richards 1995).

Motives for Trepanning

Of all samples of trepanned skulls from Peru, those from the central highlands demonstrate most clearly that many trepanations were done to treat acute head injury. Tello, Hrdlička, and others noted the high frequency of skull fractures in the central highlands and suggested that trepanation evolved there as a practical approach to treating head wounds. In our own study, we tried to quantify the relationship between head injury and trepanation and to look more closely at the frequency and location of head injuries in the large collections of non-trepanned skulls Hrdlička brought back from the Huarochirí region.

To calculate the frequency of trepanations associated with visible skull fracture, we examined a total of 506 openings made in 420 skulls; 134 of the 506 trepanations, or

Figure 4.39
(a) Cranium with an incomplete trepanation by drilling; and (b) close-up view of trepanation showing a black object (arrow), possibly stone, embedded in the wall of one of the drilled holes. Collected by Hrdlička from Matucana. San Diego Museum of Man, 1915-2-283.

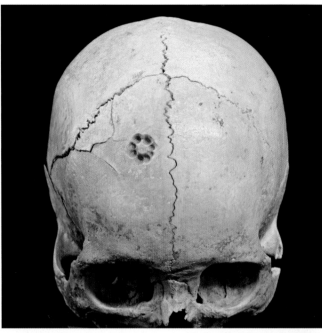

a

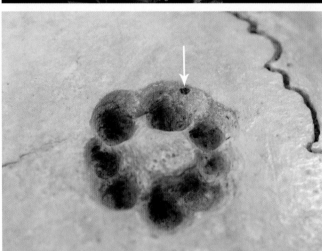

b

26.5 percent, were clearly associated with skull trauma. In many cases, these fractures were severe and were likely injuries with a poor prognosis for survival (Figures 4.40 and 4.41). In other cases, the fractures were less obvious and only identifiable by careful examination of the margins of skull defects (Figures 4.42 and 4.43). In 372 of 506, or 73.5 percent of trepanations, no evidence of skull fracture can be seen, although in some cases trepanations are located in areas of inflammation or necrotic bone, which suggests that they were meant to treat fractures and scalp injuries that had denuded the periosteum or had become infected (Figure 4.44). Our estimate of the association between trepanation and skull fracture is conservative, because it is likely that the evidence for some fractures was removed by the

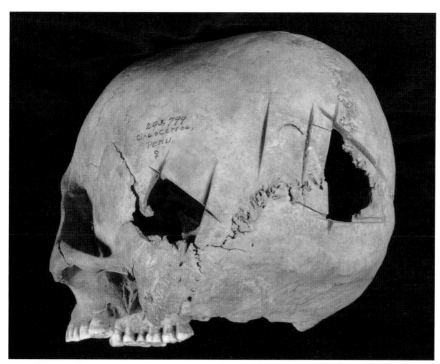

Figure 4.40
Cranium with multiple trepanation attempts placed over depressed fractures or penetrating wounds. Collected by Hrdlička from Cinco Cerros, near San Damian. National Museum of Natural History, Smithsonian Institution, 293799.

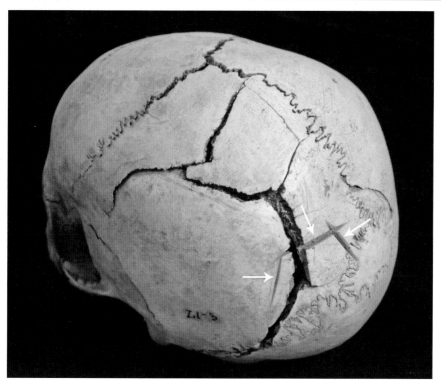

Figure 4.41
Incomplete trepanation by linear cutting on a cranium with massive blunt force injury. Collected by Tello from Llactashica. Peabody Museum of Archaeology and Ethnology 56-42-30/ N8076.0 © 2016 President and Fellows of Harvard College.

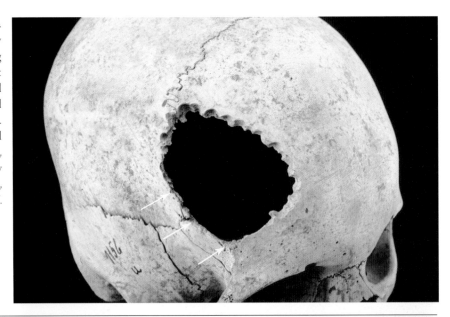

Figure 4.42
Trepanation by drilling and cutting placed adjacent to a depressed fracture with ragged margins (arrows). Museo Nacional de Antropología, Arqueología, y Historia del Perú, AF:2611, 1156U.

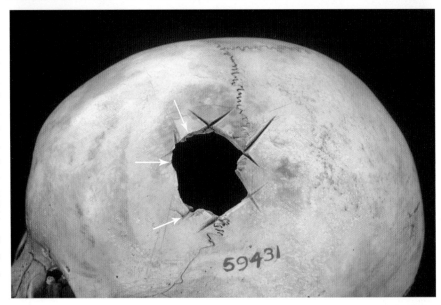

Figure 4.43
Six- to seven-year-old child with a trepanation by linear cutting placed over a depressed fracture or penetrating wound (arrows). No evidence of bone reaction. Collected by Tello from Kalwantuwi. Peabody Museum of Archaeology and Ethnology 56-42-30/59431.0 © 2016 President and Fellows of Harvard College.

procedure itself. We have recorded multiple examples of trepanations that were initiated over the site of a depressed fracture or penetrating wound but not completed. Had the circumscribed area been removed, all evidence of the injury would have been removed as well. Two examples, both children, illustrate this well. The first (see Figure 4.11) is an incomplete trepanation over a fracture site in a ten- to eleven-year-old child from Cinco Cerros. The injury is identifiable by the ragged edges and pieces of bone bent into the wound. Were the trepanation completed, these would have been removed. The second case, a skull collected by Tello from Hushana (Figure 4.45) is an incomplete trepanation on a ten- to eleven-year

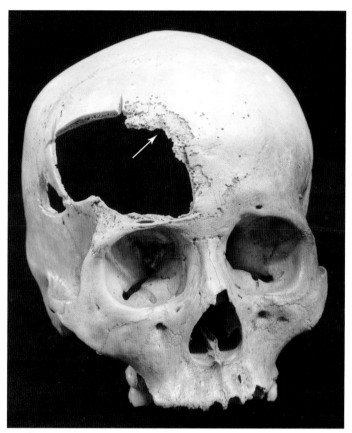

Figure 4.44
Adult male cranium showing a large trepanation by linear cutting over an area of necrotic bone and a defect with irregular margins marking a possible skull fracture (arrow). A smaller trepanation can be seen posterior to the larger one. Trepanation margins show no bone reaction. Collected by Hrdlička from Cinco Cerros. San Diego Museum of Man, 1915-2-311.

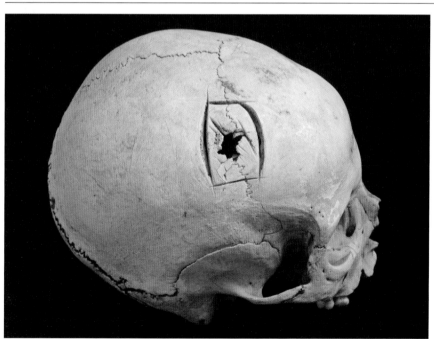

Figure 4.45
Cranium of a ten- to eleven-year-old child with an incomplete trepanation placed around a penetrating wound. Collected by Tello from Hushana. Peabody Museum of Archaeology and Ethnology 56-42-30/ N7967.0 © 2016 President and Fellows of Harvard College.

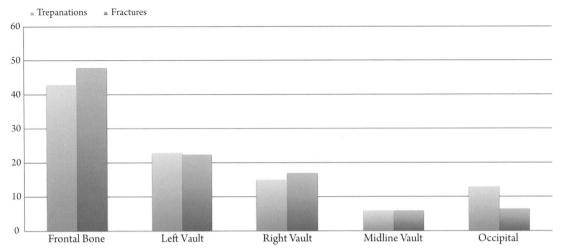

Figure 4.46 Comparison of the trepanation and skull fracture locations in the central highlands sample (%).

old child. Linear cuts were initiated around the site of a penetrating wound on the right side of the skull, defining a rectangular piece of bone that presumably was targeted for removal. The operation was aborted (perhaps because the child died), leaving the trepanation incomplete. Had it been completed and the bone removed, it would have taken with it all evidence of the wound. These two skulls serve as reminders that there are probably a number of cases in which trepanations erased the evidence for their purpose, particularly in crania where large portions of the skull vault were removed, such as in Figure 4.28. Even given the likelihood that fracture evidence was removed by some procedures, support for a strong association between skull injury and trepanation is indicated by comparing the locations of skull fractures and trepanations, both of which show the highest frequencies on the front of the skull, followed by the left side (Figure 4.46).

Fracture Incidence in Non-Trepanned Skulls

Tello's central highlands cranial collection was highly selective, as he focused on collecting trepanned skulls and examples of skeletal pathology. Thus, it is not possible to use his collections to generate statistics on the incidence of head injury or the percentage of individuals who were trepanned. Fortunately, Hrdlička's collection strategy was different, since his objective was to collect as much skeletal material as possible for the United States National Museum, with a particular interest in reconstructing Peruvian population history from skull shape. Hrdlička gathered all relatively complete skulls at the coastal and highland sites he visited, whether pathological or not (Hrdlička 1911, 1914). During his second expedition to Peru in 1913, he also sought examples of skeletal pathology to present at the 1915 Columbian Exposition, and he collected partial skulls and cranial fragments if they had fractures, trepanations, or other evidence of pathology (Tyson and Alcauskas 1980). To avoid potential bias, only complete crania were used to estimate the frequency of head injuries in the central highlands collections.

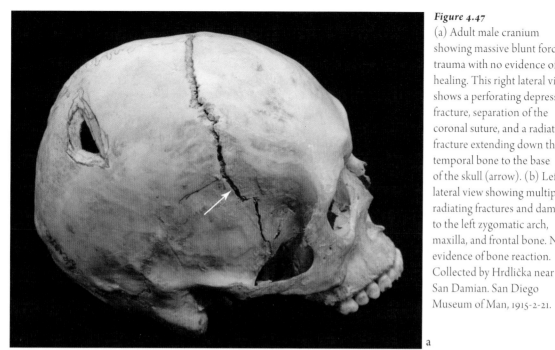

a

Figure 4.47
(a) Adult male cranium showing massive blunt force trauma with no evidence of healing. This right lateral view shows a perforating depressed fracture, separation of the coronal suture, and a radiating fracture extending down the temporal bone to the base of the skull (arrow). (b) Left lateral view showing multiple radiating fractures and damage to the left zygomatic arch, maxilla, and frontal bone. No evidence of bone reaction. Collected by Hrdlička near San Damian. San Diego Museum of Man, 1915-2-21.

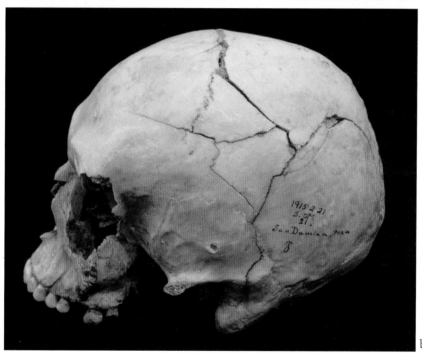

b

Figure 4.48
(a) Adult male cranium with two rectangular penetrating wounds (arrows) on the left side with radiating fractures extending anteriorly and posteriorly. No evidence of healing. (b) Superior view showing two penetrating wounds, separation of the coronal suture, and radiating fractures. No evidence of healing. Collected by Hrdlička from Cinco Cerros. San Diego Museum of Man, 1915-2-18.

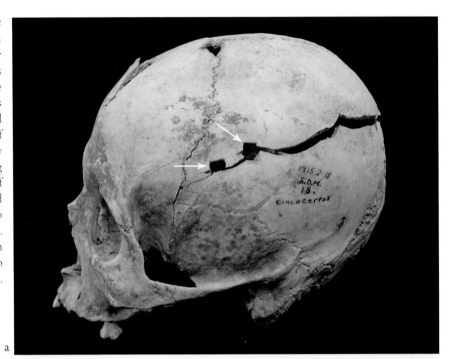

a

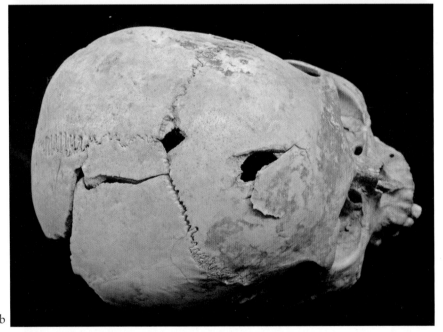

b

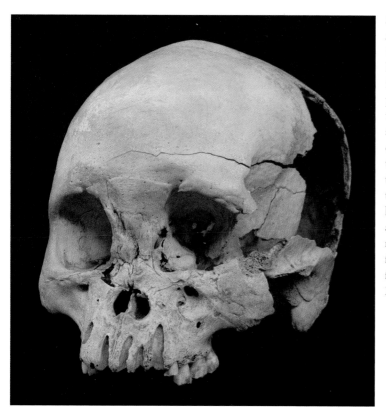

Figure 4.49
Adult male from Cinco Cerros with an extensive healed comminuted fracture of the face produced by blunt force trauma. Although he survived this injury, he later died from multiple blows to the left side and back of the skull. Partially visible in this photograph is a large hole in the left parietal and temporal bones and a radiating fracture extending forward and across the forehead. San Diego Museum of Man, 1915-2-5.

The Hrdlička collection has impressive examples of healed and unhealed skull fractures produced by clubs, sling stones, and other weapons. A number of crania show multiple unhealed blows and penetrating wounds, demonstrating a clear intent to kill rather than simply injure the victim (Figures 4.47 and 4.48). Some individuals survived massive fractures of the skull vault and face, but with deformity that would be quite visible in life (Figure 4.49). Others with healed fractures would likely have suffered from headaches and possible neurological deficits given the severity of their injuries (Figure 4.50; Chapter 10).

Not all healed fractures are as dramatic as the ones shown in Figures 4.47–4.50. Smaller, healed depressed fractures are recognizable as "dents" of varying size. Although visually less impressive, they also mark head injuries (Figures 4.51 and 4.52). To estimate the frequency of head injuries in the central highlands samples, Tulane doctoral student Brittany Dement and I examined all of the complete non-trepanned crania that Hrdlička brought back to the National Museum of Natural History and the San Diego Museum of Man. This comprises a total of 253 crania from the sites of San Damian, Cinco Cerros, Matucana, and Huarochirí. In Table 4.3, the samples are partitioned by sex and age to allow comparisons of relative risk of skull fracture in men, women, and children. Skull fractures are quite common in all groups, with the highest frequency in adult males, followed by adult females. The difference between fracture incidence in males and females is highly significant statistically, indicating that men were at greater risk of fracture than women. But children were

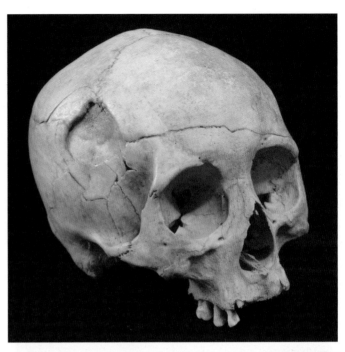

Figure 4.50
Adult female from
Cinco Cerros with a
large healed depressed
fracture of the right
temple. It shows
a central area of
impact with radiating
fractures extending out
in multiple directions.
San Diego Museum of
Man, 1915-2-348.

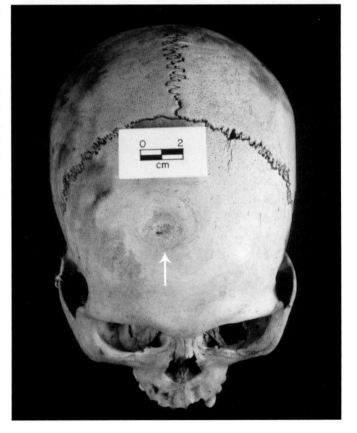

Figure 4.51
Adult male from
San Damian with
a small healed
depressed fracture
of the frontal bone
(arrow). National
Museum of Natural
History, Smithsonian
Institution, 293809.

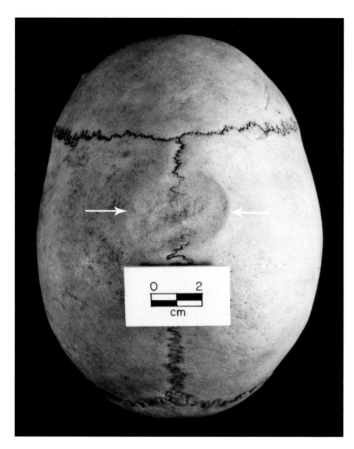

Figure 4.52
Adult male from
San Damian with
a healed depressed
fracture of the left
and right parietal
bones just posterior
to the bregma.
National Museum
of Natural History,
Smithsonian
Institution, 293813.

Table 4.3 Fractures in the central highlands sample.

SITE	N	ADULT MALES WITH FRACTURES (%)	ADULT FEMALES WITH FRACTURES (%)	CHILDREN WITH FRACTURES (%)
San Damian	160	60.9 (39/64)	31.5 (23/73)	15.0 (3/20)
Cinco Cerros	49	64.3 (18/28)	50.0 (10/20)	100.0 (1/1)
Matucana	28	69.2 (9/14)	33.3 (4/12)	75.0 (3/4)
Huarochirí	17	66.7 (4/6)	57.1 (4/7)	25.0 (1/4)
Overall	254	63.1%	36.6%	27.6 %

Combined data courtesy of Brittany Dement (Dement 2012).

not immune to head injuries: 27.6 percent of child crania had healed or unhealed skull fractures. Risk of fracture is similar among the four sites, indicating that the combined frequencies are not overly biased by one sample or another. Overall, these data indicate that populations in the central highlands of Peru had a high risk of head injury. Some of these fractures may be the result of falls or other accidents, but some are indicative of interpersonal violence.

Perhaps it is not surprising that trepanation flourished in this region given the high frequency of head injuries. Unfortunately, it is not possible to estimate what percentage of central highlanders were trepanned, given the complex history of skull collection in this region. Chullpas and burial caves were explored and disturbed many times, and it is not known how much material has disappeared into private collections or been destroyed by visitors to these sites. But the material collected by Tello and Hrdlička tells us that trepanation was widely practiced in this region.

:::

The central highlands of Peru were a major center for experimentation in trepanation, producing more than half of the trepanned skulls known from South America. Importantly, all of the known trepanation techniques are documented there. Unfortunately, the lack of dates and context for most crania precludes any regional study of the origins, spread, and evolution of trepanation. It is presumed that most trepanned skulls date to the late prehistoric period, before and after the incorporation of this region into the Inca Empire, but direct radiocarbon dating is required to confirm this. There are no descriptions of trepanation in any of the early written sources for the region, so it is unknown if and for how long the tradition continued into the colonial period. While there are scattered accounts of trepanations into modern times in the southern highlands of Peru and Bolivia (Chapter 7), none have been reported from the central highlands.

5   ORIGINS OF PERUVIAN TREPANATION

Paracas and the South Coast of Peru

LOCATED 260 KILOMETERS SOUTH OF LIMA AND SOME NINETEEN KILO-meters south of the city of Pisco, Paracas is a barren peninsula that juts into the Pacific Ocean (Figure 5.1). Its name is derived from the Quechua word *para-ako*, or "sand falling like rain," which refers to strong onshore winds that blow across the area in the afternoon hours (Paul 1991:1). In the early twentieth century, the term *Paracas* began to be applied to a distinctive style of textiles and ceramics that appeared at that time in the antiquity markets of Peru, Europe, and the United States. Paracas sites may date to as early as 900 BC in the Ica Valley, although radiocarbon dates are still relatively scarce for this time period and there continues to be some debate over Paracas chronology. Tombs on the Paracas Peninsula are believed to date from approximately 400 to 200 BC (DeLeonardis 2005; Paul 1991; Silverman 1991).

The Paracas Peninsula is extremely dry, and characterized by broad areas covered by windblown sand and a rocky hill known as "Cerro Colorado," named for its reddish color. Archaeological excavations by Tello revealed that the area around Cerro Colorado had extensive early human occupation, and that it had been an important burial site for centuries. Most importantly for the present discussion, the earliest trepanned skulls in the New World come from Paracas tombs. Trepanned skulls from Paracas are particularly important to understanding the origins and early development of cranial surgery in the New World. They document the earliest experiments with cranial surgery in the Americas, dating back to at least 400 BC (and perhaps earlier), making them contemporary with classical Greece and the Hippocratic Corpus. Although there is no evidence of contact between the Old and New Worlds at this time, it is nevertheless interesting to contemplate that at roughly the same time that Hippocrates was recommending trepanation for certain types of head injury and Greek surgeons were developing the first metal drills for making holes in skulls, similar experiments were underway across the Atlantic on the Paracas Peninsula using different tools and techniques but apparently with a similar therapeutic objective. But unlike ancient Greece, where only a few examples of trepanned skulls have been found at archaeological sites (Agelarakis 2006; Mountrakis et al. 2011; Papagrigorakis et al. 2014), more than sixty trepanned skulls have been recovered from the Paracas Peninsula cemeteries and

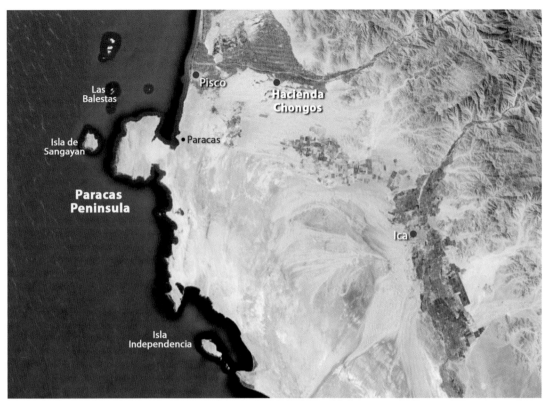

Figure 5.1 Southern coastal Peru, showing the Paracas Peninsula and the nearby site of Chongos in the Pisco Valley. Map image data from Google Earth/SIO, NOAA, U.S. Navy, NGA, Gebco, Image Landsat.

from contemporaneous sites in the nearby Pisco Valley. The Paracas Peninsula sample is important because it comes from a single archaeological site, and one with better chronological control than that of collections of trepanned skulls from the highlands of Peru, many of which lack specific information on provenance and dating.

Paracas trepanations stand out as well for their boldness. Although some skull openings are small, most are quite large. In fact, these are the largest trepanation openings found in the ancient Americas (Figure 5.2). Were there not evidence of bone reaction (and in many cases long-term healing), it would be tempting to dismiss these trepanations as simply the postmortem removal of portions of the cranium for some ritual purpose, like the perforated rondelles of cranial bone that have been found at some Neolithic sites in Europe (Clower and Finger 2001; Fletcher 1882; Piggott 1940; Prunières 1874). This can be ruled out in Paracas, because many openings show evidence of bone reaction, indicating that these were procedures done on living patients.

Interestingly, despite the importance of Paracas as an archaeological site and the extensive research that has been done on textiles from its funerary bundles (e.g., Dwyer and Dwyer 1975; Paul 1990, 1991), its trepanned skulls are less well known than those from the central and southern highlands of Peru. In fact, some recent surveys of trepanation in

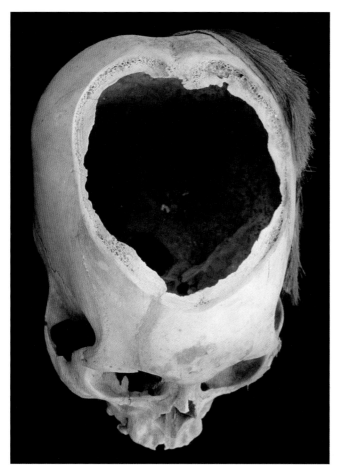

Figure 5.2
A trepanned skull from Paracas showing the removal of a large portion of the top of the skull. Museo Nacional de Antropología, Arqueología, y Historia del Perú, AF:6807, 12/5258.

ancient Peru do not include Paracas skulls at all, but focus exclusively on late prehistoric highland material (e.g., Rifkinson-Mann 1988).

The lack of attention given to Paracas trepanned skulls can be attributed to a number of factors. Because archaeological research on the Paracas Peninsula did not begin until 1925, early surveys of trepanation in Peru (Hrdlička 1914; Muñiz and McGee 1897; Tello 1913) naturally did not include this material. But another significant factor is likely the overwhelming number of mummy bundles that were excavated by Tello and his colleagues at Paracas in the late 1920s, many of which remain unopened and unstudied. While Tello and his principal collaborator Toribio Mejía Xesspe (1896–1983) opened some of the larger bundles and recorded detailed information on their contents (Tello 1929; Tello and Mejía Xesspe 1979), until recently much of these data remained unpublished and inaccessible to researchers (Daggett 1994; Gonzáles and Daggett 2005). Fortunately, the recent opening of the Tello Archives has permitted scholars to begin mining this rich data source and to create new catalogs of the materials held at the Museo Nacional de Antropología, Arqueología, y Historia del Perú and other museums (http://www.arqueologia-paracas. net/). This new research will help to better contextualize the Paracas material and clarify its chronology, which until now has been based on comparisons with ceramics and textiles from other south coast sites. A more intractable problem is that most of the trepanned crania collected by Tello were surface finds from around the looted tombs on Cerro Colorado. While they are clearly associated with tombs at the site, their original context is unknown. However, some trepanned skulls were found in intact mummy bundles and recorded by Tello and Mejía Xesspe, allowing comparisons with the material from disturbed tombs.

DISCOVERY AND EXCAVATION OF THE PARACAS PENINSULA SITES

According to Tello and Mejía Xesspe (1979), clandestine excavations on the Paracas Peninsula began around 1910, when a local fisherman discovered a burial in an area that later became known as "Arena Blanca" ("white sand") or "Cabeza Larga" ("long head") (Figure 5.3). The fisherman, a guard at a local guano factory who apparently moonlighted as a *huaquero* (grave-robber), first began to dig there secretly, searching for textiles, ceramics,

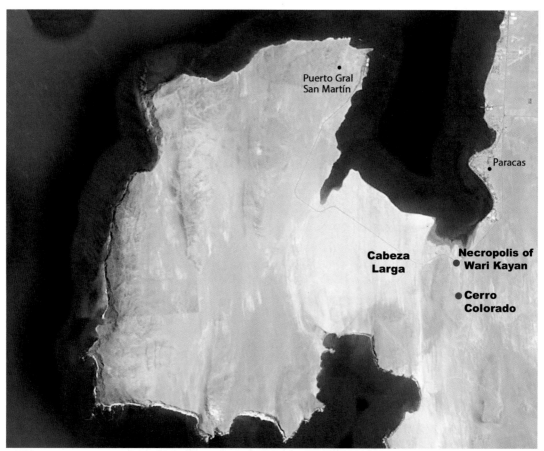

Figure 5.3 The Paracas Peninsula, with cemeteries indicated. Map image data from Google Earth © 2016 Digital Globe and Terra Metrics/SIO, NOAA, U.S. Navy, NGA, Gebco.

and other items to sell to local artifact collectors and dealers. These objects, especially the polychrome textiles wrapping the bodies (among the finest textiles ever produced in prehispanic Peru) were highly sought after by local collectors and dealers in Lima. The site soon became known to other huaqueros, who came to excavate there as well (Tello and Mejía Xesspe 1979:66). The unusual textiles also caught the attention of both Peruvian and foreign archaeologists, several of whom were able to trace their source back to a site somewhere on the south coast. Julio Tello was the one to locate the actual site, but by the time of his first visit in 1925, a great number of tombs had been disturbed, and bones, textiles, and other artifacts littered the surface of Cerro Colorado.

ARCHAEOLOGICAL INVESTIGATIONS

Tello arrived at the Paracas Peninsula on July 26, 1925, after a three-day trip from Lima. He was accompanied by North American archaeologist Samuel Lothrop, who had befriended him in Lima. Lothrop had some free time on his hands, so he offered to pay Tello for a short visit to archaeological sites of his choosing. They set off for the south coast with two of Tello's assistants in what Lothrop would describe as an old convertible with open sides and tires not much wider than those of a bicycle (Lothrop 1948; Tello and Mejía Xesspe 1979). Although not an ideal off-road vehicle, the car was equipped with wide running boards that would later prove useful for carrying a guide as well as for transporting materials collected on the expedition. The group headed south from Lima, stopping at various archaeological sites along the way, where Tello made surface collections of textiles and other materials from cemeteries that were being actively looted at the time. Upon reaching the city of Pisco, some eighteen kilometers north of the Paracas Peninsula, Tello spent a day searching for someone who could guide him to the tombs with elaborate textiles. He was fortunate to find the fisherman and huaquero Juan Quintana, who agreed to ride on the running board of the car and guide Tello to the site (Tello and Mejía Xesspe 1979).

Quintana led them from Pisco to the Paracas Peninsula, where he guided Tello to an area of looted graves that he identified as the cemetery he found in 1910. Apparently Quintana was being deceptive, because when Tello examined textile and ceramic fragments around the looted graves, he quickly recognized them as later material dating to the Chincha culture—not what he was looking for at all. Tello called Quintana's bluff and insisted he guide the car to the correct location, which he finally did (Daggett 2005; Tello and Mejía Xesspe 1979). There they found Cerro Colorado and adjacent sandy areas pockmarked with looters' pits. Human skeletal remains and scraps of textiles and sea lion skin were scattered around the holes. Tello immediately noted two unusual features of the skulls littering the area: distinctive shapes produced by intentional cranial modification and many large trepanations (Figure 5.4). Tello and his crew made a surface collection of one hundred skulls from around the looted tombs. He counted forty-four trepanned skulls, concluding that some 40 percent of the individuals buried in this area had been trepanned. This would have been an impressive number indeed, if it had been representative of the entire mortuary population.

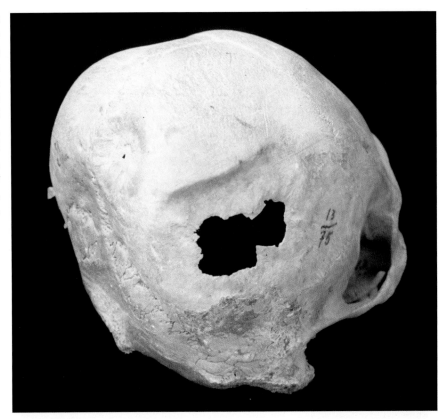

Figure 5.4
A skull from Cerro Colorado, showing cranial deformation (flattening of the occipital bone) and two healed trepanations. Museo Nacional de Antropología, Arqueología, y Historia del Perú, AF:1742, 13/75 T4.

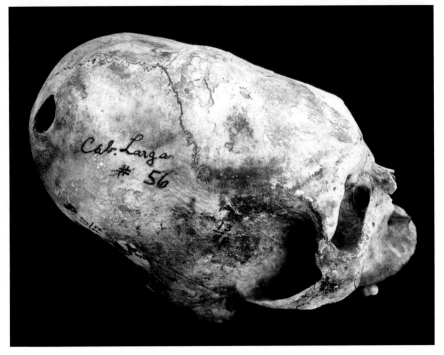

Figure 5.5
A skull from Cabeza Larga, showing a distinctive form of cranial deformation and a trepanation on the right parietal bone. Museo Nacional de Antropología, Arqueología, y Historia del Perú, AF:6867, 13/77, Cabeza Larga #56.

Exploring around the base of the west side of Cerro Colorado, in the area known locally as Arena Blanca or Cabeza Larga, Tello found other looted tombs with human skeletal remains left behind by the huaqueros. He noted that these skulls had a different form of cranial modification than did the Cerro Colorado skulls: a very distinctive elongated shape that Tello called "tabular cilíndrico" (Figure 5.5). The unusual shape of these skulls had been noted by the local huaqueros, and it was the inspiration for their naming the cemetery Cabeza Larga (Tello and Mejía Xesspe 1979:75). Here, Tello examined some fifty skulls lying on the surface, but did not see any trepanations. He noted that the textile and ceramic fragments littering this cemetery were different from those of Cerro Colorado, suggesting that the tombs might be of a distinct time period. Tello's later excavations would confirm this hypothesis.

Tello decided that excavations of intact tombs were needed to clarify the relationship between these two burial areas and to put the looted materials in some context. But this would require additional time and personnel. After gathering together the material he had collected from the surface of the cemeteries, he returned with Lothrop to Lima to seek financial support for a larger expedition. The return trip would prove to be a bit of an adventure. As Lothrop would later recount, the car was packed to the brim with four passengers and their belongings, along with various textiles and other materials that Tello had collected on the way to Paracas. Tello had selected more than fifty deformed and trepanned skulls to take back to the Universidad Nacional Mayor de San Marcos. The problem was that the car was so packed that there was not room for the skulls. Tello decided that the only way to get them back was to tie them to the running boards of the car. Lothrop does not describe exactly how this was done, but he notes in a memoir that the skulls would have been quite visible to anyone they passed on the road to Lima. Lothrop recalls wondering what people thought of this "strangely decorated car," and was relieved that it was not stopped by the police along the way (Lothrop 1948).

The trip was made more challenging by unusual weather. The 1925 El Niño, one of the strongest El Niño Southern Oscillation events in recent centuries, was descending on Peru, and constant heavy rain fell on Tello's car and its various occupants on their return trip to Lima. The road, in poor condition under normal circumstances, was transformed into a muddy morass. The car had to be pushed out of holes and ruts on numerous occasions. Lothrop notes that the last leg of the trip was twenty hours long, and that everyone arrived in Lima late at night, cold, and soaking wet. Fortunately, however, the passengers and the skulls returned safe and sound to the capital city.

On August 19, 1925, Tello made a second trip to Paracas, accompanied by Toribio Mejía Xesspe and two field assistants. Their mode of transportation presumably was more comfortable than that of their first trip south, since they were loaned the personal automobile of Dr. Roberto Levillier, the Argentine ambassador in Peru, who had developed an interest in the site and was eager to visit it. Tello set up a field camp at Paracas, where he would conduct excavations through the end of December. During this field season, they would find and excavate sixty-six graves from Cabeza Larga and five chamber tombs from Cerro Colorado. An additional one hundred crania were collected from the surface around looted tombs on Cerro Colorado.

Figure 5.6
Idealized cross-
section of a Paracas
caverna tomb (after
Carrión Cachot
1949:fig. 2).

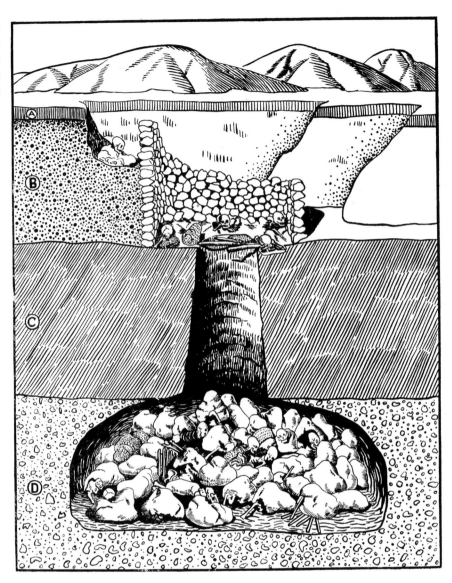

A second field season was conducted between September and December of 1927. The major achievement of this season was the discovery of another large cemetery on Cerro Colorado that contained hundreds of very well-preserved mummy bundles. This cemetery became known as the Necropolis of Wari Kayan. A total of 429 funerary bundles were excavated there (Daggett 1994; Tello and Mejía Xesspe 1979).

In 1928 and 1929, Tello conducted his final field seasons at Paracas. He excavated additional tombs at Cerro Colorado, the Necropolis of Wari Kayan, and Cabeza Larga. Unfortunately, political changes in Peru ended Tello's research at Paracas, as well as his tenure as director of Peru's national museum of archaeology (Gonzáles and Daggett 2005). In 1931, three more tombs at Cerro Colorado were excavated by a team from the museum, under the supervision of its new director, Luis Valcárcel (Yacovleff and Muelle 1932). The skeletal material recovered from this excavation (which did not include any examples of trepanation) was subsequently studied by Pedro Weiss (see below).

TELLO'S EXCAVATIONS ON CERRO COLORADO

Tello identified three large flat areas (*terrazas*) on Cerro Colorado where tombs had been excavated; he named these areas Terrazas I, II, and III. During his field seasons at Paracas, he and Mejía Xesspe excavated a number of large, bottle-shaped tomb chambers that he called "cavernas" (Figure 5.6), as well as many individual graves dug into the sand of Cerro Colorado. To locate the large tombs, Tello took advantage of the experience and skills of the old huaquero Quintana. Quintana used a time-tested tool of clandestine excavators: a T-shaped metal rod with a pointed end, known as a *vaqueta*, to probe the ground for softer, disturbed soil that might indicate the presence of a tomb shaft. Quintana also employed his gustatory senses. Tello reported that after locating a soft area, Quintana would withdraw the probe and taste it ("paladear el polvo extraído en la punta" [Tello and Mejía Xesspe 1979:127]) to judge whether the soil was natural sediment or tomb fill. Quintana explained that the two had distinct flavors. His technique apparently worked, as he was able to locate a number of tombs in this fashion.

TREPANNED SKULLS IN THE CAVERNAS TOMBS

Tello and Mejía Xesspe (1979) reported finding a total of twenty trepanned skulls in four of the cavernas tombs excavated on Terraza II. Eight mummy bundles were found in Caverna II; five of them included individuals with trepanations. Two isolated skulls found in the tomb fill were also trepanned. Grave offerings found with the mummies included seven flaked obsidian points or knives and a short club with a stone head (Figure 5.7). Tello thought these bifacially flaked obsidian tools were either dart points or knives, and that they were the type of tools used to trepan skulls at Paracas (see Tools and Techniques, below).

Caverna V contained thirty-seven mummies, eight of which showed trepanations. Five trepanned skulls were found in Caverna VI. In three cases, these came from intact mummy bundles; the other two were isolated skulls found between the mummy bundles and in the fill of the tomb shaft. In addition to the large cavernas tombs, Tello and Mejía Xesspe excavated a number of smaller individual graves on Terraza II of Cerro Colorado. There they found three more examples of trepanation.

In an attempt to systematically recover fragments of textiles, ceramics, and skeletal material left behind by looters, Tello assigned some of his museum workers to go through the substantial back dirt (some two hundred cubic meters, according to his estimate) left behind by those who had had ransacked a number of cavernas and smaller tombs on Terraza II. This exercise proved to be quite useful. A substantial amount of cultural and skeletal material was recovered, including one skull with a trepanation.

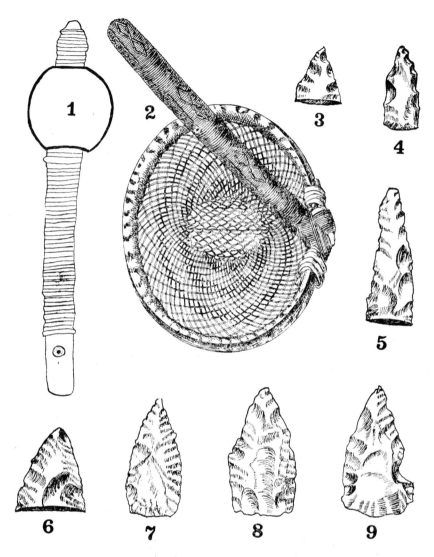

Figure 5.7
Grave offerings
from Caverna II:
a stone club with
wooden handle (1),
a colander made of
plant fiber (2), and
various obsidian
points or knives
(3–9) (from Tello
and Mejía Xesspe
1979:fig. 20).

Fig. 20. Ofrendas ceremoniales de la Caverna II: 1, porra de piedra pulida con mango de madera entorchada, 265 mm. largo y 63 mm. diámetro de la piedra; 2, colador de fibra vegetal, con mango de caña entorchada, 140 mm. diámetro de la malla; 3 a 9, puntas de obsidiana negra para cuchillo y flecha. Cerro Colorado, Paracas.

TOMBS FROM CABEZA LARGA

Tello excavated some 135 graves from Cabeza Larga. Here, graves had been dug into abandoned domestic architecture, and they included both single interments and group tombs. Tello reported that trepanations were rare, although twelve trepanned skulls in our database are identified as coming from Cabeza Larga (e.g., Figure 5.8). Apparently these were surface finds associated with looted areas, as Tello does not describe finding any trepanned skulls in undisturbed graves. As noted above, the name "Cabeza Larga" references the pronounced artificial deformation evident in many of the skulls. Indeed, most Cabeza Larga

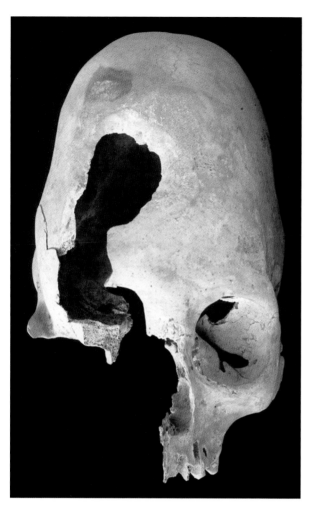

Figure 5.8
Cabeza Larga partial cranium with a healed trepanation on the frontal bone. Museo Nacional de Antropología, Arqueología, y Historia del Perú, AF:6886 P/42.

skulls show evidence of having been intentionally modified during infancy, apparently by wrapping cloth bands around the head. The result was a distinctly elongated head. Not all skulls from Cabeza Larga are deformed in this manner, however. Tello noted that some were "bilobular," with pronounced lateral bulging of the parietal bones, while others showed no artificial shaping.

THE NECROPOLIS OF WARI KAYAN

Grave pits at the Necropolis of Wari Kayan, like those of Cabeza Larga, intruded into the abandoned subterranean houses of an earlier occupation at the Paracas site. Ceramics found with these burials are of a different style from those of the cavernas tombs and are generally known as Topará. Chronologically, these ceramics postdate the cavernas tombs, falling at the end of the Early Horizon and in the early part of the Early Intermediate Period (Paul 1991; Silverman 1991). The mummy bundles at Wari Kayan and the bodies within

Figure 5.9
Skull with gold sheet found over an unhealed trepanation. Necropolis of Wari Kayan. Museo Nacional de Antropología, Arqueología, y Historia del Perú, 12/6628, Mummy 362.

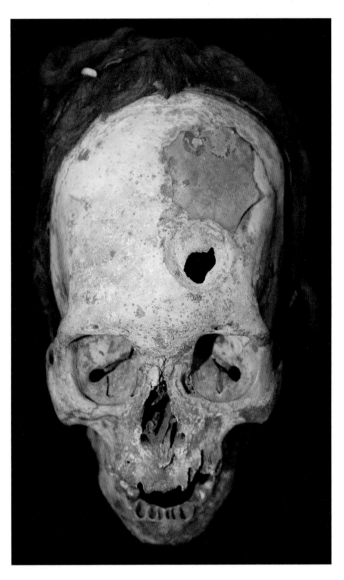

them are unusually well preserved. Many bodies are in such good condition that Tello was convinced they had been artificially mummified by smoking and the application of some preservative liquid (an acid or tar) to the skin and body cavities. Tello even suggested that the internal organs and muscles had been removed as part of the mummification process. Subsequent examination of the bodies by other researchers does not support Tello's hypothesis. In particular, no incisions or other evidence of evisceration has been found, nor signs of smoking. The excellent preservation more likely is due to the very dry burial environment and the extensive textile wrappings of the bundles that drew fluids away from the body (Allison and Gerszten 1975; Yacovleff and Muelle 1932).

Tello and Mejía Xesspe's published descriptions of their Necropolis excavations do not mention any individuals with trepanations, but three examples were found during subsequent unwrapping of mummy bundles by Tello and his assistants in the Museo Nacional de Antropología, Arqueología, y Historia del Perú. The most interesting of the three is illustrated by Tello in his publication *Antiguo Peru, primera epoca* (Tello 1929; see also Tello and Mejía Xesspe 1979). It is the mummy of an adult male with an unhealed trepanation on the left side of the frontal bone. A hammered sheet of gold, polygonal in shape, was found covering the trepanation opening (Figure 5.9). This skull has been cited by a number of writers as evidence to support the theory that ancient Peruvian trepanners placed plates of metal, gourd, or shell over trepanation openings to protect the brain (Asenjo 1963; Courville 1959; Marino and Gonzales-Portillo 2000; Sanan and Haines 1997). Attempts to find other examples of this practice have been unsuccessful (Verano and Andrushko 2010). Tello's mummy is the only well-documented case of a metal sheet directly associated with a trepanation opening. But since the patient did not survive the trepanation (there is no evidence of bone reaction), the "protection" of the covering was unsuccessful. An alternative explanation is that the gold sheet was a funerary offering rather than a surgical implant. Tello himself was conservative in his interpretation of the discovery, describing it simply as "a trepanation protected by a paper-thin plate of gold" (Tello and Mejía Xesspe 1979:pl. 12). In a later examination of the skull, Pedro Weiss doubted whether it was a true cranioplasty, and I second these doubts (Verano and Andrushko 2010; Weiss 1958).

Two more trepanned skulls from the Necropolis of Wari Kayan are noted by Mejía Xesspe in his 1968 laboratory notes on the unwrapping of mummy bundles PN 111 (12/5672) and PN 363 (12/6629). Both are described as healed trepanations (Ann Peters, personal communication 2007). Unfortunately, we did not find these skulls in our examination of the MNAAHP Paracas skeletal collection. However, even if these latter two cases are trepanations, it suggests that the practice was not common among the people buried in the Necropolis of Wari Kayan. Perhaps trepanning had an early fluorescence and then declined during the Late Paracas–Early Nasca transition.

CHALLENGES WITH THE PARACAS SAMPLE

As described above, Tello and other excavators found human skeletal material littering the surface of the Paracas cemeteries because of looting. Most trepanned skulls from Paracas were surface finds, without specific context. Others were found in the back dirt of looters' pits. In his excavations of tombs on Cerro Colorado, Tello also found evidence of prehistoric disturbance of human remains—human bones were found around the entrances to the caverna tomb chambers, as well as dispersed in tomb fill (depicted schematically in Figure 5.6). The disarticulated remains probably represent earlier burials that were disturbed during the digging of new tombs, or perhaps during reentry into tombs to bury additional bodies. Tello found some trepanned skulls in tomb fill, and he concluded that they belonged to earlier burials. How much earlier is not clear, as they lacked associated cultural material that could date them. Thus, contextual information on the majority of trepanned skulls from Paracas is limited, although, as noted above, some individuals with trepanations were found in intact funeral bundles.

Tello and Mejía Xesspe carefully unwrapped and recorded a number of the larger Paracas funerary bundles at the Museo Nacional de Antropología, Arqueología, y Historia del Perú (MNAAHP). They made observations on cranial modification and trepanation, but their published descriptions, photographs, and illustrations focus more on the textiles, ceramics, and other grave goods found with the bodies (Tello and Mejía Xesspe 1959, 1979). Although Tello reportedly planned a publication on trepanation at Paracas, it never appeared. To this day, study of the osteological material from Paracas has been sporadic and limited in scope. Photographs of selected Paracas skulls have been included in a number of publications on cranial modification and trepanation, but they appear as isolated examples included in more general reviews of trepanation in ancient Peru. No data have been published, for example, on the total size of the sample, its demographic characteristics, or on the location, success rate, or possible motivations for trepanning.

STUDIES OF PARACAS HUMAN REMAINS

Pedro Weiss and T. Dale Stewart were among the first to be given access to Paracas skeletal and mummified material for study. Weiss was invited to analyze a small set of burials and disassociated skeletal remains excavated in 1931 by Eugenio Yacovleff and Jorge Muelle from Cerro Colorado (Weiss 1932). He made observations on physical characteristics and cranial morphology, including cranial deformation and evidence of skeletal and dental pathology, and conducted microscopic study of hair and skin samples. Weiss noted only one skull with a lesion that resembled a healed trepanation, but concluded that it was more likely a case of bone infection (osteomyelitis).

Some years later, Weiss was able to do a larger study of Tello's osteological collections at the MNAAHP, presumably including all of the trepanned crania Tello had brought back from Paracas. In a series of publications on trepanation in ancient Peru, Weiss includes descriptions and photographs of some of the Paracas skulls to illustrate surgical techniques and possible motivations for trepanation, but he does not provide details on the sample as a whole (Weiss 1949, 1953, 1958).

T. Dale Stewart, a curator at the National Museum of Natural History at the Smithsonian Institution, was primarily interested in cranial deformation and recording bone measurements for estimating the living stature of the Paracas people (Stewart 1943). Tello gave him access to a small sample of skeletal material for this purpose, but Stewart was only able to make brief observations on trepanned crania on exhibit in the national anthropology and archaeology museum in Lima (Stewart 1943). Additionally, several important books on ancient Peruvian trepanation written by Peruvian neurosurgeons and medical historians include photographs of Paracas skulls, but they do not provide any details on the sample or its context (Graña et al. 1954; Lastres 1951; Lastres and Cabieses 1960). The only general overview of Tello's collection of skeletal material from Paracas is a photographic catalog of crania in the MNAAHP collections compiled by the biologist Arturo del Pozo in the mid-1980s (Pozo 1988). Also included are photographs and descriptions of a sample of roughly contemporary crania from the Pisco Valley curated at the Museo Regional de Ica.

Although Del Pozo notes the presence or absence of cranial modification and trepanation, he focuses on description of morphological traits of the crania. He does provide museum catalog numbers for each skull and divides his sample into "Cavernas," "Necrópolis" (in which he includes crania from both the Necropolis of Wari Kayan and Cabeza Larga), and "Regional Ica," but he does not provide any additional information on the collections.

LABORATORY STUDY
OF THE PARACAS TREPANNED SKULLS
Sample Size and Characteristics

In 1989, I examined the large human osteological collection of the MNAA in Lima, where I photographed and collected detailed data on all trepanned skulls in the department of physical anthropology. I was able to locate and record a total of fifty-nine trepanned skulls in Tello's collection from Cerro Colorado and Cabeza Larga. I made assessments of age and sex for each skull and recorded observations on the presence or absence and form of cranial modification. The sample includes both males and females ranging in age from adolescents to older adults. All but four show intentional cranial modification of the cavernas or necropolis type. Although there are no data on the overall frequency of cranial modification at Paracas, Tello and Mejía Xesspe's descriptions suggest that nearly all skulls were modified. I also examined all non-trepanned Paracas skulls for evidence of skull fractures and other pathology, and recorded data on nineteen skulls that had healed or unhealed fractures but were not trepanned.

No examples of trepanation were observed in infants or children. Apparently this is not simply a reflection of sampling or collection bias, as Tello and Mejía Xesspe excavated many infant and child burials from these sites, particularly from tombs on Cerro Colorado, and they did not observe any cases of trepanation in this age group (Tello and Mejía Xesspe 1979). It is possible that some Paracas adults with healed trepanations received them in childhood. But if infants or children were trepanned with any frequency, then one would expect to see some who died following unsuccessful operations, since only 39 percent of trepanations at Paracas show long-term healing (see Success Rates, below). The absence of any unhealed trepanations in children suggest that they were not subjected to such procedures.

The youngest individuals with trepanations are teenagers. Two examples were found on Cerro Colorado, one in a caverna tomb (13/33 Tumba VI) and one on the surface (P/2 Paracas "U"). The first, a late adolescent male, has a trepanation that appears to have treated a skull fracture, as indicated by a broken edge on the left side of the skull that shows jagged edges. Fresh scrape marks on the margins of the trepanation and a lack of any visible bone reaction suggests that the patient died during or shortly after surgery (Figure 5.10). The second individual has a trepanation that shows short-term healing (porous areas around the margins of the opening mark early stages of bone remodeling), suggesting survival of perhaps several weeks (Figure 5.11). In this case, there is no indication of why the trepanation was executed. Two other adolescents from Paracas have unhealed penetrating injuries of the skull. One of these (MNAAHP AF:6843, 12/9100) shows multiple cut marks around

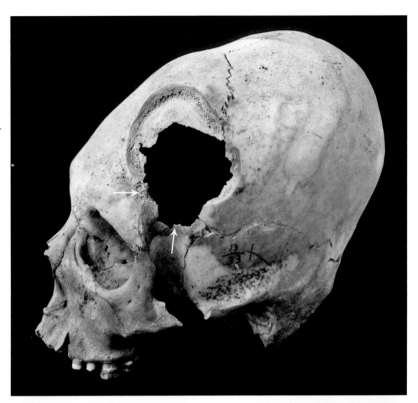

Figure 5.10
Late adolescent male with an unhealed trepanation. Jagged fractures of the sphenoid, frontal, and parietal bones (inferior margin of the opening) and an irregular porous area at the anterior margin (arrows) mark a depressed skull fracture, probably the reason for the trepanation. Museo Nacional de Antropología, Arqueología, y Historia del Perú, Cerro Colorado 13/33, Tumba VI.

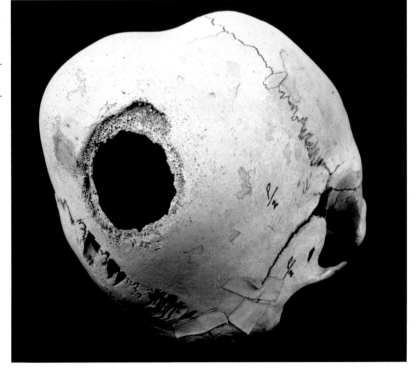

Figure 5.11
Adolescent, probably female, with a trepanation on the right parietal bone. The margins of the defect show bone remodeling indicative of short-term survival. Museo Nacional de Antropología, Arqueología, y Historia del Perú, Cerro Colorado P/2, Paracas "U".

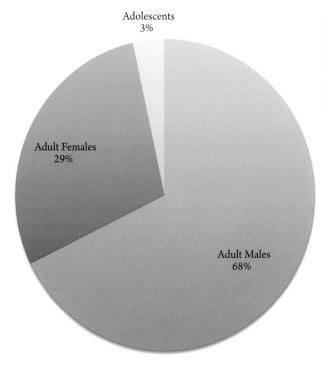

Adolescents
3%

Adult Females
29%

Adult Males
68%

Figure 5.12
Age and sex
distribution
of trepanned
individuals at
Paracas.

the edges of the wound, suggesting that some attempt was made to treat it. The other shows no evidence of intervention.

Among Paracas adults, men were trepanned substantially more often than women (Figure 5.12). Of the fifty-seven adult skulls for whom sex could be assessed with some confidence, forty (68 percent) are males and seventeen (29 percent) are females. This difference is highly significant ($\chi^2 = 9.281$, $d.f. = 1$, $p = 0.0023$). This may reflect the fact that Paracas males had a higher frequency of skull fractures than did females, and thus were more likely to receive trepanations to treat these injuries (see Motivations for Trepanning, below).

Trepanation Locations

Paracas trepanations are most commonly found on the frontal bone (43 percent), followed by the occipital (21 percent), and the left side of the skull and the midline (14 percent) (Figure 5.13). The least common location is the right side of the skull (8 percent). Perhaps not coincidentally, the frontal bone and left side of the skull are also the most frequent locations for skull fractures at Paracas (see Motivations for Trepanning, below). The relatively high frequency of trepanations on the occipital bone is unusual, as most other samples from Andean South America exhibit a low frequency in this region. The area of the occipital bone that is covered with heavy musculature (the nuchal region) was avoided, however, and no trepanations were executed there. The temporal region, also covered by significant muscle, appears to have been avoided as well, as only 10.5 percent of Paracas trepanations are located in this area. Apparently no attempt was made to avoid cranial sutures, however, since 45.6 percent of Paracas trepanations cut through them.

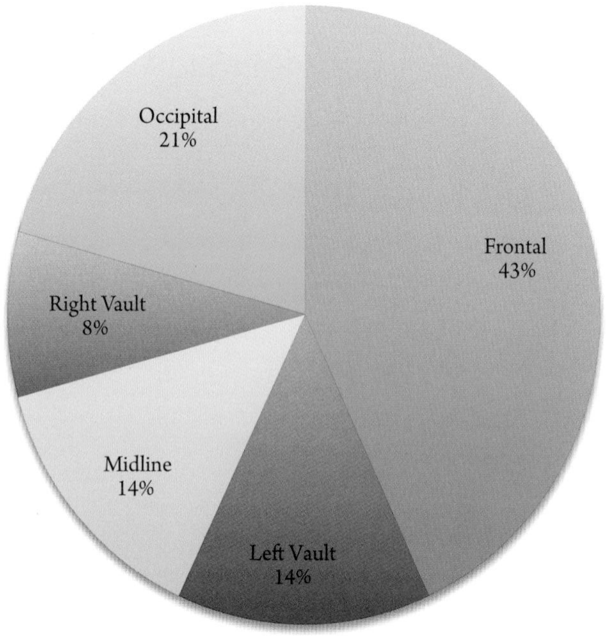

Figure 5.13
Locations of
trepanations
at Paracas.

Occipital
21%

Frontal
43%

Right Vault
8%

Midline
14%

Left Vault
14%

Tools and Techniques

Metal tools have not been found at Paracas or other southern coastal Peruvian sites dating to this time period, and thus they can be ruled out as instruments used to make the openings found in these skulls. Metallurgy on the south coast of Peru during this time was limited to hammered gold sheets that were used as personal adornment and placed as offerings in some of the larger mummy bundles at the site. Bifacially chipped obsidian knives and points, however, were found with a number of Paracas burials. These are the tools Tello believed were used to trepan skulls. Due to the excellent preservation conditions at the site, a number of these knives were still hafted to wooden handles (Figure 5.14). These sharp-edged tools would have served well for scraping and cutting bone (Paul Broca and others did experimental trepanations with flint knives on dog and human cadaver skulls and found that they worked; see Chapter 8). Unhealed Paracas trepanations show fine striations consistent with the marks that would be made by repeated scraping and grooving with a stone tool (Figure 5.15). A unique example of a Paracas skull with an unfinished trepanation was illustrated by Pedro Weiss in his 1958 publication *Osteologia cultural: Prácticas cefálicas* (Weiss 1958:599, pl. 23). I was able to find the skull in 1990 (Figure 5.16). Unfortunately, it had suffered some damage since it was first photographed by Weiss and portions of bone are now broken or lost. Nevertheless, it is useful for showing how Paracas trepanners made large openings in skulls. After grooving the boundaries of the area to be trepanned, the outer table and spongy bone were gradually scraped from the outside in toward the center, leaving only a thin portion of the inner table that was then carefully broken and removed. In this case, a small island of bone at the center remained (originally still attached by a thin plate of the inner table, now broken), suggesting that the procedure

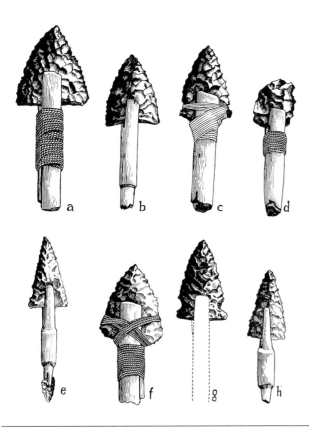

Figure 5.14
Hafted stone knives
from Paracas (after
Carrión Cachot
1949:pl. XXIV).

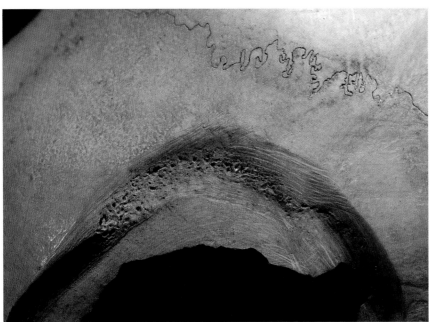

Figure 5.15
Close-up photo of the
margin of a Paracas
trepanation. Numerous
scrape marks on the
bone of the outer table,
spongy bone, and inner
table are visible. There
are no signs of bone
reaction, indicating
death during or shortly
after the operation.
Museo de la Nación,
12/7508, Caverna II, 14.

Figure 5.16
Incomplete trepanation showing the technique of grooving and scraping. The large separate piece of bone in the center of the hole was originally attached by a thin plate of the inner table that has broken away, but its location in the photo approximates its original position. Museo Nacional de Antropología, Arqueología, y Historia del Perú, AF:1725, 13/35, Caverna VI.

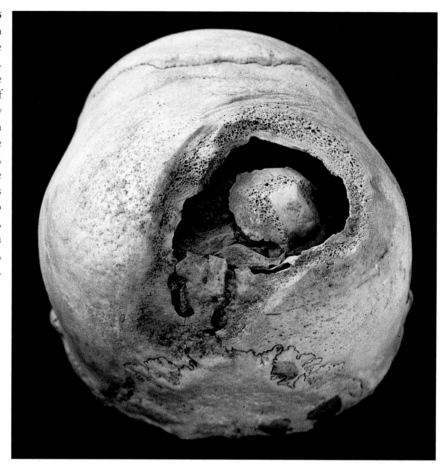

was prematurely halted. Based on this unique specimen and careful examination of others, Paracas trepanations can best be described as employing a mixed technique involving initial grooving followed by scraping.

First in a 1929 publication (*Antiguo Perú, primera epoca*) and later in his 1959 monograph *Paracas: Primera parte*, Tello describes a surgical "kit" that he found in one of the Paracas cavernas tombs. It was a packet that contained obsidian knives of various sizes fitted with wooden handles and stained with blood, along with a small spoon or curette made from a whale tooth (which he suggested was used for denuding the periosteum), cotton pads, bandages, and thread used to suture wounds (Tello 1929:147–148; Tello and Mejía Xesspe 1959:204). Unfortunately, Tello did not publish a photograph or drawing of this assemblage of objects, although in *Antiguo Perú* he includes a photo of a trepanned skull with preserved hair and scalp, which he asserts shows thread used to suture the scalp following the operation (Tello 1929:fig. 101). Unfortunately, the quality of the photograph is poor, and it is difficult to interpret. I examined the specimen in the MNAAHP in 1989, but at that time no soft tissue or hair remained. No other cases of sutured wounds are known from Paracas. In fact, in modern medicine suturing of wounds in non-sterile environments is not advised, due to the risk of trapping bacteria within a wound and encouraging the formation of an abscess. In a review of the Paracas case as well as claims of sutured trepanations in other pre-Hispanic mummies in Peru, Lastres and Cabieses (1960:152–153) found the evidence unconvincing.

Trepanation by drilling was also practiced at Paracas, although this was uncommon. Tello and Mejía Xesspe (1979) describe only one case: Mummy 38 (13/605) from Caverna V on Cerro Colorado. It shows a cluster of eight small holes drilled on the left parietal bone just superior to the osteometric landmark of the asterion (Figure 5.17). This skull is reported to have been found with a cloth bandage over the drilled area. Pedro Weiss (1958) examined and published photographs of this skull, in addition to five other drilled trepanations from Paracas. I was able to locate two of these in the collections of the MNAAHP: one from Cerro Colorado (12/5091) and one from Cabeza Larga (AF:2615, P/21). The Cerro Colorado skull shows a series of complete and partial holes drilled into the right side of the frontal bone, anterior to the coronal suture (Figure 5.18). The holes are adjacent to or cutting across an irregularly shaped opening, apparently a penetrating wound or depressed fracture. Four of the holes are complete and lie anterior and superior to the defect. Three holes cut through the medial margin of the defect, forming incomplete circles. Given the direct association between the irregular defect and the drilled holes, it is likely that the latter were placed there in an attempt to treat the wound. The lack of remodeling indicates that the operation was unsuccessful. The skull from Cabeza Larga shows four drilled holes on the right occipital bone (Figure 5.19). As in the previous case, the holes are associated with a lesion, in this case an irregularly shaped opening (resembling the rear leg of a deer running from right to left) that penetrates the inner table of the skull. The opening has smooth edges, suggesting it might be a drainage channel or a fractured area that was in the process of remodeling at the time of death. Fine cut marks are visible above the drilled holes, and a curved area was scraped or cut out below the largest drilled hole on the left. Like the previous case, the holes seem to have been drilled in an attempt to drain a preexisting injury. The attempt was unsuccessful, as in the three cases illustrated here, as well as the three additional drilled trepanations illustrated in Weiss (1958:pl. 20).

It is unclear what tool was used to make these perforations. Tello thought that they might have been punched out with a sharp instrument. This seems unlikely, given the difficulty of driving a sharp point through bone without penetrating the dura mater. Moreover, the cross-sectional shape of the holes is conical, wider on the external surface of the skull and narrower on the internal surface, with horizontal striations on the walls typically seen in ancient drilling of beads and other artifacts. Weiss suggested that Paracas trepanners drilled the holes with a small obsidian point (Weiss 1958:585–586), but given the brittle nature of obsidian, this seems unlikely as well. Microscopic study of the margins of the drilled holes could clarify the issue.

Trepanation by drilling and cutting would be tried later in the central and northern highlands and cloud forest of northern Peru but with a similar lack of success. The poor survival rate probably was due to the fact that the dura mater could be perforated easily with this method, resulting in an infection of the meninges.

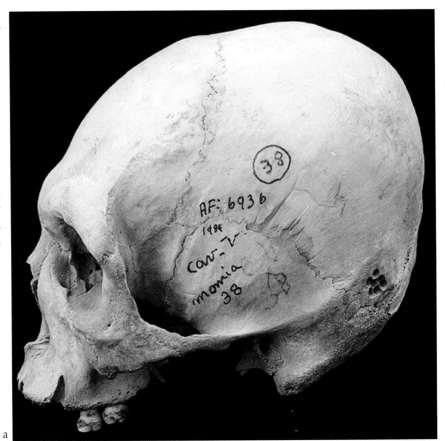

Figure 5.17
(a) Skull of Mummy 38, Caverna V, with drilled holes on the left parietal bone, just superior to the asterion; and (b) close-up of drilled holes. Museo Nacional de Antropología, Arqueología, y Historia del Perú, AF:6936, 13/605.

a

b

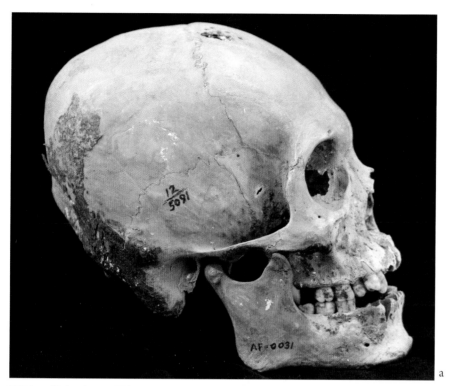

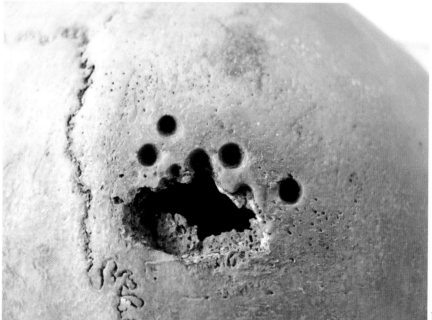

Figure 5.18 (a) Skull of an adult male with drilled holes on the frontal bone, visible at the top of the photograph; and (b) close-up of drilled holes. Museo Nacional de Antropología, Arqueología, y Historia del Perú, AF:0031, 12/5091.

Figure 5.19
(a) Skull of an adult male from
Cabeza Larga with drilled holes
on the right occipital bone
(technically the drilling is located
on a large lambdoid ossicle, or
"Inca bone"); and (b) close-up
of drilled holes surrounding
a small defect with smooth
margins. Museo Nacional de
Antropología, Arqueología, y
Historia del Perú, AF:2615, P/21.

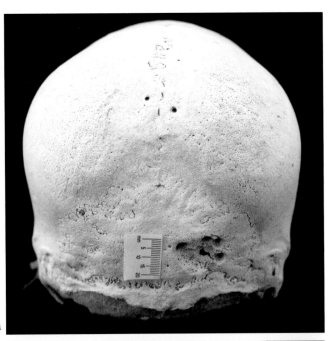

a

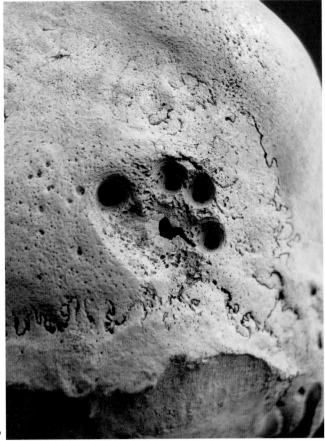

b

Success Rates

The success rate of Paracas trepanners was evaluated by examining bone reaction following the procedure. No bone reaction can be found in 39 percent of Paracas trepanations. In these cases, scraped or cut bone still shows the striations left by the instrument used to make the holes (Figure 5.20), and there is no smoothing of edges, closing off of the exposed spongy bone (diploë), or surrounding porous areas, which would indicate hyperemia and osteoclastic activity. In these cases, the patients would have died during the procedure or shortly afterward. On the other hand, 23 percent of Paracas trepanations show some remodeling of the exposed spongy bone and margins of the opening, marking the initial phases of bone healing and indicating survival of at least several weeks (Figure 5.21). Finally, nearly 40 percent show extensive remodeling of their margins (Figures 5.22 and 5.23), marking long-term survival. While the long-term survival rate of Paracas trepanations does not equal that of later Peruvian skull surgeries, it is nevertheless an impressive achievement, given that these represent the earliest experiments in skull surgery in the New World and that some of these trepanations treated head injuries and their complications. Even modern neurosurgeons cannot guarantee survival of a patient with a severe depressed fracture, penetrating wound, or hematoma. As will be shown below, the ancient inhabitants of the Paracas Peninsula appear to have had a substantial risk of head injury.

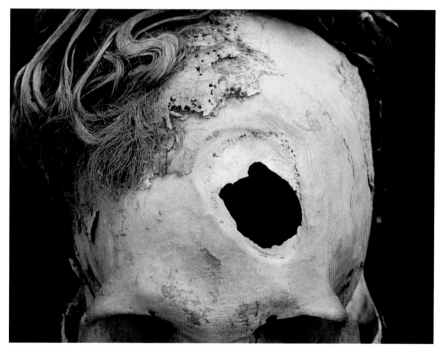

Figure 5.20 Trepanation on the frontal bone showing fresh striations from scraping and no sign of bone reaction. Museo Nacional de Antropología, Arqueología, y Historia del Perú, AF:6852, 13/76, Caverna VI.

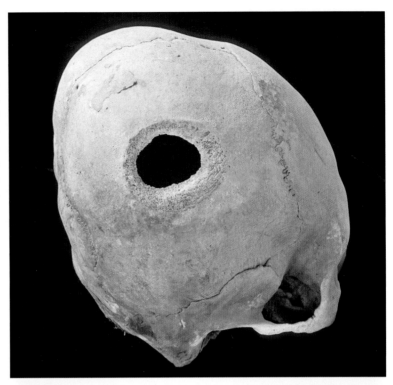

Figure 5.21
Paracas trepanation showing partial remodeling of the margins of the opening, indicating short-term survival following the procedure. Museo Nacional de Antropología, Arqueología, y Historia del Perú, AF:6923.

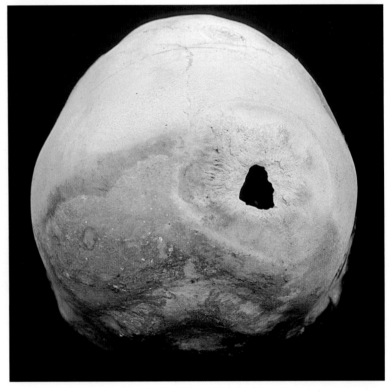

Figure 5.22
Skull from Cabeza Larga with a well-healed trepanation. Museo Nacional de Antropología, Arqueología, y Historia del Perú, AF:6859, Paracas IV A.

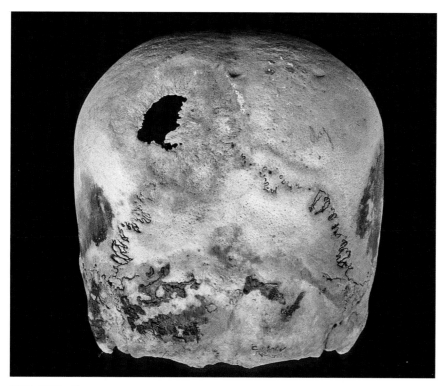

Figure 5.23
Skull from Cerro
Colorado (Mummy 22,
Cavernas V) with a
well-healed trepanation.
Museo Nacional
de Antropología,
Arqueología, y Historia
del Perú, AF:1783.

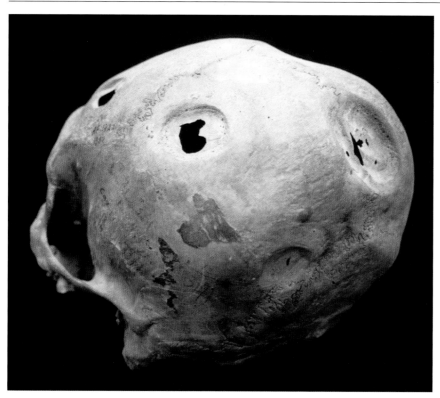

Figure 5.24
Skull from Caverna IV,
Cerro Colorado, with
four trepanations,
none of which
show bone reaction.
Museo Nacional
de Antropología,
Arqueología, y
Historia del Perú,
AF:1722, Cav IV 13/34.

Multiple Trepanations

Most Paracas trepanations (with the exception of drilled examples) are single openings, but a few individuals have multiple holes. Those with more than one trepanation show mixed success. In one case, a skull has four trepanations that appear to have been executed at the same time. Unfortunately for the patient, none show evidence of bone reaction (Figure 5.24). One individual has a well-healed trepanation on the left parietal, but a second, later procedure on the right parietal shows only short-term healing (Figure 5.25). Two individuals were more fortunate in having two well-healed trepanations each. The first has two healed openings on the right parietal bone (see Figure 5.4). The second also has two well-healed openings. While the opening on the back of the skull is relatively small, the other is truly impressive in size, one of the largest prehistoric trepanations I have seen anywhere in the world (Figure 5.26). Cases like these may represent either a return for a second operation after the first healed or perhaps a single operation in which multiple holes were made. The difficulty in establishing chonology lies in the fact that well-healed trepanations are difficult, if not impossible, to assess. Only if the openings show different stages of healing can one make a reliable judgment. It can be assumed that the four unhealed openings shown in Figure 5.24 were executed at the same time. Perhaps a trepanner made repeated openings in search of something, such as a blood clot or other problem, that led the patient to seek help. Alternatively, perhaps a Paracas trepanner was practicing his technique on a cadaver, analogous to what is done in the training of modern neurosurgeons. This scenario is purely speculative, however, given that there is no other evidence of experimental trepanning of skulls at Paracas.

Motivations for Trepanning

Tello initially claimed not to have found any evidence of skull fractures at Paracas (Tello and Astuhuamán González 2005:203), although subsequent unwrapping of mummy bundles and examination of skeletal remains revealed a number of examples. In my own study of the collection, I have identified many cases of healed (Figures 5.27 and 5.28) and unhealed skull injuries (Figure 5.29). Of the seventy-one Paracas skulls I was able to examine at the MNAAHP, a total of fifty-four fractures were observed in thirty-seven individuals (twenty-five males, eight females, and four of uncertain sex), yielding a fracture incidence of approximately 52 percent. Most of these are healed depressed fractures of the vault, although several unhealed penetrating wounds and five cases of nasal bone and facial fractures were also found. What caused these injuries? Slings (*hondas* or *warakas*) are common items in mummy bundles of the Peruvian south coast, and a number have also been found in Paracas tombs (Tello and Mejía Xesspe 1979:figs. 9, 63, 95). Similar slings are still made and worn by men in many areas of the Andean highlands today. In addition to hunting, one of their common uses today is in ritual battles (*tinku*) between highland villages (Orlove 1994; Urton 1993). Capable of propelling an egg-sized stone over a substantial distance (Brown Vega and Craig 2009), these weapons can produce serious and sometimes lethal head wounds (McIntyre 1975:157). Wooden clubs with stone heads have also been found in Paracas graves and at other contemporary sites (see Figure 5.7). Clubs also would have been effective implements for skull bashing. Finally, Paracas people used

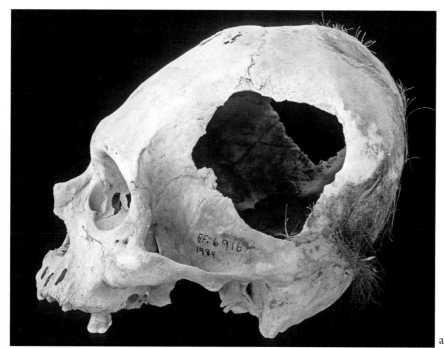

a

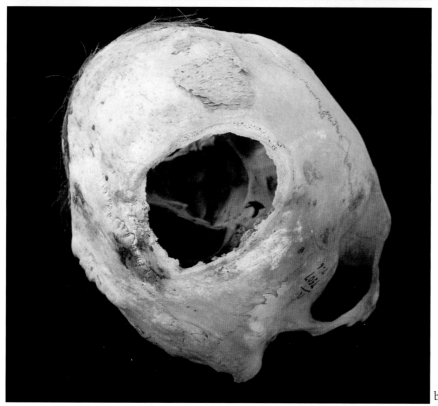

b

Figure 5.25
(a) Healed trepanation of the left parietal bone (with postmortem breakage of the inferior portion); and (b) trepanation of the right parietal bone of the same individual, showing only initial stages of bone remodeling. Museo Nacional de Antropología, Arqueología, y Historia del Perú, AF:6916, 12/7507 T-6.

Figure 5.26
(a) Skull from Cerro Colorado with two healed trepanations, the larger of which involved removing much of the left parietal bone. Part of the left temporal bone was broken postmortem. (b) Posterior view of the skull, showing the smaller healed trepanation on the right parietal and occipital bone. Museo Nacional de Antropología, Arqueología, y Historia del Perú, AF:2641, P/13 U.

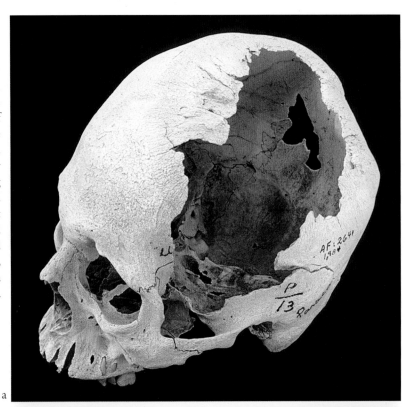

a

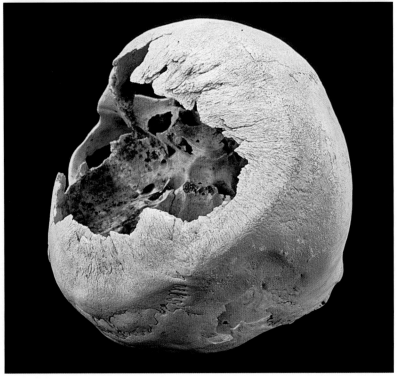

b

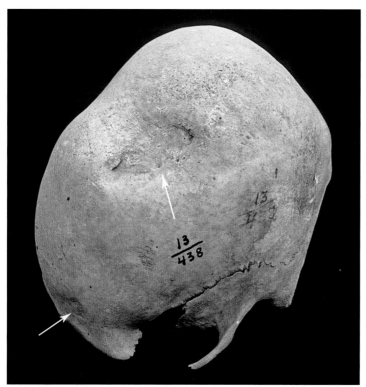

Figure 5.27
Partial skull with two healed depressed fractures (arrows), one on the left forehead and a larger one at the junction of the frontal and left parietal bones. Museo Nacional de Antropología, Arqueología, y Historia del Perú, AF:1757, 13/438.

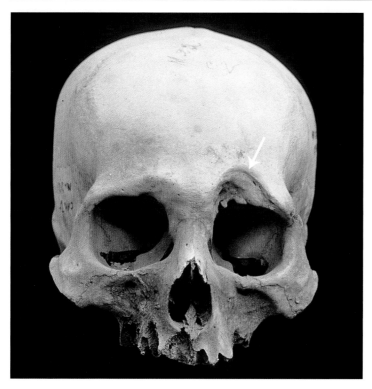

Figure 5.28
Skull with a healed depressed fracture (arrow) of the left superior orbital margin. Museo Nacional de Antropología, Arqueología, y Historia del Perú, AF:1783, Caverna V, M-22.

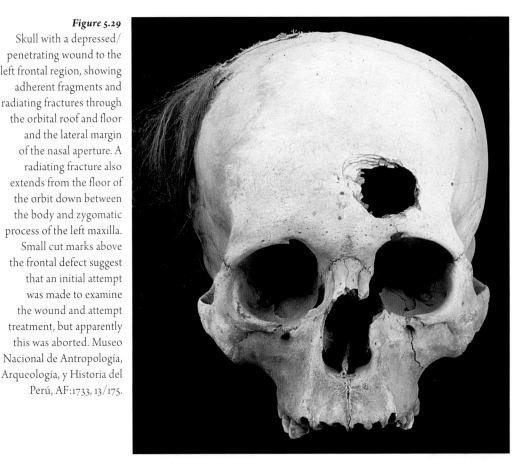

Figure 5.29
Skull with a depressed/penetrating wound to the left frontal region, showing adherent fragments and radiating fractures through the orbital roof and floor and the lateral margin of the nasal aperture. A radiating fracture also extends from the floor of the orbit down between the body and zygomatic process of the left maxilla. Small cut marks above the frontal defect suggest that an initial attempt was made to examine the wound and attempt treatment, but apparently this was aborted. Museo Nacional de Antropología, Arqueología, y Historia del Perú, AF:1733, 13/175.

spear-throwers (*estólicas*)—wooden shafts with hooks at one end that were designed to propel darts with greater velocity and range than possible by simply throwing with the arm (Tello and Mejía Xesspe 1979:figs. 40, 68). Presumably these darts could produce penetrating wounds to the skull if they struck at the proper angle and with sufficient force.

Because skull fracture is one of the most frequent reasons for trepanning worldwide, the possible association between the two was examined in the Paracas sample. Only seven of sixty-eight total trepanations (10.3 percent) are clearly associated with skull fractures. In such cases, the evidence consists of one or more of the following: fracture lines radiating out from the margin of a trepanation, such as in the case of Figure 5.30; scraping around the margins of a penetrating wound (Figures 5.31 and 5.32); and one border of an otherwise smoothly cut opening that shows a ragged, fractured edge that appears to mark the site of injury, as in the case of crania shown in Figures 5.10 and 5.33.

A significant challenge in attempting to interpret the motive for Paracas trepanations is their generally large size. While some openings are small, others are amazingly large, in several cases reflecting the removal of nearly half of the superior portion of the skull vault (Figure 5.34). In these examples, any evidence of small depressed fractures, penetrating wounds, or other lesions could easily have been removed by the trepanation itself. A

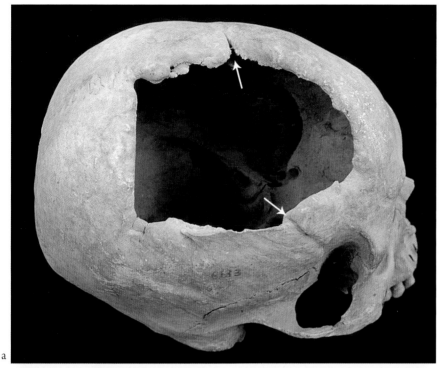

a

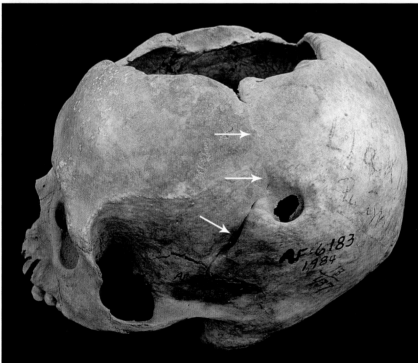

b

Figure 5.30

(a) Skull with a healed trepanation associated with a major skull fracture. Fracture lines can be seen radiating laterally and downward from the left and right margins of the opening (arrows). (b) Left lateral view showing a fracture line (arrows) extending down to the squamosal suture. The small smooth-walled defect on the left parietal bone is of unknown origin, but presumably is related to the skull fracture. Smoothing of the margins of the trepanation and partial obliteration of the radiating fracture lines indicates long-term survival. Museo Nacional de Antropología, Arqueología, y Historia del Perú, AF:6183, 13/437.

Figure 5.31
A skull from Cabeza Larga that shows cut marks and scraping around the margins of a depressed/penetrating wound on the left frontal bone. Porous areas and the irregular margins of the defect indicate some period of survival and early bone remodeling of the fracture margins, but the cut and scrape marks show no evidence of bone reaction, suggesting that death occurred during or shortly after the surgical intervention. A curved concentric fracture can be seen extending out from the anterior margin of the defect (arrow), supporting the interpretation of a fracture, rather than a lytic lesion of some other origin. Museo Nacional de Antropología, Arqueología, y Historia del Perú, AF:10001, P/6.

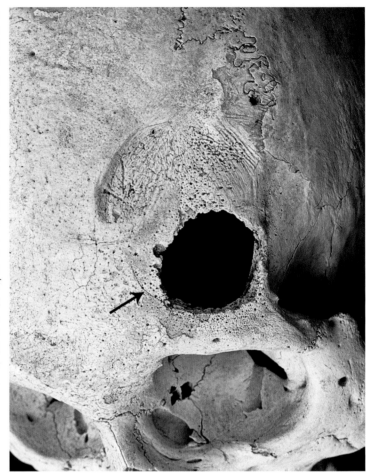

number of cases of unfinished trepanations placed over or near the site of a skull injury are known from the central highlands of Peru (Chapter 4), but few have been found at Paracas. But some indirect support for an association between skull injury and trepanation can be derived by comparing the locations of skull fractures and trepanations in Paracas skulls. In both cases, the highest frequencies are on the front of the skull (Figure 5.35).

Openings as large as those found on some Paracas skulls have long raised doubts about whether such large portions of the skull could be removed successfully from a living patient. The skeletal evidence from Paracas confirms that it was done, in some cases successfully. One skull with a large trepanation shows short-term healing, as indicated by initial remodeling of the margins of the opening, and bone reaction on the external table surrounding the opening, confirming that the patient was alive (Figure 5.36). As described above, others show extensive healing, indicating long-term survival.

I am aware of only a few other examples in which prehistoric individuals with such large trepanations survived. Among the modern Kisii of Kenya, which is one of the only traditional societies in the world that still performs such procedures in a non-medical

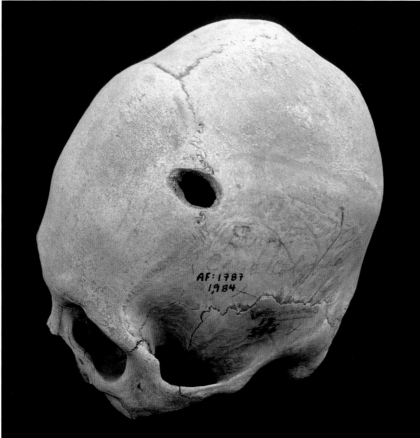

Figure 5.32
(a) Partial skull from Cerro Colorado that shows a penetrating wound of the left frontal and parietal region. This was confirmed by examining the endocranial surface, which shows beveled fracture margins typical of penetrating wounds. (b) The margins of the external defect show fine cut and scrape marks, indicating that some attempt was made to clean the wound and smooth the margins of the hole. The treatment was unsuccessful, as there is no evidence of healing. Museo Nacional de Antropología, Arqueología, y Historia del Perú, AF:1787, 13/506 Superficie.

a

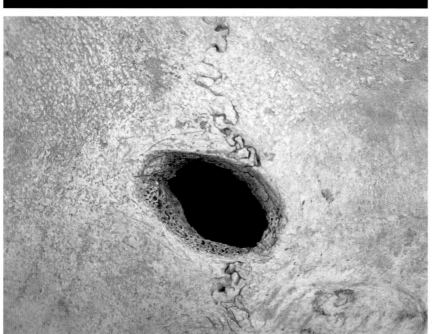

b

Figure 5.33
(a) A trepanation placed adjacent to a preexisting fracture of the superior border of the left orbit, marked by irregular and jagged edges. (b) Oblique view from below. Patches of subperiosteal bone showing hemorrhage or inflammatory response are visible on the roof of the affected orbit. The trepanation margins show no healing. Museo de la Nación, Paracas Cavernas 13/216, #5.

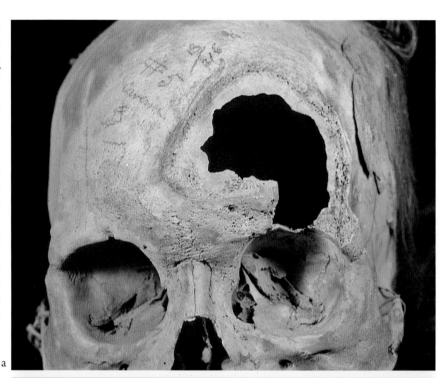

a

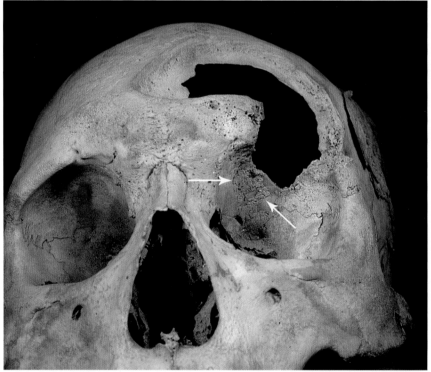

b

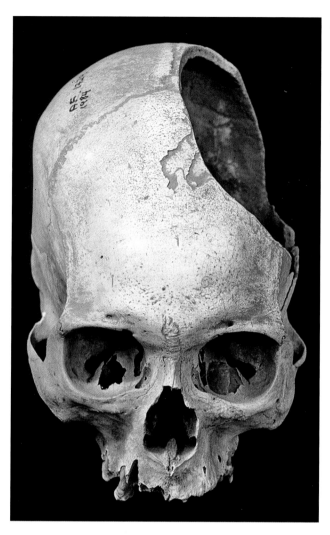

Figure 5.34
Paracas skull with
a large trepanation
showing no healing.
Museo Nacional
de Antropología,
Arqueología, y Historia
del Perú, AF:1729, "U."

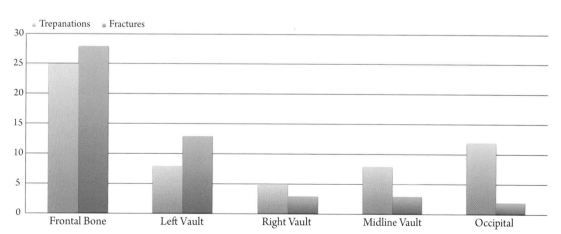

■ Trepanations   ■ Fractures

Figure 5.35 Comparison of the location of trepanations and skull fractures at Paracas.

Figure 5.36
Paracas skull with a large trepanation showing short-term healing. The trepanation cuts across an old healed depressed fracture on the left parietal bone. Perhaps this was a source of headaches the patient wished to have treated. Museo Nacional de Antropología, Arqueología, y Historia del Perú, AF:1724, 12/9080.

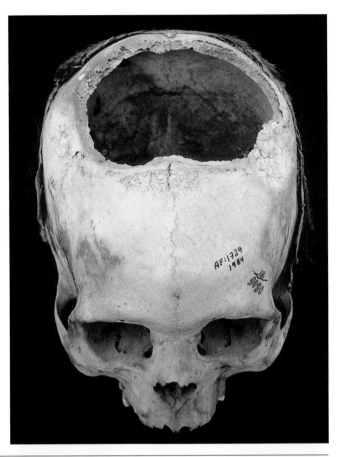

Figure 5.37
Skull from Cabeza Larga with inflammation and lytic destruction of the left mastoid process and adjacent bone. A trepanation placed posterior and superior to the area of active infection shows no bone reaction. Museo Nacional de Antropología, Arqueología, y Historia del Perú, AF:10002, P/5.

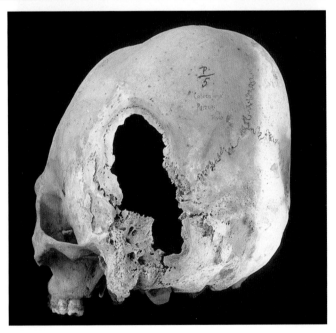

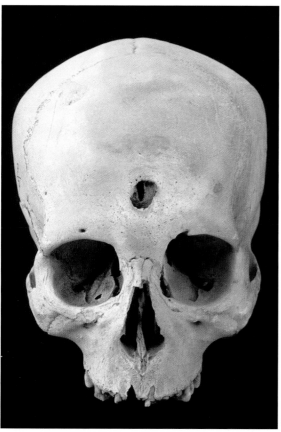

Figure 5.38
(a) Skull from Cabeza
Larga with an oval
defect on the frontal
bone that penetrates
the inner table; and
(b) close-up of oval
defect. Museo Nacional
de Antropología,
Arqueología, y Historia
del Perú, AF:2515, P/23
U Cabeza Larga.

a

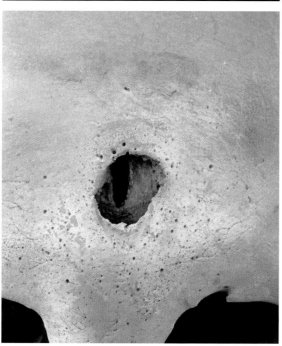

b

setting with simple tools (see Chapter 8), some cases of very large skull defects (usually resulting from multiple trepanations) have been documented photographically and radiographically. Kisii patients who lose large portions of their skull vault sometimes wear special protective headgear (Furnas et al. 1985). No doubt some members of the ancient Paracas culture with large healed trepanations would have felt the need for protection, although no examples of protective head coverings have been found.

Four skulls in the Paracas sample stand out as unusual cases based on trepanation location. In two, individuals openings were placed near the mastoid process (Figures 5.17 and 5.37). The other two cases are irregular holes located over or near the frontal sinuses (Figures 5.38 and 5.39). In the example shown in Figure 5.37, pain associated with middle ear or mastoid infection may have been the stimulus for trepanning. Middle ear infections are common in children today, and probably also were in the past. A chronic middle ear infection can sometimes spread to the mastoid air cells, resulting in mastoiditis (Roberts and Manchester 1995). The Cabeza Larga skull appears to be such a case. The left mastoid area shows inflammation and lytic destruction, with multiple drainage channels to its external surface. A trepanation was placed posterior and superior to this inflamed area, presumably in an attempt to treat the infection. It was not successful, judging from the lack of bone reaction around the margins of the trepanation. In fact, this approach to treating an externally draining mastoid infection was probably a bad idea, as it might allow pus draining from the infected area to come into contact with the exposed dura, spreading the infection to the meninges. In the second case of trepanning near the mastoid process (Figure 5.17), the motivation is less obvious. There is no visible sign of mastoiditis or of chronic middle ear infection. Nevertheless, the placement of multiple drilled holes above and posterior to the mastoid area suggest an attempt to treat some complaint in this area.

The two cases of defects over or near the frontal sinuses (see Figures 5.38 and 5.39) are more difficult to interpret because they may be either trepanations or penetrating wounds. Both are quite similar in appearance: oval holes that penetrate the outer and inner tables of the skull and open into the frontal sinuses. Bone resorption on the edges of the defects and halos of porous bone surrounding the holes indicate short-term survival. No clear cutting or scraping marks can be seen on the bone, making it possible that these were penetrating wounds and not trepanations, but the similarity in their location and general features, along with the fact that both skulls were found at a site where trepanation was practiced, suggest that these may be healing trepanations. Three examples of trepanation involving the frontal sinuses are known in the Hrdlička collection from the central highlands of Peru (Burton 1920; Tyson and Alcauskas 1980). All appear to be associated with skull fractures, and the involvement of the frontal sinus might simply be coincidental. In the Paracas cases, there are no obvious skull injuries associated with these defects. If these were indeed experiments in treating sinus headache, they were not successful, as they only show short-term healing.

A final specimen is interesting but enigmatic (Figure 5.40). This skull from Caverna V of Cerro Colorado has three small trepanations located in the middle of a circular area of dead bone. Perhaps the openings were made to encourage healing in an area that had lost its external blood supply due to an injury that had caused a sub-periosteal hematoma or

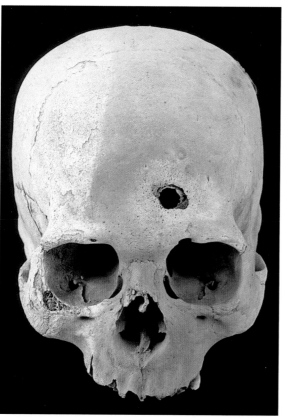

Figure 5.39
(a) Skull from Cerro Colorado with an oval defect on the frontal bone that penetrates the inner table. This specimen also has healed fractures of the nasal bones. (b) Close-up of oval defect. Museo Nacional de Antropología, Arqueología, y Historia del Perú, AF:2519, P/7 U Cerro Colorado.

a

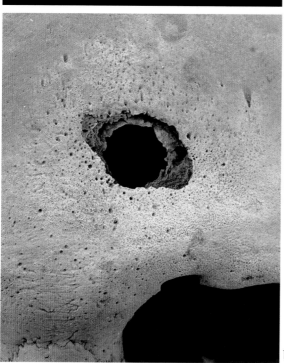

b

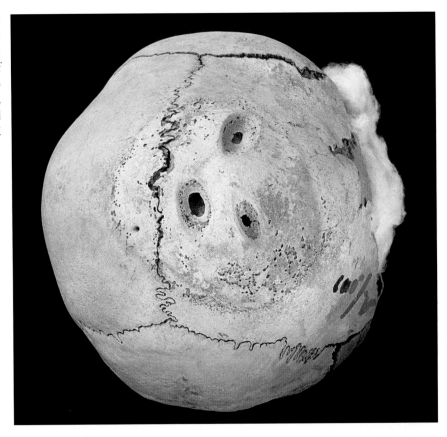

Figure 5.40
Skull from Cerro Colorado
with three trepanations
placed in an area of
necrotic bone. Museo
Nacional de Antropología,
Arqueología, y Historia del
Perú, AF:6920, Caverna V.

scalp necrosis in this area. In the Western medical tradition, scraping and drilling through areas of dead bone has been practiced by surgeons since the time of Hippocrates; it is done to help stimulate scar tissue and healing in head wounds where the bone has been exposed and has lost its blood supply (for a review of historic cases of the treatment of scalping victims, see Bruesch 1974). This case from Paracas may represent such an attempt, although the lack of healing indicates that the surgery was not successful.

Defects in the Skull of Uncertain Origin

Two Paracas skulls have large defects with ragged edges and porous margins (Figures 5.41 and 5.42). Possible diagnoses for these defects include metastatic carcinoma or bone infection (pyogenic osteomyelitis). Both can produce defects of the skull vault with ragged, "moth-eaten" edges (Kaufman et al. 1997; Ortner 2003). Given the rarity of cancer in ancient human remains, metastatic carcinoma is possible but unlikely. Head injuries, however, were common at Paracas, and some of these likely resulted in open wounds of the scalp, which would be prone to infection. Trepanation, of course, would be another potential source of infection, since it involved cutting through the scalp and exposing the bone. In these skulls it is unclear whether the infection might have resulted from head injury, surgery, or both. None of the defect margins show evidence of cutting or scraping,

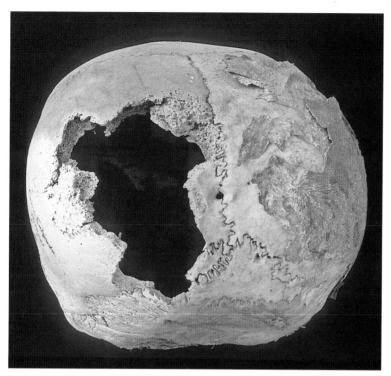

Figure 5.41
Skull from Cerro Colorado with
a large erosive (lytic) defect
on its posterior aspect. Edges
are irregular and sharp, and the
bone shows no visible blastic
response. Some postmortem
breakage is visible on the
medial side of the opening,
complicating diagnosis. Museo
Nacional de Antropología,
Arqueología, y Historia del
Perú, AF:9997, P/33.

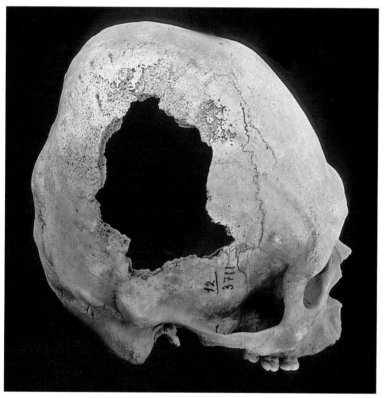

Figure 5.42
Skull from Cerro Colorado with
a large erosive defect on the right
side of the vault. Unlike the skull
in Figure 5.37, there is extensive
active bone remodeling above
the defect. Museo Nacional
de Antropología, Arqueología,
y Historia del Perú, AF:6834,
12/3711 "Desmonte."

although the aggressive bone destruction associated with these lesions might have erased such evidence. Whatever the cause and diagnosis of these lesions, it is clear that neither individual survived them, as they were active at the time of death.

Surgical Skill and Anatomical Knowledge

How skilled were early Paracas trepanners, and how much did they know (or learn) about the anatomy of the skull and brain? Given the size of some of the holes they made in skulls, and the apparent frequency with which they trepanned (based on Tello's original estimate of 40 percent), they could certainly be characterized as "radical" surgeons. Weiss commented as follows (my translation from the Spanish):

> *Febris operatis*, which is the eternal disease of surgeons, reached its maximum level at Paracas, where one finds a great number of enormous craniotomies that would have had no possibility of survival and which seem to be the work of an insane surgeon, and many other cases in which one cannot find a rational reason for the operation. The exaggeration in the art of trepanning at Paracas is paralleled by their pronounced forms of cranial deformation (Weiss 1953:31).

Weiss's point is well taken, yet a substantial proportion of their patients did survive, indicating that Paracas trepanners were in many cases able to avoid infections, severe bleeding,

Figure 5.43
Skull from Cerro Colorado with two large trepanation openings on either side of the sagittal suture, leaving a bridge of bone between them. Museo Nacional de Antropología, Arqueología, y Historia del Perú, AF:6954, 30/334 1926.

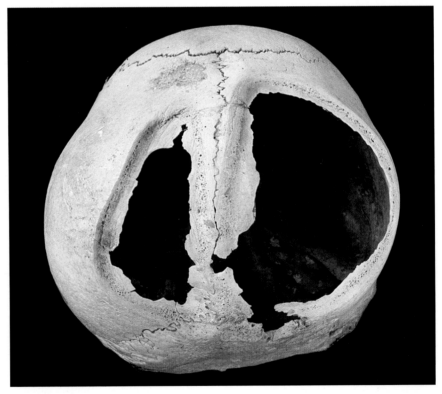

and other complications associated with cutting into the scalp and bone. Based on the location of trepanations in the Paracas sample, areas with thick muscle and rich blood supply, such as the temporal fossa and nuchal area, were avoided. But was there an understanding of other areas of the skull that one should avoid?

Weiss argued that Paracas trepanners knew to avoid cutting through bone over the sagittal suture because of the underlying superior sagittal sinus that drains blood from the brain, which if torn could cause fatal bleeding. Several neurosurgeons have told me that they avoid doing craniotomies over the sagittal sinus for this reason. Weiss's evidence for such knowledge among Paracas trepanners are two skulls with trepanations on both sides of the sagittal suture, leaving a small bridge of bone between them (Weiss 1958:pl. 26). I was able to locate only one of these in the collections of the MNAAHP (Figure 5.43). Weiss's inference that it demonstrates knowledge of the location of the sagittal sinus may be correct, although it is also possible that Paracas trepanners were simply avoiding the sagittal suture, which would be quite visible once the scalp was removed. The data do not suggest, however, that Paracas trepanners systematically avoided cutting across cranial sutures, since twenty-nine out of sixty-six (43.9 percent) trepanations do cut across sutures. Whether or not the sagittal sinus was avoided, neither skull illustrated by Weiss shows any evidence of bone reaction, perhaps making this a moot question. And it should be noted that there are other skulls from Paracas where trepanations are placed over the sagittal sinus. Some of these patients survived; others, such as the skulls in Figures 5.2 and 5.36 did not. Although Weiss's hypothesis is an interesting one, and has been cited by other authors (Lastres 1951; Lastres and Cabieses 1960), it is based on a very small sample (n=2).

Trepanation by drilling was also practiced at Paracas, and the presence of this technique demonstrates that there was some active experimentation in trepanation methods. The drilled trepanations differ from the large scraped openings in that they are focused on small areas. They may represent exploratory probing of inflamed areas or the location of a patient's complaint. Similar drilled trepanations were done in later time periods in the northern, central, and southern highlands of Peru, although the method never seems to have been very popular or successful.

How Frequent Was Trepanation at Paracas?

Estimating what percentage of Paracas individuals were trepanned is difficult for a number of reasons. Tello estimated that approximately 40 percent of the skulls he collected from looted tombs on Cerro Colorado were trepanned. If this were characteristic of the entire mortuary sample, it would be impressive indeed. But clearly there was selective collection of trepanned skulls by Tello and his colleagues, which would inflate their relative frequency. Additionally, many mummy bundles in the national museum of anthropology and archaeology have never been opened or radiographed. Mummies and skeletal remains from Paracas were exchanged with other museums in Peru and other countries, and detailed records are lacking in most cases. Several ongoing projects are now reviewing Tello and Mejía Xesspe's field and laboratory notes and museum catalog records to better document the location and content of museum collections, but this is not a simple task. A crude estimate of the frequency of trepanation at Paracas can be made by counting the number of skulls in Arturo del Pozo's 1988 catalog and dividing the number of trepanned skulls by the total sample. It is an imperfect count, because a number of trepanned skulls mentioned by Tello and Mejía Xesspe are not illustrated by Del Pozo.

Del Pozo's catalog illustrates forty-five skulls that he classifies as coming from cavernas and forty-five from the Necropolis. One skull in his Necropolis sample (Cráneo No 41, AF:1705) is labeled "La Puntilla," a cemetery on the Paracas Peninsula that dates to a later period (ca. AD 1100–1450), so it will be excluded from the count here. Removing this individual, his Paracas sample comes to eighty-nine skulls, of which sixteen are trepanned. This yields a frequency of 18 percent, substantially lower than Tello's estimate. However, for some reason thirty-six of the trepanned skulls I recorded at the MNAAHP are not included in Del Pozo's catalog. This makes a total of fifty-two trepanned skulls, which when divided by 125 (89 + 36), suggests that 42 percent of adults at Paracas were trepanned. This is very close to Tello's original estimate, based on his initial surface collection in 1925. But there are still reasons to suspect them numbers. If 40 percent of Paracas adults were trepanned and only 39 percent of them survived the procedure, then the social and demographic impact of such high mortality would have been devastating. I think it more likely that the numbers reflect collection bias rather than a true estimate of how many Paracas adults were trepanned.

Trepanned Skulls from Coastal Valleys near Paracas

The Paracas Peninsula is located just south of the mouth of the Pisco River. There are numerous archaeological sites in the Pisco Valley, some of which are contemporary with cemeteries on the Paracas Peninsula. Trepanned skulls have been found at some of these sites, in particular at Hacienda Chongos, located on the south side of the Pisco River. The Museo Regional de Ica began excavations at Hacienda Chongos in 1962, excavating a cemetery that covered an area of approximately 200 × 120 meters (Pezzia 1969). The cemetery appears to be contemporaneous with the Paracas tombs, based on grave goods and similar forms of cranial modification and trepanation technique (Pezzia 1968, 1969).

The Museo Regional de Ica also has osteological remains (almost exclusively crania) from other sites in the Pisco and Ica Valleys. Most of this material was surface-collected from cemeteries, which like Paracas were seriously damaged by looting activity beginning in the late nineteenth century. As a result, osteological material from the Pisco Valley and adjacent south coast valleys has little contextual information. In most cases, all that is known is the archaeological site or hacienda name. Very little has been published on this material. There is one general article on the frequency of skull fracture and trepanation in the Ica museum's osteological collection, published in 1976 by paleopathologist Marvin Allison and archaeologist and museum curator Alejandro Pezzia (Allison and Pezzia 1976). It provides a summary, in tabular form, on skull fracture and trepanation in the Ica collection, but no information on the specific sites from which the material was collected or the contexts in which they were found, although they were claimed to be of a "known cultural association and cemetery." Some of the data are problematic, in that they describe trepanned skulls that are dated to the later Nasca, Huari, and Ica cultures. I am not aware of trepanned skulls ever being reported from Nasca sites, nor are any of the Nasca specialists with whom I have spoken. Recent studies of large Nasca skeletal collections have not reported any examples (Drusini 1991; Drusini et al. 2001; Kellner 2002). An explanation for this apparent anomaly can be found in Allison and Pezzia's article, in which they note that four of the trepanned skulls they date as Nasca were executed with a "crosscut technique" (intersecting linear cuts) and "were from a highland location rather than a coastal one." Indeed, this trepanation technique is found only in highland Peru, indicating that these skulls do not come from a Nasca site. I am also not aware of any trepanned skulls from well-dated Wari or Ica sites on the south coast of Peru, although a small number of trepanned skulls have been found at highland Wari sites (see Chapter 7). It thus appears that the cultural affiliation of some of the trepanned skulls in the Ica museum are less secure than claimed by Allison and Pezzia.

Skulls at the Museo Regional de Ica and Museo de Sitio Paracas Julio C. Tello

In the summer of 2013, I had the opportunity to examine and record data on trepanned skulls of the osteological collections of the Museo Regional de Ica and the Museo de Sitio Paracas Julio C. Tello. Allison and Pezzia's 1976 study identifies twenty-four skulls in the Ica collection as trepanned, but I was only able to confirm fourteen cases. The remaining ten, which were recorded on museum catalog cards as trepanned skulls, included three trophy heads (identified by a perforation on the frontal bone and breakage of the base of the skull) and seven examples of skull openings caused (in my opinion) by taphonomic processes, including postmortem breakage, wind or sand erosion, and rodent damage (see Chapter 3, Figures 3.16 and 3.17). The skulls that I believe can be confidently identified as trepanned come from Chongos (n=5), Topará (n=1), Tunga (n=2), Parausa (n=1), and Laramate, Palpa Valley (n=1). Four skulls have no provenance information, but their trepanations are of the same technique and form as the skulls at Paracas (scraping of large circular or oval openings). In fact, some or all of them may be from the Paracas Peninsula, but collected by archaeologists other than Tello. Alternatively, they may be from Chongos, which, as noted below, is contemporary with the Paracas cavernas and the Necropolis.

HACIENDA CHONGOS

Based on their trepanation technique, the five trepanned skulls from Chongos would fit seamlessly into the Paracas collection (Figures 5.44–5.47). A bifacial stone knife with a wooden handle was discovered there as well (Figure 5.48). It is made of a fine-grained stone (probably chert) rather than obsidian, but is otherwise similar to the hafted knives found at Paracas.

Skulls from Chongos also show the two common forms of cranial modification at Paracas: the tabular oblique or "cuneiform" style characteristic of the cavernas of Cerro Colorado (Figure 5.44b), and the pronounced annular deformation and elongated head typical of Cabeza Larga (Figure 5.45). This evidence, along with similarities in ceramic and textile styles, suggests close contact between the people of Hacienda Chongos and those buried on Cerro Colorado at Paracas (Peters 1987; Pezzia 1969). In fact, some scholars have suggested that Paracas was primarily a mortuary site used by elites from the Pisco Valley and other nearby south coast valleys. Tello did not agree, arguing that domestic architecture and refuse deposits on and around Cerro Colorado demonstrated that there

Figure 5.44
(a) Skull from Hacienda Chongos with a large unhealed trepanation along the midline of the skull. A postmortem fracture extends outward from the left side. A healing lesion (depressed fracture?) is present on the left frontal bone above the sphenoid. (b) Lateral view showing cranial deformation similar to the form commonly found in Paracas skulls. Museo Regional de Ica, 00291-12, 37, Chongos Superficie.

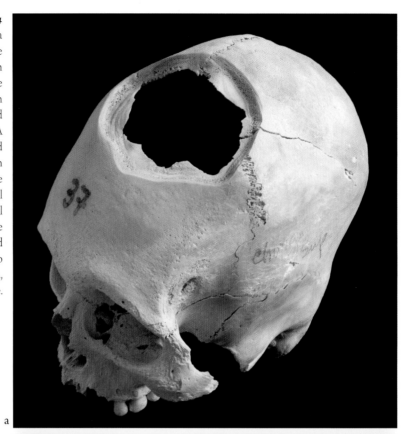

a

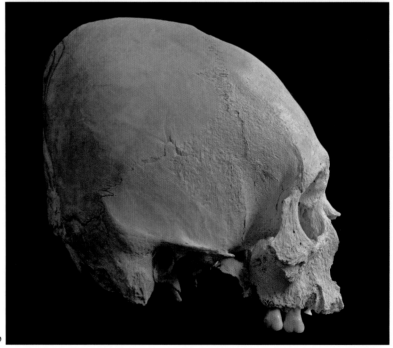

b

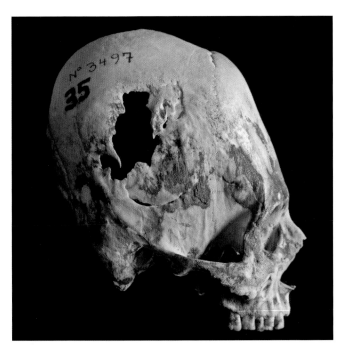

Figure 5.45
Lateral view of a Chongos skull with cranial deformation similar to that seen at Cabeza Larga. It has a large healed skull fracture that may have been surgically treated, although there is no visible evidence of cutting or scraping. Museo Regional de Ica, DB-4397, 00293-12, Tumba 35 4° Expl. Hda. Chongos.

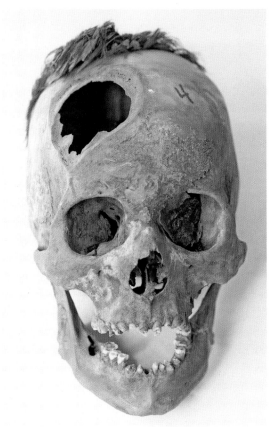

Figure 5.46
Skull from Hacienda Chongos with an unhealed trepanation on the right frontal bone. The nasal bones show healed fractures. Museo Regional de Ica, 00853-12, 4.

Figure 5.47
Skull from Hacienda
Chongos with an
unhealed trepanation
on the left parietal bone.
MP/535, MSP-0660-04,
T-9 No 3397 2nda Exped.

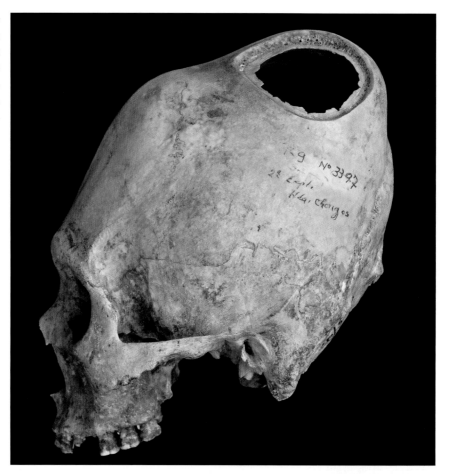

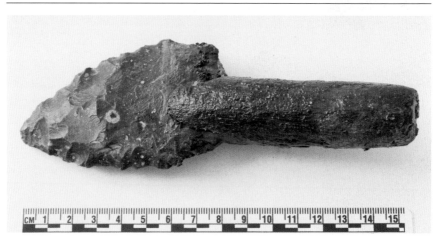

Figure 5.48 Hafted stone knife from Hacienda Chongos. Museo Regional de Ica, 00297-07, DB 3598.

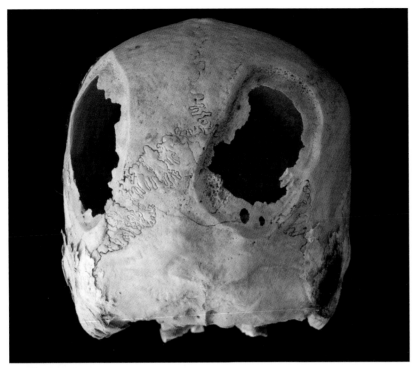

Figure 5.49
Skull from the
Museo de Sitio
Paracas Julio
C. Tello with
two unhealed
trepanations. MSP-
0831-12.

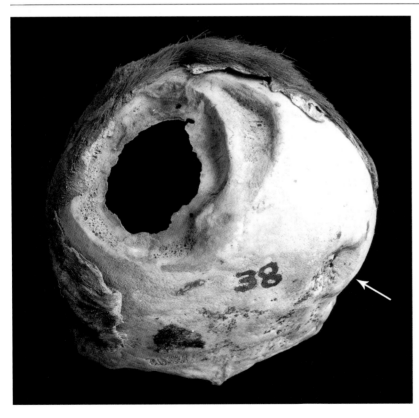

Figure 5.50
Unprovenanced
skull with two
trepanations, one
healed (arrow) and
one with no evidence
of healing. Museo
Regional de Ica,
00294-12, 38.

was a substantial population living on the peninsula (Tello and Mejía Xesspe 1979). Most Paracas scholars concur with Tello's assessment, although there has been some debate about how large a population could be supported by the limited resources of the peninsula (for a review of the debate, see Silverman 1991).

One skull from the Museo de Sitio Paracas Julio C. Tello and one from the Museo Regional de Ica collection show trepanations in the Paracas style, and may be from the Paracas Peninsula, although catalog cards were not available for them during my visit in 2013. The first is a skull with two unhealed trepanations on either side of the mid-sagittal plane (Figure 5.49). The second also has two trepanations. One is healed and the other shows no evidence of bone reaction (Figure 5.50).

Disappearance of Trepanation on the South Coast

After its early and brief fluorescence at Paracas and nearby sites, trepanation disappears from the archaeological record of the south coast of Peru. While there have been claims of trepanned skulls found at later south coast sites (Allison and Pezzia 1976), this remains unconfirmed. Destruction of sites by looting has been a continuing problem since the late nineteenth century, but there have been extensive archaeological surveys and excavations at later south coast sites in the twentieth and early twenty-first centuries that have produced hundreds of burials from Nasca, Wari, and Chincha sites (Drusini 1991; Drusini et al. 2001; Kellner 2002). A number of museums have large collections of skulls from looted cemeteries, and these have been examined extensively by researchers as well. None of these studies have reported trepanned skulls, so it is safe to assume that the practice indeed disappeared from the south coast of Peru during the late Paracas period.

Evidence of trepanation first appears at archaeological sites in highland regions of Peru and Bolivia in the Early Intermediate Period (ca. AD 100–600) and then spreads widely. Did highlanders originally learn of trepanation from contact with the Paracas culture? Evidence of trade with the highlands and more distant tropical regions is evident from the presence of exotic items in Paracas graves, such as obsidian (from sources in the Peruvian highlands), Spondylus shell (from coastal Ecuador), and tropical bird feathers (from the rainforest). Iconography influenced by Chavín de Huántar in northern highland Peru also appears in some phases of Paracas art. Whether this long-distance trade was limited to physical objects or it also included the spread of some south coast cultural traditions such as trepanation is unknown, but such exchange is certainly possible. What is puzzling is that trepanation disappeared from its place of origin only to flourish later elsewhere. After Paracas, trepanation was limited largely to the highlands. Only a handful of trepanned skulls are known from all of coastal South America, and these appear to be introductions by the Inca Empire, which spread from the southern highlands of Peru to dominate all of the central Andean highlands and coast in the late fifteenth century.

6 THE NORTHERN HIGHLANDS AND CLOUD FOREST

JOHN W. VERANO,
ANNE R. TITELBAUM,
BEBEL IBARRA ASENCIOS,
and MELLISA LUND VALLE

THE ANCASH REGION OF THE NORTHERN HIGHLANDS IS CHARACTERIZED
by two large valleys that run from the southeast to the northwest: the Callejón de Huaylas
and the Región de los Conchucos (Figure 6.1). These valleys mark the drainages of the
Santa River, which flows north then west to the Pacific coast, and the Marañón River,
which flows north and then east to the Amazon Basin. The Cordillera Blanca, the eastern range of the Andes, divides the Callejón de Huaylas and Región de los Conchucos,
although a series of small canyons provide routes of communication between the two.
The southern boundary of highland Ancash is defined by a mountain chain (the Cordillera
Huayhuash) and a series of deep canyons that appear to have limited travel and interaction
between the central and northern highlands (Lau 2011). To the north of Ancash are today's
Departments of La Libertad and Cajamarca.

Numerous prehistoric archaeological sites are known from both sides of the Cordillera
Blanca. Fortified hilltop settlements became common in the Early Intermediate Period
(ca. AD 100–600) with the emergence of the Recuay culture, and continued into later time
periods as well, indicating that defense was a long-term concern in this region. Trepanation
was practiced during the Late Intermediate Period (ca. AD 1000–1400) and perhaps earlier,
during the Middle Horizon Period (ca. AD 600–1000). Trepanned skulls have been found
in burial caves and chullpas on both the western and eastern slopes of the Cordillera Blanca.

These caves and burial structures, like similar examples found in the central and southern highlands and Altiplano region, contain largely disassociated skeletal remains and few
diagnostic grave goods. In some cases, however, artifacts and radiocarbon dating of skeletal material permit the tombs to be assigned to specific archaeological periods. Only a
few of these mortuary sites have been systematically investigated. The most extensive
research has ocurred at the site of Marcajirca, located at an elevation of 3,800 meters in the
Conchucos Region near the modern town of Huari, and at Keushu, located at a similar
altitude on the western side of the Cordillera Blanca above the modern town of Yungay
(Gerdau-Radonić and Herrera 2010a, 2010b). Recently, field research has also been undertaken at Hualcayán, located on the western flanks of the Cordillera Blanca near the modern
town of Caraz, by the Proyecto de Investigación Arqueológico Regional Ancash (PIARA).

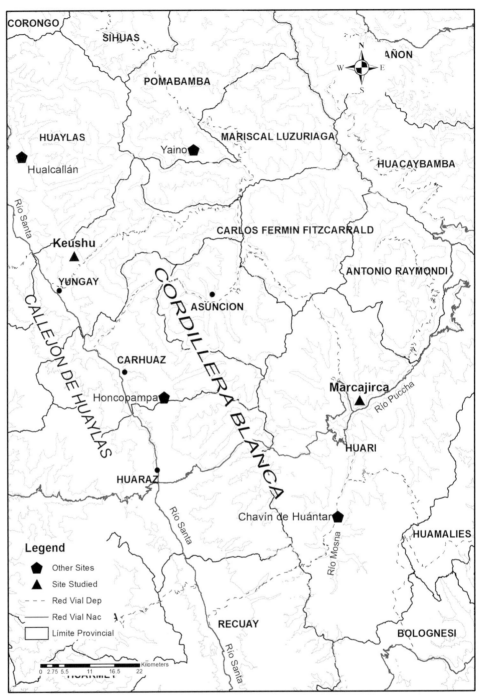

Figure 6.1 Map of the northern highlands of Peru. Archaeological sites with trepanned skulls are marked by triangles, modern towns and cities by circles. Map by Bebel Ibarra Asencios.

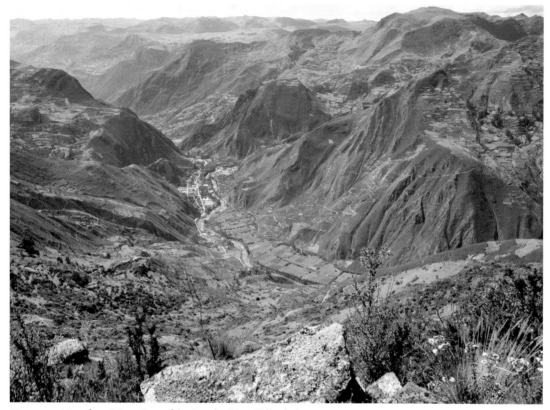

Figure 6.2 View from Marcajirca of the Puccha River Valley below.

All three sites have yielded trepanned skulls. Most appear to date to the Late Intermediate Period, but one from Hualcayán may be associated with the earlier Recuay culture (Emily Sharp, personal communication 2014).

MARCAJIRCA

Marcajirca is a Late Intermediate Period to Early Historic Period site located in the Department of Ancash, about 550 kilometers (342 miles) northeast of Lima (see Figure 6.1). Extending over four hectares, the site sits on a rocky ridge at the top of a steep-sided mountain in the Cordillera Blanca, at an elevation of 3,800 meters (12,500 feet) (Figure 6.2). Marcajirca is located in a region that, during the Middle Horizon Period, apparently was not under the influence of the Wari state. Field survey of various archaeological sites in the Puccha Valley have found no evidence of Wari pottery or architecture (Ibarra Asencios 2014), in contrast to later evidence of Inca influence in the region and at the site of Marcajirca.

Archaeological testing at Marcajirca has been underway since 2004 as part of an annual bioarchaeological field school directed by Bebel Ibarra Asencios. Excavation has revealed that the site includes residential, public, and funerary sectors. The residential sector contains the foundations of houses, while public areas include a standing tower and a large amphitheater-like structure. The funerary component includes twenty-two caves and thirty-five chullpas that contain human skeletal remains. Some areas appear to have a mixed function, as houses and chullpas are found in close proximity (Figure 6.3).

At Marcajirca, the earliest burials appear to have been interred in the caves (Figure 6.4). Later, chullpas were constructed for burial. Built from locally available stone and roofed with wood, chullpas are typically square in plan and accessed by a small opening (Figure 6.5). There is no apparent consistency in the placement or orientation of chullpas, although most are associated with low-walled courtyards that appear to have served as private spaces for funerary activities (Figure 6.6). Calibrated radiocarbon dates from wood samples from the chullpas and from human remains from both caves and chullpas average around AD 1200, with a range from AD 1000 to 1640, placing them within the Late Intermediate, Late Horizon, and early colonial periods.

Some caves and chullpas at Marcajirca have been fully excavated, while others have only been tested. Based on the minimum number of individuals in each burial context, it is apparent that the bodies were not all interred at the same time, but that tombs were reused over time. Excavations have revealed remains of hearths or fires in front of chullpa entrances, suggesting offerings were burned. Some disturbance of material in the caves and chullpas likely occurred over their period of active use. Additional disturbance has occurred as a result of visitors and artifact hunters. Other than minor surface disturbance, however, the chullpas are structurally intact and very well preserved.

It is interesting to ponder why people chose to live at Marcajirca. The site is difficult to access, requiring a two- to three-hour arduous hike from the river below (see Figure 6.2). Its high altitude environment is subject to harsh conditions with wide fluctuations in daily temperatures and relatively little rainfall. The site is located in the ecological zone known as the *puna*, where there are abundant high-altitude grasses suited to camelid herding, but the zone is not well suited to agriculture, which today is practiced at lower elevations where there are better soils and a more hospitable climate. To farm and to obtain food and water, the inhabitants would have needed to descend the mountain and transport materials back up to the site.

Given knowledge of the cultural climate of the Late Intermediate Period, we may speculate that the remote site location was chosen for defensive reasons. Supporting this inference are walls on the lateral borders of the site, as well as both indirect and direct evidence of violence in the form of weapons (sling stones, mace heads, and ground stone projectile points; Figures 6.7–6.9), and healed (Figure 6.10) and unhealed skeletal trauma, including cranial fractures (Figures 6.11–6.13). Two distinct ethnic groups were present in the region—the Huaris and the Pincos—and there appears to have been a history of conflict between them, as indicated by the fact that the Inca built separate administrative centers and storage areas for the two groups: Huari Tambo and Pincos Tambo, located less than a day's walk from one another. Variation in forms of intentional cranial deformation suggest that the Marcajirca sample itself contains members of distinct ethnic groups, some of whom deformed the heads of their infants using cloth bands, producing a distinctive head shape, and others who did not practice head shaping. Among those who practiced cranial deformation, at least two quite distinct forms are present (Figures 6.14 and 6.15).

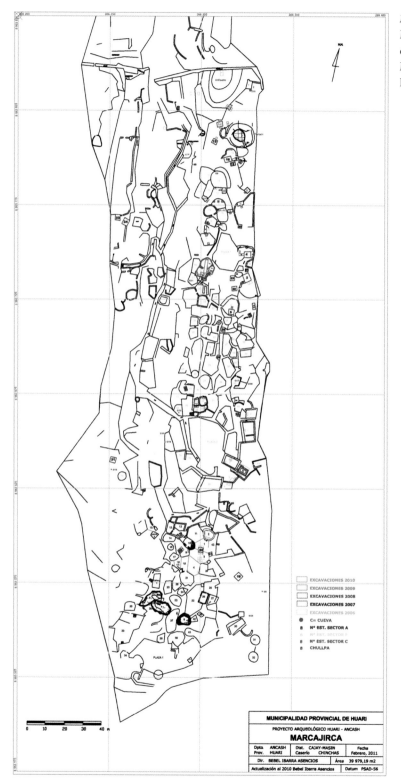

MUNICIPALIDAD PROVINCIAL DE HUARI

PROYECTO ARQUEOLÓGICO HUARI - ANCASH

MARCAJIRCA

Dpto.	ANCASH	Dist.	CAJAY-MASIN	Fecha
Prov.	HUARI	Caserío	CHINCHAS	Febrero, 2011
Dir.	BEBEL IBARRA ASENCIOS		Área	39 979,19 m2
Actualización al 2010 Bebel Ibarra Asencios			Datum	PSAD-56

Figure 6.3
Map of the site
of Marcajirca.
Map by Bebel
Ibarra Asencios.

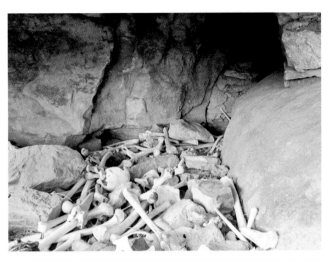

Figure 6.4
A funerary cave with jumbled bones on the surface.

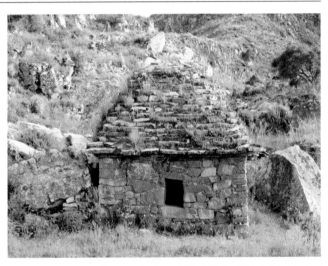

Figure 6.5
A typical chullpa, with its small rectangular entrance.

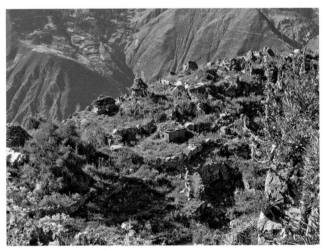

Figure 6.6
A cluster of chullpas in the northeast portion of the site.

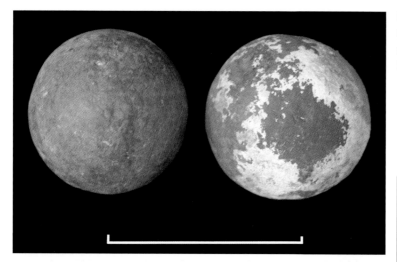

Figure 6.7
Sling stones found
at Marcajirca. Scale
is 5 cm.

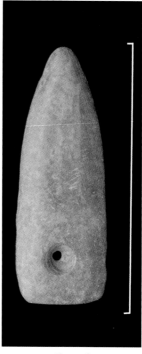

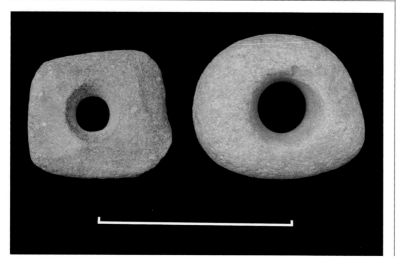

Figure 6.8 Stone club heads. Scale is 10 cm.

Figure 6.9 Ground stone
projectile point. It is perforated,
possibly to be worn as a pendant.
Scale is 5 cm.

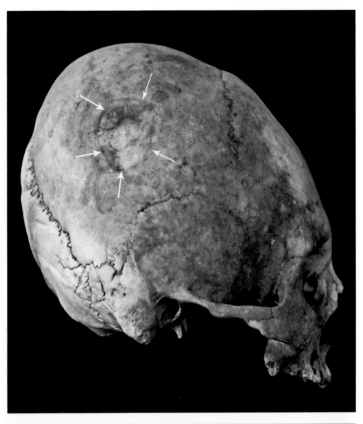

Figure 6.10
Healed depressed skull fracture (arrows), probably produced by a sling stone or stone mace head. Cueva 19, 49-C19-B2-1621.

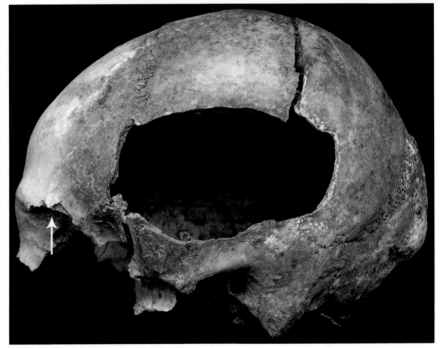

Figure 6.11
Unhealed skull fracture, showing a large broken out area and radiating fractures extending from its superior margin and inferiorly through the sphenoid bone. Fractures are also visible on the left superciliary arch (arrow). Chullpa 8, 49-CH8-1.

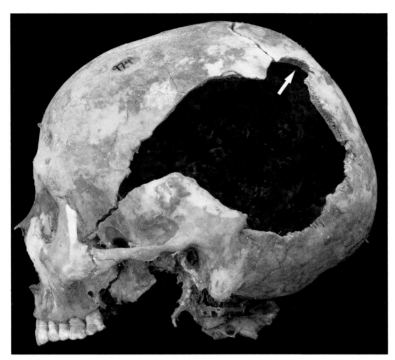

Figure 6.12
Massive perimortem blunt force trauma to the left side of the skull with multiple radiating fractures. A semicircular broken out area (arrow) may mark the impact scar of a star-headed mace. Cueva 3 (2008).

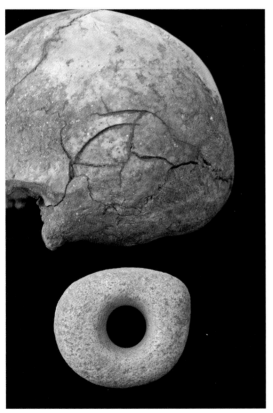

Figure 6.13
Perimortem blunt force trauma compared with a stone mace head, the kind of weapon that may have produced fractures like this one. Cueva 3 (49-C3-F3-1043).

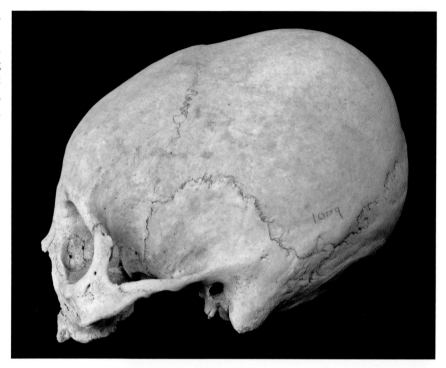

Figure 6.14
Annular (circumferential) cranial modification in an adult female, producing an elongated, flattened head shape. Cueva 19, 49-C19-B2.

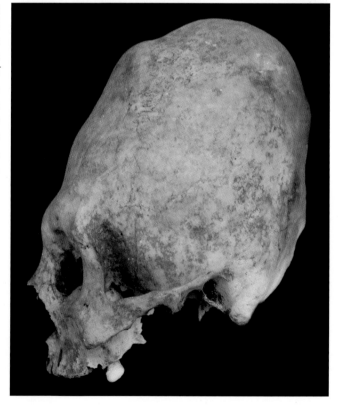

Figure 6.15
Annular cranial modification in an adult male. This form is distinct from that of Figure 6.14: a shorter and taller head with a pronounced bulge at the top of the forehead. Cueva 19, 49-C19-B1-1010.

Trauma

The frequency and location of trauma at Marcajirca was examined in a sample of twenty-four adult crania and 835 adult upper and lower limb bones (clavicles, humeri, radii, ulnae, femora, tibiae, and fibulae) representing a minimum of ninety individuals from four chull-pas. Evidence was found of injuries due to both the challenges of the terrain and interpersonal conflict (Titelbaum et al. 2013). Of the long bones examined, 1.6 percent show healed fractures. These include three Colles's fractures of the right radius, styloid process fractures in two ulnae, two humeral shaft fractures, one fracture of the lateral clavicle, two tibial plateau fractures, one proximal tibial shaft fracture, one of the medial malleolus of the tibia, and one fibular shaft fracture. Most of these injuries were likely sustained by falls on the uneven terrain.

Eight crania (33 percent; five male, one possible female, two indeterminate) have healed or unhealed fractures, and five of the eight have multiple injuries. In total, twenty antemortem and perimortem injuries were identified, 60 percent of which were found on the left side of the cranium, most located on the frontal bone (55 percent). Fractures of the nasal bones were common as well. Of the fourteen healed cranial wounds, nine (64.3 percent) are located on the frontal bone, four (28.6 percent) involve the nasal bones, and one is on the right parietal bone (7.1 percent). Most antemortem wounds are ovoid in shape and shallow, perhaps having been inflicted by a star-shaped mace head or sling stone (Lovell 1997). The six perimortem wounds are located on the frontal bone (33.3 percent), the nasal bones (33.3 percent), and on the left parietal bone (33.3 percent). The majority of the observed healed and unhealed craniofacial trauma is present on the front left side of the skull. In contrast, there are relatively few injuries on the sides or back of the head. This pattern of injury is suggestive of face-to-face conflict, especially considering that a right-handed assailant with a club would deliver most wounds to the left side of the head (Stewart 1958).

Comparing frequencies of cranial trauma with data from other Late Intermediate Period sites, we find that head injuries are relatively frequent, although not as common as reported for a Late Intermediate Period sample from the former Middle Horizon Period Wari capital, where there is a 71 percent prevalence (Tung 2008). However, at the former Wari capital, both males and females were affected, which may be indicative of a massacre event. Unlike the Wari capital, there are trepanations at Marcajirca, including well-healed ones, suggesting that there were people who survived their wounds, had their injuries surgically treated, and survived for long periods afterward.

Trepanations

To date, there are nine crania from three caves and three chullpas that have a total of eleven trepanations. Based on robust cranial morphology, all nine appear to be males. Three are young adults, two are middle adults, five are older adults, and one cranial fragment is of indeterminate age. Trepanation methods include scraping (n = 4) (Figure 6.16) and cutting (n = 4), both linear cutting with angular intersections (n = 2) and cutting with rounded borders (n = 2). Due to the extent of healing, it is not possible to determine the technique used in three of the trepanations (see, for example, Figures 6.17 and 6.18). The smallest of the cranial openings is 10 × 10 millimeters, whereas the largest is 90 × 57 millimeters. Ten

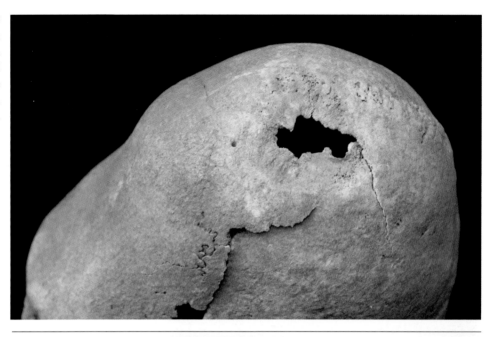

Figure 6.16
Adult male with a healed trepanation on the left parietal executed with the scraping method. Chullpa 15, U2/C1.

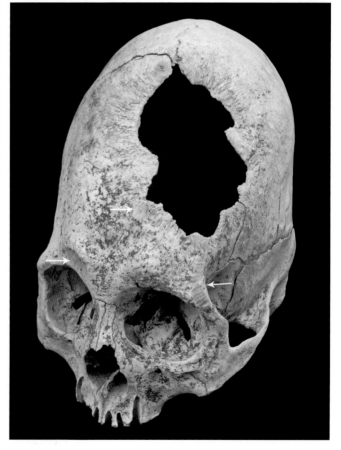

Figure 6.17
Young adult male with a large healed trepanation of the frontal and parietal bones. Healing of the margins makes it unclear which trepanation method was used. Arrows in the photo indicate areas of postmortem rodent gnawing. Cueva 19, 49-C19-B2-1000.

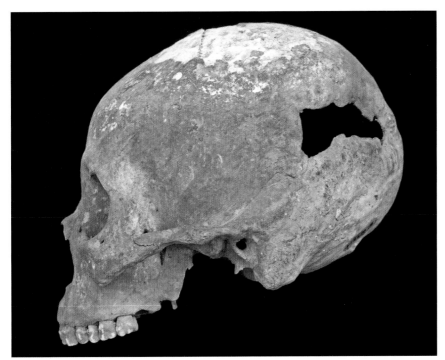

Figure 6.18
Young adult male with a healed trepanation on the left parietal bone. Healing of the irregularly shaped opening makes it unclear which trepanation method was used. Cueva 7B, 49-C7B-5.

of the trepanations (91 percent) show long-term healing, whereas only one indicates short-term survival. None show evidence of infection or inflammation.

Eighty-two percent of the trepanations are located on the left side of the cranium—on the left side of the frontal bone (n = 4) and on the left parietal (n = 5)—and 73 percent of the trepanations are found on the anterior part of the cranium—on the frontal bone (n = 6) and anterior portion of the parietal (n = 2). The placement of trepanations on the front left side of the cranium is consistent with the previously noted pattern of injuries suffered in face-to-face conflict with a right-handed assailant.

Skull Fractures and Trepanation

Of the trepanned crania, six (67 percent) have antemortem depressed fractures or penetrating wounds. Of the six, five demonstrate long-term healing of both the trauma and the trepanation, whereas one shows only short-term healing. Two individuals appear to have had surgery to treat wounds inflicted by star-shaped maces. Most of the fractures (65 percent) were located on the left side of both the head and face (Table 6.1).

The cranium of an older adult male from Cueva 7B has healed antemortem trauma to both nasal bones, a small, ovoid, healed depression above the left supercilliary arch, and two healed trepanations on the frontal bone (Figure 6.19). Both are found just anterior to the coronal suture, and one is located to the right of the midline (14 × 16 mm), while the other is to the left of the midline (16 × 7 mm). Both trepanations show similar healing, suggesting that they may have been made at around the same time. If that is the case, then the surgery may have been done to treat the impact of a star-headed mace.

Table 6.1 Trepanation and skull fracture locations at Marcajirca.

	FACIAL BONES	FRONTAL BONE	LEFT VAULT	MIDLINE VAULT	RIGHT VAULT	OCCIPITAL
Trepanations (n=11)	0 (0%)	6 (55%)	5 (45%)	0 (0%)	0 (0%)	0 (0%)
Fractures (n=17)	9 (53%) (4L, 5R)	5 (29%) (4L, 1R)	3 (18%)	0 (0%)	0 (0%)	0 (0%)

Figure 6.19
Old adult male with healed fractures of the nasal and left frontal bone and two healed trepanations by the scraping method. Section F, Cueva 7B.

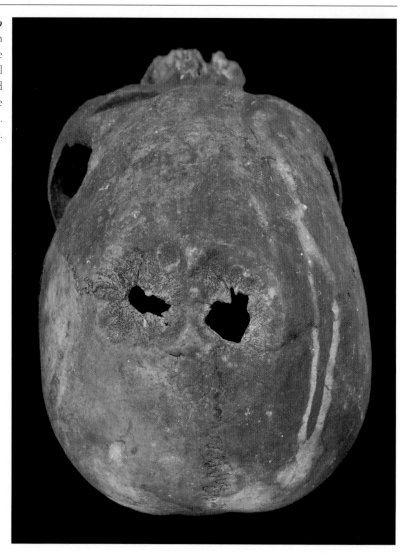

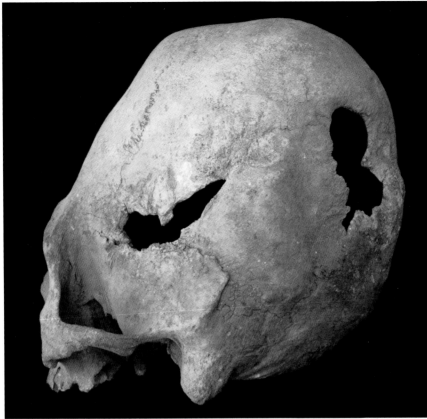

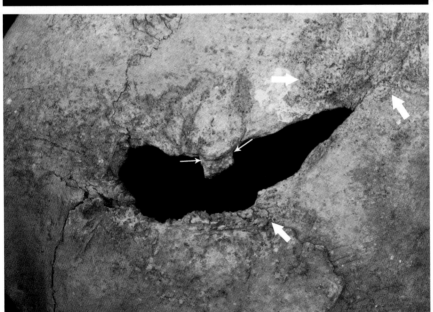

Figure 6.20
(a) Old adult male with two trepanations. Both show healing, although the trepanation on the temple still shows active bone remodeling, suggesting that it was made later than the first. (b) A close-up of the trepanation in the temple region shows areas of active bone remodeling (large arrows) and a possible cut mark along the superior margin of the defect (small arrows). Cueva 7B, 49-C7B-3.

Figure 6.21
(a) Young adult male with a trepanation associated with skull fracture; and (b) close-up showing a radiating fracture extending down the coronal suture (large arrows) and small cavities and a "line of demarcation" (small arrows) marking the early stages of remodeling of necrotic bone (Barbian and Sledzik 2008). Sector F, Chullpa 14.

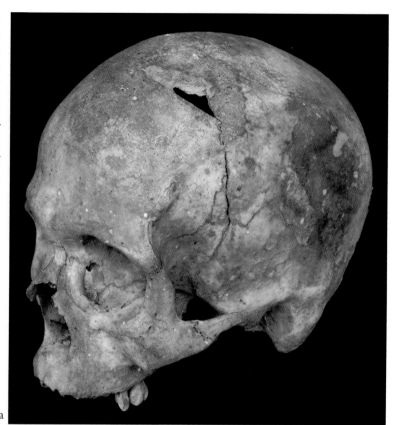

a

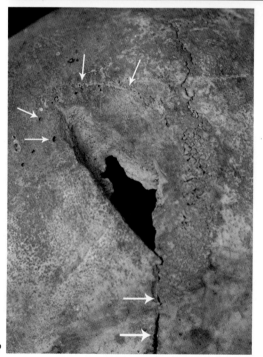

b

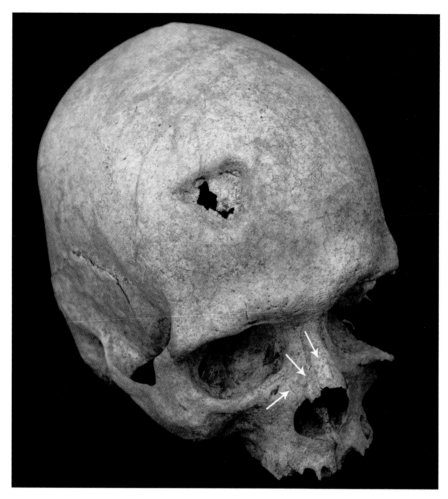

Figure 6.22
An old adult male with
a healed triangular
depression and small
irregular opening.
It appears to be a
trepanation by the
cutting method that
primarily removed the
outer table and spongy
bone. Also visible in
the photo are healed
fractures of the nasal
bones and right maxilla
(arrows). Chullpa 7,
49-CH7-7.

Another older adult male from Cueva 7B also has healed trauma to both nasal bones and two healed trepanations (Figure 6.20a). The first is located on the anterior-inferior portion of the parietal, just above the squamosal suture, measuring 54 × 14 millimeters. It seems to show bone healing still in process, as indicated by incompletely remodeled subperiosteal bone deposited around the opening. A possible cut mark is still visible on its superior margin (Figure 6.20b). The second trepanation is located on the posterior portion of the parietal adjacent to the lambdoid suture, a bilobular opening measuring 43 × 23 millimeters. Both of these older adult males were found in the same burial cave (Cueva 7B).

A young adult male from Chullpa 14 has a partly healed triangular trepanation (36 × 14 mm) on the left side of the frontal bone (Figure 6.21a). Cut marks and grooves are visible around the margins of the opening, as are small cavities created by osteoclasts breaking down necrotic bone (Figure 6.21b). The surgery appears to have been executed to treat complications from a skull fracture. Beginning at the lateral margin of the triangular cut, a linear fracture line runs inferiorly along the coronal suture, travels through the left parietal, and then along the sphenotemporal suture.

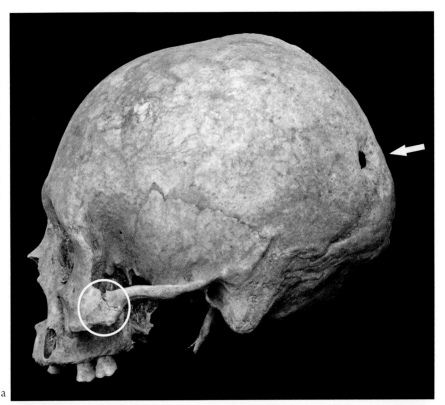

a

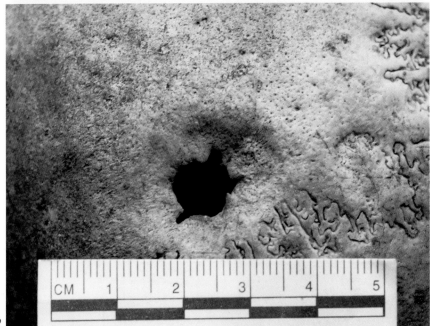

b

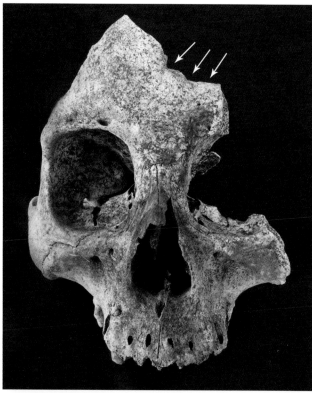

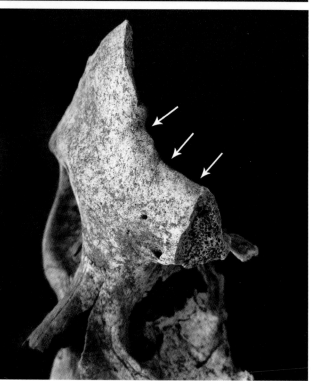

Figure 6.24
(a) Fragmentary cranium
of an adult male that shows
the rounded border of a
trepanation on the left frontal
(indicated by white arrows).
(b) Detail of the preserved
trepanation margin, indicated
by white arrows. Chulpa
26, skull 15. Photographs
by Anne R. Titelbaum.

An older adult male from Chullpa 7 has a well-healed triangular depression on the right side of the frontal bone with a small irregular opening in its center. Measuring 26 × 22 millimeters, it appears to be a healed trepanation. The cranium has healed fractures of both nasal bones, a linear fracture on the right maxilla that travels from the inferior edge of the orbit to the nasal aperture, and a healed non-union fracture between the frontal bone and the left zygomatic (Figure 6.22).

The cranium of a middle adult male from Cueva 2 has a small, well-healed, rounded trepanation on the posterior superior quadrant of the left parietal measuring 10 × 10 millimeters (Figure 6.23). There is also a well-healed fracture of the zygomatic process of the left temporal bone.

The fragmentary cranium of an adult male from Chulpa 26 preserves the anterior margin of a well-healed circular trepanation on the left side of the frontal bone, about 1.6 centimeters from the glabella (Figure 6.24). This individual also has a well-healed fracture of the right nasal bone.

KEUSHU

At Keushu, located on the western side of the Cordillera Blanca, recent excavations have recovered eight trepanned crania from two communal burial structures, one dated on the basis of associated ceramics to about AD 700–900, the other to the Late Intermediate Period (about AD 1200–1470) (Gerdau-Radonić and Herrera 2010a, 2010b). Some crania have multiple openings, producing a total count of sixteen trepanations. Three trepanation techniques have been identified: scraping, linear cutting, and drilling and cutting. The success rate was high, as twelve of the sixteen openings have evidence of long-term healing, representing a success rate of 75 percent. Possible motivations for trepanning have been identified in two crania (skull fracture and infection), but the remainder have no evidence suggesting why the procedure was done.

CAJABAMBA (CAJAMARCA)

North of the Callejón de Huaylas and west of the land of the Chachapoya (see below) lies the Department of Cajamarca. The Museo Nacional de Antropología, Arqueología, y Historia del Perú has a single trepanned cranium from this region, cataloged as coming from Cajabamba, approximately 80 kilometers southeast of the city of Cajamarca. The cranium is interesting because it has two trepanations executed by different techniques. The first, which shows extensive healing, is located near the joining of the metopic and coronal sutures and appears to have involved the scraping method. It is marked by a large area (54 × 72 mm) of remodeled bone and a small opening (Figure 6.25a). The second trepanation, located on the occipital bone, was executed with the drilling and cutting method, and it shows no healing (Figure 6.25b). In addition to the drilled holes, this trepanation shows fine cut marks around the margin of the opening, which indicate that perpendicular cuts were made, probably to retract flaps of scalp and expose the bone.

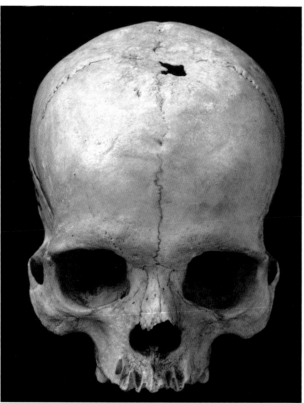

a

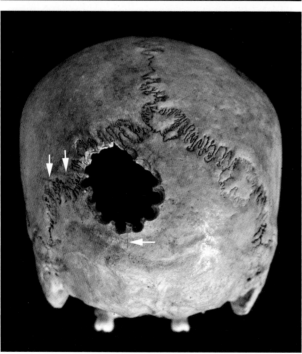

b

Figure 6.25
(a) Cranium of a young adult male from Cajabamba showing a healed trepanation by scraping near the joining of the metopic and coronal sutures. (b) Posterior view of cranium showing an unhealed trepanation (40 × 39 mm) made with the drilling and cutting method. Cut marks around the margins of the opening (arrows) appear to mark where the scalp was cut to expose the bone. Museo Nacional de Antropología, Arqueología, y Historia del Perú, AF:1388, MNAA/012, INC-75.

CHACHAPOYAS

The Chachapoyas region, located in the modern Department of Amazonas, is a roughly oval or trapezoidal area of the northeastern Peruvian Andes, defined on the west and north by the Marañón River and on the east by the Huallaga River (Figure 6.26). Its southern boundary is a constricted area where the Marañón and Huallaga Rivers lie only a hundred miles apart. It is a rugged region characterized by steep mountains and diverse microenvironments. Traversing the Chachapoyas region from west to east, one passes from the dry tropical forest along the Marañón to high grasslands and eventually snow-capped peaks that reach elevations of over fifteen thousand feet, and then down into the cloud forest of the eastern slopes of the Andes.

The origins of the ancient Chachapoya culture can be traced back to around AD 800 (Schjellerup 1997; Von Hagen 2002). Chachapoya sites are recognizable by their distinctive circular stone houses and elaborate mortuary structures built on inaccessible cliffs. Many Chachapoya ruins can be reached today only by foot or on mule. The remoteness and difficulty of access to major sites such as Gran Pajatén, Kuélap, and Laguna de los Cóndores have contributed to their mystique (Kauffmann Doig and Ligabue 2003; Muscutt 1998; Savoy 1970; Von Hagen 2002). The Spanish chroniclers Cieza de León and Garcilaso de la Vega described the Chachapoya people not as a single ethnic group, but as a number of distinct peoples who united when threatened by external forces (Cieza de León 1941 [1553]; Garcilaso de la Vega 1960 [1604]). Despite unified resistance, the region was conquered by the Inca around AD 1470 in what was described as a difficult and bloody campaign. Inca reprisals were severe, including executions and forced resettlement of many of the Chachapoya in other parts of the empire. Given their treatment by the Inca, it is not surprising that the Chachapoya chose to ally themselves with the Spanish after the capture of Atahualpa in 1532, and they willingly assisted them in the conquest of their enemy (Schjellerup 1997).

History of Discoveries

Modern interest in the ancient inhabitants of the Chachapoyas region is generally traced to the "rediscovery" of the impressive citadel of Kuélap in 1843 by Crisóstomo Nieto, a judge from Chachapoyas. In 1892, he published a description of the site, and shortly afterward the ruins were visited by a number of explorers, including Adolf Bandelier, Ernst Middendorf, Charles Wiener, and Antonio Raimondi (Von Hagen 2002). Accounts of these expeditions encouraged others to visit the Chachapoyas region in search of this "lost civilization," and such interest continues to the present day (González and León 2002; Kauffmann Doig and Ligabue 2003; Muscutt 1998; Savoy 1970).

Although some early explorers photographed and mapped sites like Kuélap (Bandelier 1909), the first scientific excavations at Chachapoya sites were not conducted until 1948, when French archaeologists Henry and Paule Reichlen explored a number of sites in the region and conducted limited excavations at Kuélap, Revash, and other locations (Reichlen and Reichlen 1950). Importantly, the Reichlens collected artifacts and human skeletal remains from some of these sites. Their skeletal collection can be found today at

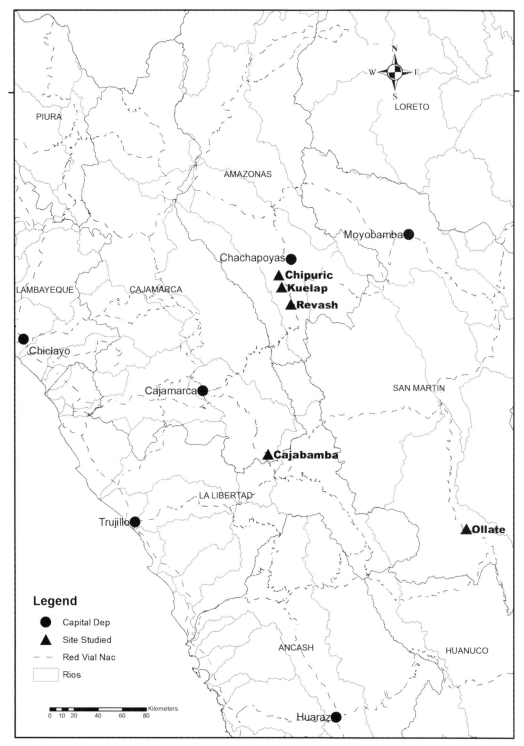

Figure 6.26 Map of the Chachapoyas region, indicating the locations of major archaeological sites. Map by Bebel Ibarra Asencios.

the Museo de la Nación in Lima. Other Chachapoya skeletal and mummified remains are curated in a number of smaller regional museums. Presently, the largest collection of Chachapoya human remains and funerary offerings is from the Laguna de los Cóndores and is housed in the newly constructed Museo Leymebamba near the modern city of Chachapoyas (Guillén 2007). The collection includes numerous mummies, as well as skeletal remains from ossuaries at the site. Curiously, no evidence of trepanation has been reported from Laguna de los Cóndores, although trepanned skulls are known from a number of other sites in the Chachapoyas region.

The Reichlen Collection

The Museo de la Nación curates the skeletal material from the Reichlens' 1948 expedition. It includes a total of ninety-eight crania from the mortuary complex of Revash, and one cranium each from the sites of Kuélap and Chipurik. In addition, there is a trepanned cranium from Ollate (marked "Ollate 3"). Ollate is not mentioned in the Reichlens' 1950 publication, but the skull is marked in a similar fashion to the others, and thus it appears to belong to their collection. Of the total sample, eleven crania have trepanations and ten have visible fractures (mostly healed) but no trepanations. Most of the trepanned skulls came from Revash 2, a large funerary cave that the Reichlens estimated contained more than two hundred mummies. Unfortunately, due to transportation difficulties they were able to collect only a small portion of the material, primarily crania. Of the trepanned crania they collected from Revash, Chipurik, and Ollate, two were children and nine were adults. Among the nine adults, six were judged to be male and three female.

Revash Children

The two trepanned children are of particular interest because it is rare to find trepanations in this age group. The first skull, from the Revash 2 funerary cave, belonged to a child of about seven or eight years of age, based on dental development. A partially healed trepanation of uncertain technique is on the left frontal bone (Figure 6.27). Externally, the opening is surrounded by a roughly rectangular area of superficial bone resorption that marks an area of necrotic bone that was in the process of remodeling at the time of death. There is also periosteal reaction surrounding the trepanation site and extending down the bones of the face to the alveolar area. Internally, there is a large area of new bone deposited over the inner table of the frontal bone that extends to but does not cross the coronal suture. These areas of new bone deposition presumably mark the spread of an infection from the trepanation site, a serious complication.

The second child, also from Revash 2, was between eight and ten years of age at the time of death, based on dental development. It has a healed depressed fracture on the left parietal bone, adjacent to the sagittal suture, and an oval-shaped trepanation on the same bone, just superior to the squamosal suture (Figure 6.28). There is no clear relationship between the fracture and trepanation, although it is possible that that surgery was executed in an attempt to treat headaches or other posttraumatic symptoms. The margins of the trepanation are smooth and remodeled, indicating survival for a substantial period of

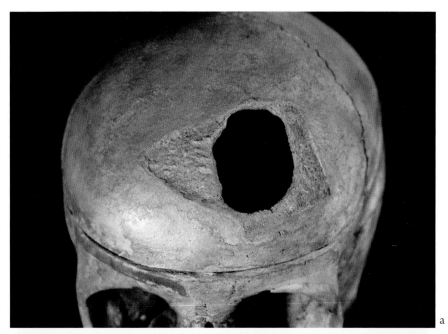

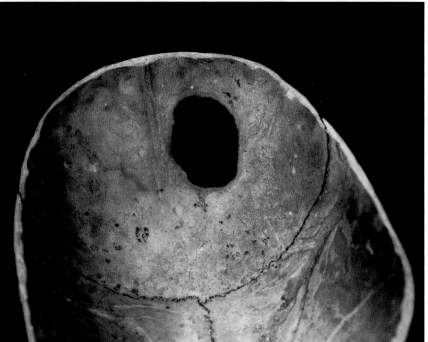

Figure 6.27 (a) A seven- to eight-year-old child with a partially healed trepanation on the frontal bone. (b) Internal view, showing extensive bone reaction surrounding the trepanation opening. The reaction extends to but does not cross the coronal suture. Revash 2, Cráneo 5. Museo de la Nación, Cráneo 70, MPCS 005.

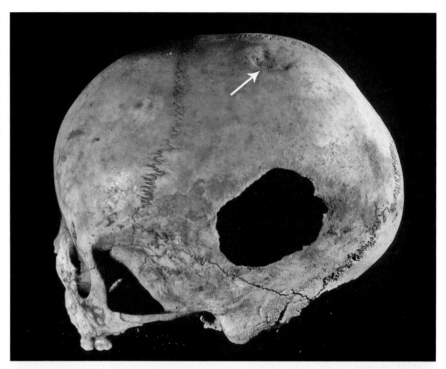

Figure 6.28
An eight- to ten-year-old child with a healed depressed fracture (arrow) and a healed trepanation on the left parietal bone. Revash 2, catalog number 00203. Museo de la Nación.

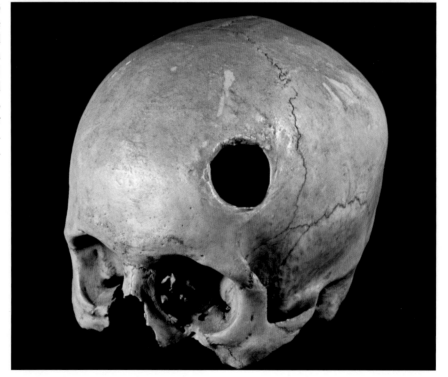

Figure 6.29
An adult male with a healed circular trepanation (diameter: 30 mm) on the left frontal bone. Revash 5, catalog number MP-2050 00151. Museo de la Nación.

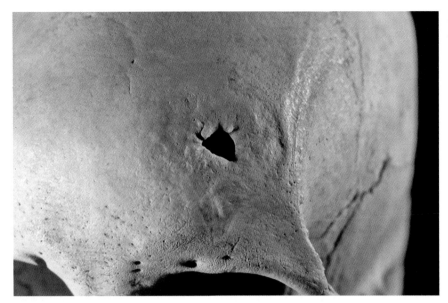

Figure 6.30
An adult female with
a healed trepanation
by the scraping
technique on the
left frontal bone.
Revash 2 (Grotte),
Cráneo 83. Museo
de la Nación.

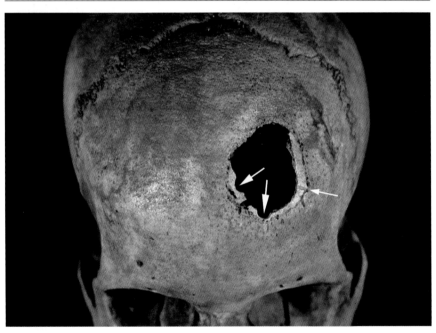

Figure 6.31
An adult male with a partially healed trepanation by the drilling and cutting method on the
left frontal bone. Arrows pointing downward mark two partial drill holes; an arrow pointing
to the left indicates cut marks. Revash 2 (Grotte), Cráneo 73. Museo de la Nación.

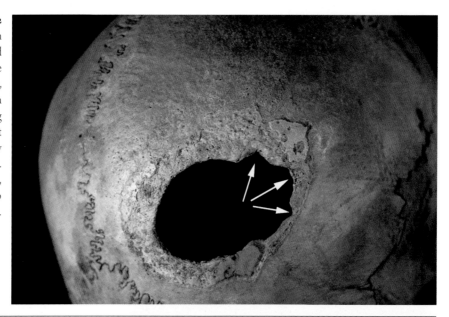

Figure 6.32
An adult male with
a partially healed
trepanation on the
right parietal bone,
possibly made with
the drilling and cutting
method. Arrows point
to what may be largely
remodeled drill holes.
Revash 2 (Grotte),
Cráneo 75. Museo
de la Nación.

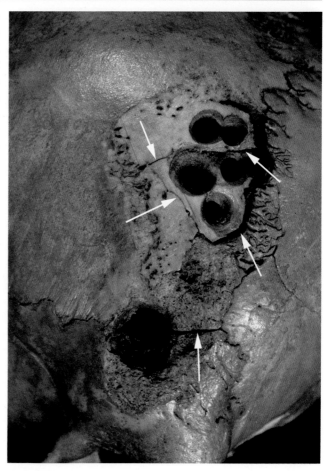

Figure 6.33
Young adult female
with multiple drilled
holes over an apparent
skull fracture. Arrows
point to fracture lines.
Revash 2 (Grotte),
Cráneo 72. Museo
de la Nación.

time, obliterating any indication of what technique was used to make the opening. Given the state of healing and lack of obvious inflammation around the trepanation margins, it is likely that the child's cause of death was not related to the trepanation procedure or postoperative complications.

Revash Adults

Seven adults (four males and three females) from Revash 2 and one adult from Revash 5 have trepanations. Three (43 percent) show long-term survival, while four (57 percent) exhibit short-term healing only. Of the three trepanations with long-term healing, one is of uncertain technique, one appears to have been done by the circular grooving technique (although it lacks the beveling normally seen in this type of trepanation; Figure 6.29), and one appears to have been done by scraping (Figure 6.30). Of the trepanations with short-term healing, one is of uncertain technique (possibly drilled), and the other three are either clearly or probably executed by the drilling and cutting method. The probable cases are two openings that are partially remodeled but have scalloped defects on their margins that appear to be drill holes. The first case (Figure 6.31) is the most suggestive. It has a roughly circular defect on the left frontal bone surrounded on three sides by a narrow strip of necrotic bone. Two semicircular cuts can be seen on the medial and inferior edges of the defect as well as two fine cut marks on the necrotic bone on the lateral aspect. Had healing continued and the remaining necrotic bone been resorbed by osteoclastic activity, these tell-tale marks would have been lost, supporting Fernando Cabieses's assertion that healing of trepanations often obliterates evidence of how the cuts were made (see Chapter 4). In the second case of partial healing (Figure 6.32), the evidence is more ambiguous. Here again, there is a partially healed opening, with segments of necrotic bone still present around the margins. One located anterior-superior to the opening shows several fine cut marks on its surface. The anterior margin of the defect has three scalloped areas that might represent drill holes that are largely resorbed, although this is not as clear as in the previous case. Alternatively, they could represent irregular margins of a skull fracture. Had healing continued, these irregular edges presumably would have smoothed.

The final example of a partially healed trepanation from Revash (Figure 6.33), the cranium of a young adult female, is unambiguous as to trepanation technique: six conical drill holes are present on the left side of the skull. Five are located in a cluster on a roughly rectangular area of necrotic bone just anterior to the lambdoid suture. The sixth hole, slightly larger and partially remodeled by osteoclastic activity, is located just above the left mastoid process. That it is also a drill hole and not a drainage channel (cloaca) is indicated by the fact that it shows similar beveling to the other drill holes. The holes are not arranged in a circle, so the objective does not seem to have been to drill around an area and then cut the bridges between them. Close examination of the drilled areas suggests that the motivation for the procedure involved the multiple fracture lines extending across the areas where holes were drilled. Thus, the motive here appears to have been to treat a depressed skull fracture, perhaps an attempt to drain an intracranial hematoma or abscess. The attempt was not successful, judging by the evidence of inflammation and incomplete healing.

Skull Fractures at Revash

In addition to the cases described above, five adult male and three adult female crania have fractures. Including three cases of healed fracture in the trepanned skulls, this produces a relatively low fracture rate of eight out of ninety-eight (8 percent) in the Revash sample. Half of these fractures were simple circular or oval depressions in the outer table of the skull, representing what must have been relatively minor injuries. Only one case of significant blunt force trauma with radiating fractures was found, although two of the partially healed trepanations show ragged, irregular margins, which suggest that the surgery treated a fracture. Overall, the fracture incidence seems fairly low, as Kenneth Nystrom noted in his study of this collection (Nystrom 2004, 2007). But some indication of interpersonal violence is suggested by the fact that three individuals—one female and two males— have healed nose fractures, an injury commonly associated with interpersonal violence (Walker 1997). The one skull the Reichlens collected from the site of Kuélap (Kuélap 3 Muro Central, MPCS 017) has healed concentric and radiating fractures on its right temporal and parietal bones, reflecting a serious blow to the temple.

Chipurik

Five crania were collected by the Reichlens from burial structures at the site of Chipurik, located on the River Luya near the modern city of Chachapoyas. Only one of the five crania (Chipurik 3, Groupe A, Cráneo 15, MPCS 026) has a trepanation. Mellisa Lund Valle and I recorded data on it, but apparently no photographs were taken. The trepanation is circular in form, approximately 30 millimeters in diameter, and surrounded by a rectangular area of roughened bone, presumably marking where the periosteum was removed during the procedure. The trepanation shows long-term healing. We also observed a small, healed, depressed fracture just medial to the trepanation and healed fractures of the left nasal and nasal process of the left maxilla.

Ollate

As noted above, a single skull in the Reichlen collection is recorded as coming from Ollate 3 (Figure 6.34), a site quite distant from the others described above. It is the cranium of a young adult male with a large, well-healed trepanation located along the midline of the vault, extending from the bregma to just above the external occipital protuberance. A small oval opening is also present just anterior to the bregma, associated with a depressed area that may mark a fracture. This is one of the more impressive examples of a substantial trepanation that did not cause the death of the patient. Given its large size, this opening may represent multiple operations, although the degree of healing appears consistent throughout.

TREPANNED SKULLS FROM OTHER CHACHAPOYA SITES

Trepanned skulls have been collected by explorers and anthropologists from a number of Chachapoya sites, including Kuélap (Figure 6.35), and examples can be found today in regional anthropology museums and private collections. Unfortunately, most of these

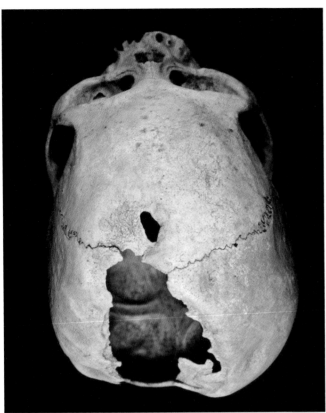

Figure 6.34
(a) Superior view of a young adult male cranium with a large well-healed trepanation along the midline of the vault. A smaller, oval-shaped opening is also present on the frontal bone just anterior to the bregma.
(b) Posterior view of the cranium. Ollate 3, catalog number 52086. Museo de la Nación.

a

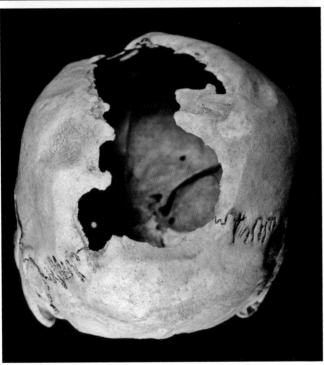

b

Figure 6.35
(a) Left parietal bone from a cranium found near the entrance of the outer wall of Kuélap (Ruiz Estrada 2013:37) that has a trepanation done by the drilling and cutting method. On the external surface, a roughly rectangular area of necrotic bone can be seen delimited by shallow grooves (arrows). (b) On the inner surface, a ring of light color surrounded by pitting marks the early stages of bone remodeling. Both inner and outer table bone changes indicate short-term survival. Museo Nacional de Antropología, Arqueología, y Historia del Perú, AF:8574, AM4-1 Ix.

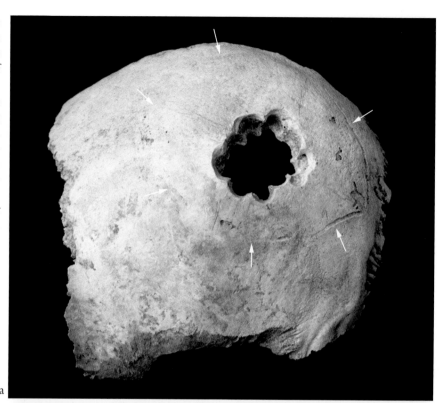

a

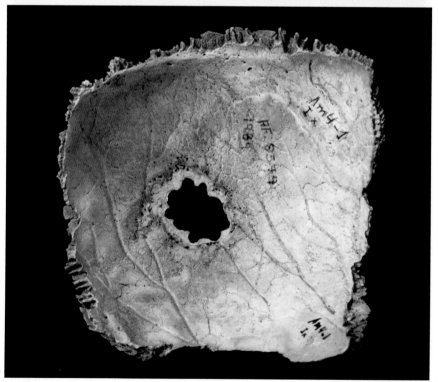

b

crania lack reliable provenance information, although they are often attributed to particular sites (Gaither 2010; Nystrom 2007; Ruiz Estrada 2013). Recent archaeological surveys of rock shelters in the province of Luya by the Jucusbamba Archaeological Project have recovered four crania with healed trepanations (Koschmieder and Gaither 2010). In other cases, skeletal material has been examined and photographed during archaeological site surveys, but then left where discovered in funerary structures and caves. One such survey, which includes information on skull fractures and trepanation, was published by Danish archaeologist Inge Schjellerup and colleagues (Jakobsen et al. 1987; Jørgensen 1988; Schjellerup 1997). Their study of skeletal remains from five Chachapoya sites (Huepón, Runashayana, Tibababmo, Achil, and Salsipuedes) found fractures, both healed and unhealed, in 33 of 153 skulls (22 percent) they examined. Small, healed, depressed fractures were most common in female skulls, while more severe injuries (often unhealed) were found only in males. Trepanations were found on three skulls. In two cases, they were directly associated with skull fractures, thus appearing to have been performed for therapeutic purposes. In the first example, three small (four millimeters in diameter) holes were drilled in the frontal bone, surrounded by a circular depressed fracture. The three holes are not arranged in a line, but instead define the points of a triangle. Their purpose may have been to test for the presence of a hematoma and to drain it, but Jakobsen and colleagues (Jakobsen et al. 1987) note that the drill holes do not penetrate the inner table of the skull, suggesting that the patient died before the operation was complete. In the second case, a series of six holes were drilled along the posterior margin of a circular punched-out fracture located on the top of the skull near the bregma. In this skull, the bridges of bone between the holes were cut and a piece of bone was removed, as is typical of the drilling and cutting method. In both cases the surgery was unsuccessful, as no evidence of healing can be observed. The third trepanned skull has a well-healed, roughly circular hole located over the sagittal suture, just posterior to the bregma. Healing of the margins makes the choice of trepanation technique unclear, but it may have been drilling and cutting (Jørgensen 1988).

Intersite Variability in Skull Fractures and Trepanation

The skeletal samples reviewed above suggest that there was substantial variability in the risk of skull fracture among the Chachapoya. This probably reflects both regional and temporal variability in the frequency and nature of interpersonal conflict (Jakobsen et al. 1987; Nystrom 2004, 2007) Unfortunately, most Chachapoya skeletal samples lack precise dating and provenance, making it difficult to test for regional or temporal differences. Trepanned skulls have been found at some sites but not at others. Is this also a sampling problem, or was the practice of trepanation limited in space and time? Again, the lack of secure dating for trepanned skulls from the Chachapoyas region makes it difficult to know. While trepanned skulls can reasonably be placed somewhere in the Late Intermediate Period (ca. AD 800–1450), none have been securely dated. But there is some potential for at least partially resolving these questions. Recent archaeological excavations at the site of Kuélap have encountered abundant human skeletal remains in documented archaeological contexts. These demonstrate a relatively high frequency of skull fractures and other indications of trauma and violent death (Nystrom and Toyne 2014). Recent excavations at Kuélap have recovered eighteen trepanned crania, and report a relatively high success rate of 70 percent (Toyne 2014). Trepanned crania from the other Chachapoya sites described above show variable success rates, ranging from 30–50 percent. Clearly, more archaeologically excavated samples are needed to better understand the practice of trepanation in the Chachapoyas region.

The Southern Highlands and Altiplano

AT THE TIME TELLO AND HRDLIČKA WERE PUBLISHING THE FIRST REPORTS on trepanned skulls from the central highlands, Yale University was conducting anthropological expeditions in the southern highlands of Peru, exploring a series of Inca sites northwest of Cuzco (Figure 7.1). The expeditions were funded in part by the National Geographic Society, and articles published in their magazine brought worldwide attention to Inca ruins in this area. Most dramatic, of course, is Machu Picchu, which Yale professor Hiram Bingham first publicized in 1912. As part of his study, Bingham and his research team explored more than one hundred small caves and crevices on the hillsides surrounding the site, and made a large collection of human and faunal skeletal remains and grave offerings (Eaton 1916; Miller 2003). Mammalian osteologist George Eaton, who wrote a monograph on the human remains (Eaton 1916), concluded that the great majority were of women. Bingham used these data to support his hypothesis that Machu Picchu was an *acclawasi*, where chosen women ("Virgins of the Sun") lived out their lives in relative solitude. Subsequent research on Machu Picchu called this rather imaginative scenario into question, and it is now clear that Machu Picchu was one of the Inca Pachacuti's royal estates (Burger and Salazar 2004; Rowe 1990). A recent review of the skeletal remains concluded that the Machu Picchu burials contained not only women but also a significant proportion of men, infants, and children (Verano 2003b). It appears that those buried in the hillsides around Machu Picchu were neither Virgins of the Sun nor natives of the area, but servants drawn from different parts of the Inca Empire, brought there to tend the estate. Thus, the burial population at Machu Picchu is not representative of the local inhabitants of the Cuzco region (Turner 2009; Turner and Armelagos 2012). Their skeletal remains confirm that they were an atypical group: skull fractures were uncommon, and no examples of trepanation were found (Verano 2003b). This contrasts sharply with Inca skeletal remains from other sites in the Cuzco region, where both skull fractures and trepanations are common.

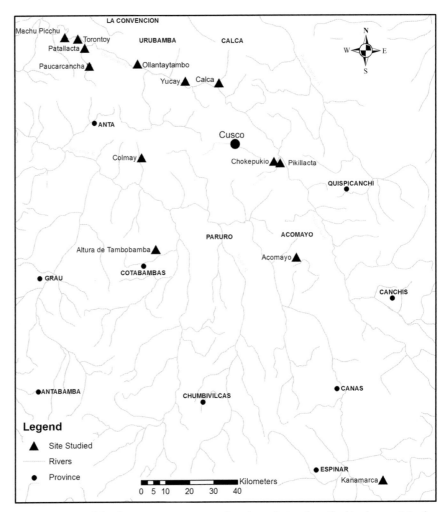

Figure 7.1 Map of the Cuzco region, noting archaeological sites described in the text. Map by Bebel Ibarra Asencios.

1914 AND 1915 YALE EXPEDITIONS

During the subsequent 1914 and 1915 Yale expeditions, skeletal remains were collected from a number of Inca sites, including Patallacta, Paucarcancha, Torontoy, Huata, Yanamanchi, Sillque, Huispan, and Huarocondo (see Figure 7.1). The expedition team gathered approximately 330 human crania, many postcranial elements, and a few mummies. According to George MacCurdy, who was in charge of analyzing and describing the material, of 273 relatively complete skulls, forty-seven (17 percent) had trepanations. Many examples of skull fractures, both healed and fresh, were also found, and MacCurdy judged that about 28 percent of the trepanations were performed to treat such fractures (MacCurdy 1918, 1923). With regard to skull injuries and trepanation, MacCurdy concluded: "the high percentage of both marks a period of warfare among the Incas of the region in question" (1923:288).

MacCurdy noted that trepanned skulls from the Cuzco area differed from those of the central highlands in surgical technique. No examples were found of trepanations by linear incisions; instead, all appear to have been done by circular or oval grooving. Another distinctive feature was the number of skulls with multiple trepanations, often showing long-term healing. The most impressive of these is a skull from Patallacta with five healed circular trepanations of nearly identical size (described below).

Little in the way of culturally diagnostic material was found in the burial caves of the Cuzco region, so their age and length of use is uncertain. MacCurdy reported isolated finds of ceramic vessels and fragments, as well as a few bone and metal pins, but he did not publish photographs of them. Many mummies were found, and their wrappings and body position were recorded. All, according to MacCurdy, were originally placed in a seated position with the legs tightly flexed against the chest. The majority were tied with plant fiber rope and seated atop a woven fiber base. A few had textile wrappings, but these seem to have been rare (MacCurdy 1923). The burial caves were all located near Inca residential sites, so it is reasonable to assume their use dates to this time period.

The caves from which skeletal material was collected no doubt had been visited prior to the Yale expeditions and grave offerings had been removed. MacCurdy reported that mummies and skeletal remains in the caves he explored were in a state of disorder, suggesting disturbance of their original positions. He noted that one burial cave at Torontoy had become home to vampire bats that harassed pack mules stopping to rest in the nearby town. To drive out the bats, local residents had set fire to the mummy bundles in the cave. MacCurdy reported that not much skeletal material was salvageable from this location (MacCurdy 1923:224).

Diversity in Head Shape

Cultural modification of skull shape (cranial deformation) is common in remains from these caves. MacCurdy noted that nearly half of the skulls (147 of 341) show intentional modification of the "Aymara" form (a term commonly used in the early twentieth century to refer to a head shape first seen in Aymara skulls from Bolivia). This form of cranial modification, more commonly known today as annular or circumferential head shaping, was produced by wrapping infants' heads with cloth bands. Other skulls show no modification, except for a few cases that appear to have mild flattening of the occipital bone. MacCurdy was less certain about these, noting that "in only a very few crania was there even a suspicion of the coastal or occipital-frontal type of deformation" (1923:287). This is in contrast to Machu Picchu, where a few skulls were found with unmistakable occipital flattening, suggesting coastal origins (Verano 2003b). The presence of both culturally modified and unmodified skulls in the same burial caves provides support for ethnohistoric accounts stating that multiple ethnic groups inhabited the Cuzco area in Inca times (Rostworowski de Diez Canseco 1999; Rowe 1946).

Museum Curation and Study of the Collection

Following MacCurdy's study, the skeletal remains collected by the 1914–1915 Yale expeditions were deposited in the Museo Nacional de Antropología, Arqueología, y Historia del

Perú, where they can be found today. In my examination of the material in 1989, I was not able to find all of the trepanned skulls published by MacCurdy. This may be explained, in part, by his classification of trepanations. Reviewing his photographs of forty-five specimens, some lesions that he described as trepanations are more likely healed depressed fractures or scalp wounds (e.g., MacCurdy 1923:pls. 22, 23, 31, 33, and 34). MacCurdy himself classified a number of these cases as only "possible" healed trepanations. Others that clearly are trepanned skulls were not found in the museum's main storeroom. These specimens may have lost their original catalog numbers, or they may be stored elsewhere. As a result it was only possible to locate and record seventeen trepanned skulls from this collection, along with six other skulls that show fractures but no evidence of surgical intervention.

Patallacta Skulls

The most impressive skull in the collection came from a burial cave near the ruins of Patallacta. Patallacta was first mapped by Hiram Bingham in 1912, and it was studied subsequently by Ann Kendall, who identified it as an Inca administrative center consisting of carefully laid out residences, work areas, and terraced agricultural fields (Gasparini and Margolies 1980:77–79; Kendall 1985). The Yale expedition recovered ninety-two crania and some postcranial remains from caves near the ruins. In one of these caves, they found the cranium of an adult male with five healed trepanations (Figure 7.2). The five openings are circular in form and very consistent in size, ranging between thirty and thirty-five millimeters in diameter. The openings have smooth and inwardly beveled edges. All are well healed, indicating long-term survival. Since they are all healed, it is unclear whether the openings were made in a single operation or as sequential interventions. There are no fractures or other indications of why the trepanations were executed. One opening was made along the midline of the skull, directly over the sagittal sinus, a location avoided even by modern neurosurgeons because of the risk of fatal bleeding. In this case, the surgeon was sufficiently skilled or fortunate to avoid tearing the sinus.

I found six other trepanned skulls recovered by the Yale expedition from burial caves at Patallacta. One skull has one, possibly two, healed trepanations (Figure 7.3); the others have single openings (Figure 7.4). In some cases, trepanations appear to be associated with skull fractures or penetrating wounds, while in others there is no obvious association. Skull fractures are common in the Patallacta sample: a total of eighteen healed and unhealed fractures were found in the nine skulls I examined. MacCurdy considered one of these healed fractures to be a possible trepanation, but it appears more likely to have been a head wound that healed spontaneously (Figure 7.5).

Material from Other Inca Sites

The Yale expeditions also found trepanned skulls at the sites of Paucarcancha, Torontoy, Huata, and Yanamanchi. Additionally, these sites produced dramatic examples of skull fractures, some lethal, some healed. An adult male from Huata is the most dramatic, showing multiple healed skull fractures and two trepanations (Figure 7.6). This unfortunate individual appears to have been struck repeatedly, perhaps with a star-headed mace, which left a series of depressed and penetrating wounds on the skull vault. The two trepanations

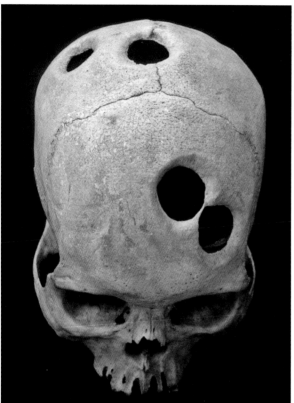

a

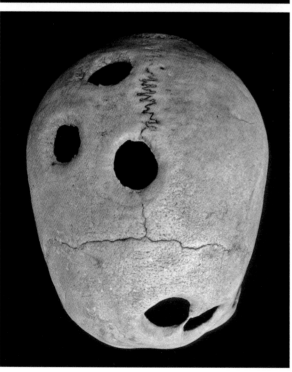

b

Figure 7.2
Adult male from
Patallacta with five
healed trepanations:
oblique view (a); and
superior view (b). Museo
Nacional de Antropología,
Arqueología, y Historia
del Perú, original catalog
number 628.

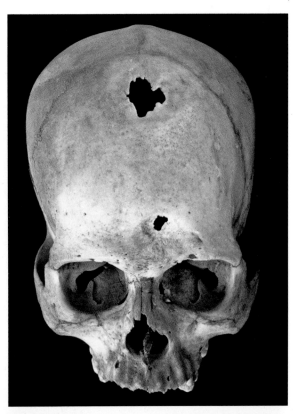

Figure 7.3
Adult male from
Patallacta with a healed
trepanation on the frontal
bone near the bregma
and a second possible
trepanation over the left
orbit associated with
a depressed fracture.
Museo Nacional
de Antropología,
Arqueología, y Historia
del Perú, AF:6918, 629.

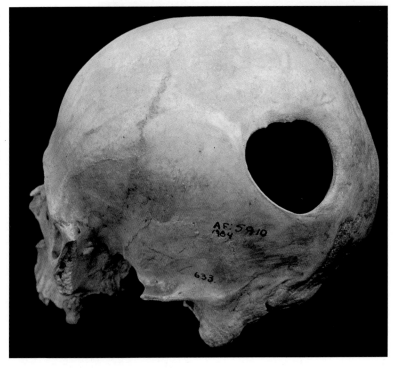

Figure 7.4
Adult male from
Patallacta with a
healed trepanation on
the left parietal bone.
Museo Nacional
de Antropología,
Arqueología, y
Historia del Perú,
AF:5910, original
catalog number 633.

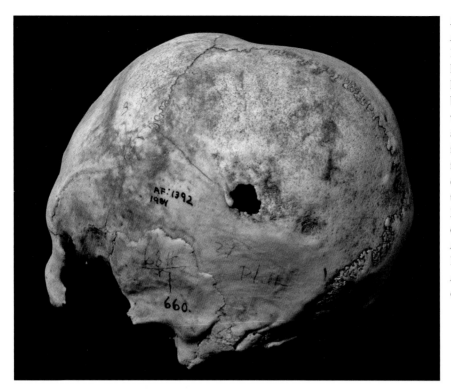

Figure 7.5
Adult male from
Patallacta with a
healed injury on the
left parietal marked
by a depressed area
with a small opening
and a radiating
fracture extending
from the anterior
edge of the opening
to the coronal suture.
Museo Nacional
de Antropología,
Arqueología, y
Historia del Perú,
AF:1392, original
catalog number 660.

may mark impact sites as well, although the cutting or scraping of their centers makes it hard to judge. Large abscesses are present around the roots of several upper teeth. While unrelated to the skull injuries, the combined effects of these issues must have made his last days extremely uncomfortable. Others who suffered head injuries did not survive long. Two women from Paucarcancha have massive vault fractures with no sign of bone reaction (Figures 7.7 and 7.8). One (Figure 7.8) has multiple fine cut marks around the fractured area, suggesting that the scalp was cut in preparation for treatment of the wound, but there is no indication that a trepanation was attempted. Other attempts at trepanation and wound treatment were unsuccessful as well, such as an adolescent male with an unhealed trepanation on the right parietal bone (Figure 7.9), and a child of about twelve or thirteen years with a penetrating wound with scrape marks around its margins (Figure 7.10) The wound is unusual for its small size. Apparently a sharp weapon with a pointed end less than nine millimeters in diameter penetrated the back of the skull. Numerous cut and scrape marks can be seen around the margins of the hole, and its edges have been smoothed, indicating an attempt at treating the wound. There is no evidence of bone reaction, however, suggesting that the child died during or shortly after treatment.

Another clear example of a trepanation following a skull fracture involves a young adult male from the site of Torontoy (Figure 7.11). In this case, a large opening was cut on the left temple. A preexisting fracture is marked by radiating lines that extend forward across the zygomatic process of the frontal bone and downward across the squamous portion of the temporal bone. Fractures in this region of the skull are particularly dangerous

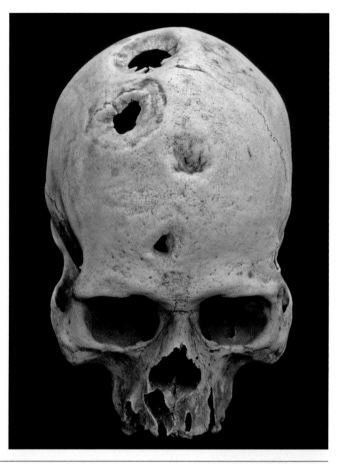

Figure 7.6
Adult male from Huata with multiple healed depressed fractures (four recorded, three visible in photo) and two healed trepanations. There is also a large abscess above the right upper incisors. Museo Nacional de Antropología, Arqueología, y Historia del Perú, original catalog number 877.

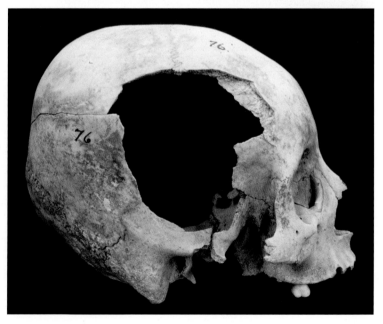

Figure 7.7
Adolescent female from Paucarcancha with massive blunt force trauma to right side of the skull. No evidence of surgical intervention. Museo Nacional de Antropología, Arqueología, y Historia del Perú, AF:0837, original catalog number 76.

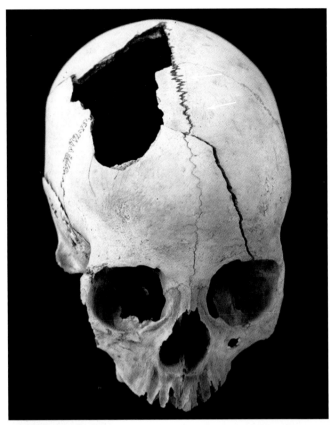

Figure 7.8
Young adult female from Paucarcancha with blunt force trauma to the right frontal and parietal bones. Museo Nacional de Antropología, Arqueología, y Historia del Perú, AF:0388, original catalog number 77.

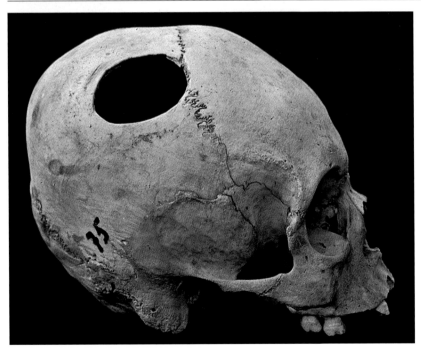

Figure 7.9
Adolescent male from Paucarcancha with an unhealed oval trepanation (34 × 46 mm) on the right parietal bone. Cut marks are visible around the margins of the opening, particularly on its posterior aspect. No indication of why the trepanation was done. Museo Nacional de Antropología, Arqueología, y Historia del Perú, AF:0369, original catalog number 75.

Figure 7.10
(a) A twelve- to thirteen-year-old child from Paucarcancha with a small unhealed penetrating wound on the occipital bone (arrow). (b) Close-up of the wound. Museo Nacional de Antropología, Arqueología, y Historia del Perú, AF:1381, original catalog number 136.

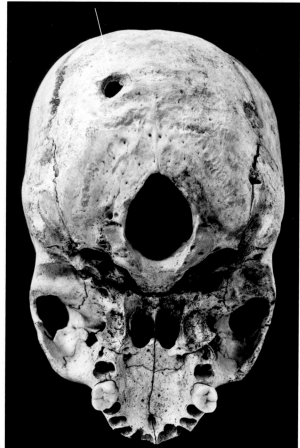

a

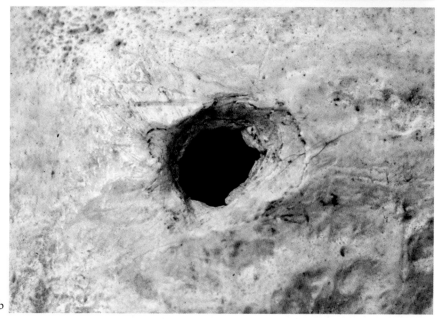

b

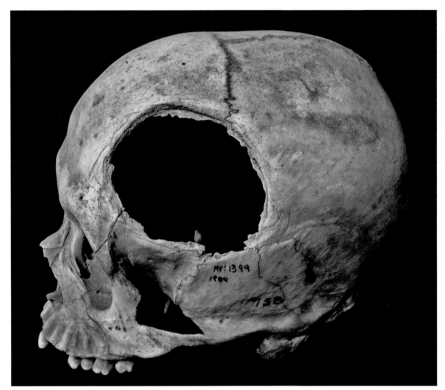

Figure 7.11
Young adult male from Torontoy with blunt force trauma to the left temple area and a large trepanation (56 × 72 mm) placed over it. Museo Nacional de Antropología, Arqueología, y Historia del Perú, AF:1399, original catalog number 758.

because branches of the middle meningeal arteries lie just under the bone and they can easily tear when the temporal bone is fractured, producing a life-threatening extradural hematoma (see Chapter 10, Figure 10.2). Such was probably the case here; fresh scratches around the margins of the trepanation and the lack of bone remodeling indicate that the patient died during or shortly after the operation.

Motivations for Trepanning

The trepanned skulls collected by the 1914 and 1915 Yale expeditions from burial caves in the Cuzco region show some variability in technique, as well as evidence for possible motivations. Some are clearly associated with skull fractures, and thus can be assumed to be practical attempts to treat acute head injuries. Their technique seems to conform to the necessity of the moment, as indicated by openings of variable shape and size. While not all trepanations were successful, examples of skulls from the same burial caves with massive untreated fractures illustrate the kinds of severe head wounds that a trepanner might have faced.

In contrast to trepanations associated with skull fracture, the skull from Patallacta with five openings of consistent size and shape (see Figure 7.2) suggests some other motivation for the procedures. Perhaps this patient had recurring headaches or other neurological symptoms and sought definitive relief through repeated surgeries. Whether relief was eventually found is unknown, of course. What is most striking is the uniformity of the openings and the successful healing of all five, even the one placed in a particularly hazardous location. As we will describe below, other skulls with multiple healed trepanations were later found at other sites in the Cuzco region, so this case is not unique.

TREPANNED SKULLS FROM OTHER INCA SITES

Table 7.1 lists the total sample of trepanned skulls from the southern highlands examined in this study. Most museums have only small samples of trepanned skulls from this region. The exception is the Museo Inka in Cuzco, which holds the largest collection of skeletal material and mummies from the Cuzco region, including nearly 150 trepanned skulls. Most of these crania come from burial structures and caves at Ollantaytambo and several ossuaries at Calca (see Figure 7.1). The specific provenance of others is unknown; many simply are cataloged as coming from the Cuzco area. Most of the material from identified sites was excavated by the Museo Inka from Ollantaytambo and Quimsarumiyoc (Calca), under the direction of Luis Llanos (Llanos 1936, 1941). The skeletal material was subsequently analyzed by Sergio Quevedo, who published a series of articles focusing on the Calca material with observations on some of the Ollantaytambo skulls (Quevedo 1941, 1943b:201). Quevedo's Calca sample was relatively small—he described a total of fifty-five adult skulls from the site, eleven of which (20 percent) are trepanned. Oddly, in his 1941 publication on excavations at Quimsarumiyoc, Llanos reports finding twenty-one trepanned skulls, nearly twice the number reported by Quevedo. The reason for this discrepancy is not clear. Quevedo noted that all of the trepanations from Calca were circular or oval, with no examples of linear cutting, drilling, or scraping. He thus considered the circular/oval technique to be characteristic of the Cuzco region, although he did find some scraped trepanations at Ollantaytambo (Quevedo 1943b:202). He also noted the consistent and small size of the Calca trepanations, most with diameters of about four to five centimeters.

Trepanations by Linear Incisions (Quadrilateral)

In a broader study of skulls from sites throughout the Cuzco region, Quevedo noted that he had seen only one skull with a quadrilateral trepanation like that of the Squier skull from Yucay. In fact, he concludes that this skull is a fake, a modern "trepanation" done on an ancient skull to bring a higher price from a collector (Quevedo 1943b:201). The origin of the skull is unknown, but it was originally housed in a private museum. Quevedo describes the "trepanation" as a rectangular opening (2 × 1.5 centimeters) located on the left parietal bone. In 2002, I located the skull in the Museo Inka collections (Figure 7.12). It has an opening that clearly was created by a modern saw, with long cuts unlike anything I have ever seen in ancient trepanations. The cuts appear fresh, with no evidence of bone reaction. When I first saw this specimen, I thought it might represent a legitimate scientific experiment attempting to replicate an ancient trepanation technique, but after reading Quevedo's 1943 description, I became convinced this was the skull he wrote about. Quevedo was a surgeon and a bit of an experimental trepanner himself, as will be seen in Chapter 8, but evidently he knew a fake when he saw one.

Table 7.1 Trepanned skulls from the southern highlands of Peru.

SITE NAME	NUMBER OF TREPANNED SKULLS	COLLECTION
Acomayo	4	Museo Inka
Alturas de Tambobamba	6	Museo Inka
Calca	2	Museo Inka
Chokepukio	5	Museo Inka
Cochahuasi-Huancalli	3	Phoebe A. Hearst Museum of Anthropology
Colmay	16	Phoebe A. Hearst Museum of Anthropology
Cuzco region	12	British Museum of Natural History, National Museum of Natural History, AMNH, MNAAHP, Museo Inka
Huata	2	MNAAHP
Incamanchi	1	MNAAHP
Ollantaytambo	63	Museo Inka
Pachar	1	Museo Inka
Patallacta	7	MNAAHP
Paucarcancha	6	MNAAHP
Pikillacta	2	Museo Inka
Sacsahuaman	3	Museo Inka
Sauma	1	Phoebe A. Hearst Museum of Anthropology
Torontoy	2	MNAAHP
Yucay	1	AMNH
no provenance	45	Museo Inka

The Museo Inka does have one adult male cranium with a legitimate quadrilateral trepanation. It was on exhibit when I first visited the museum in 1992, and I was able to photograph and examine it. It is reported to have been found in the Cuzco area, but no more specific provenance is known. It has an unhealed rectangular trepanation (30 × 40 millimeters in maximum dimensions) on the right parietal bone (Figure 7.13). Until recently, it was only the second example of this form of trepanation known from the southern highlands of

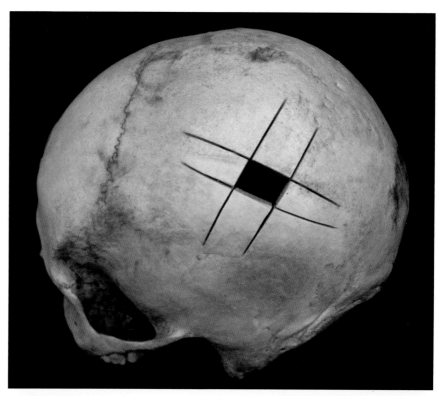

Figure 7.12
Cranium with a "trepanation" made with a modern saw. Museo Inka 2592/ MO-H 344.

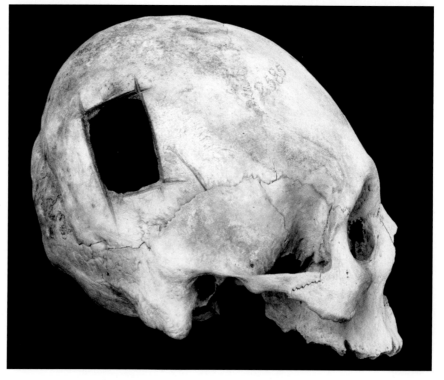

Figure 7.13
Adult male cranium with a quadrilateral trepanation on the right parietal bone. (30 × 40 mm) No sign of bone reaction. Museo Inka 2585.

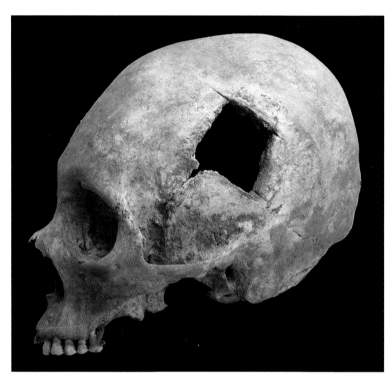

Figure 7.14
Cranium of a woman from Kanamarca who died around the age of forty-five. She has an unhealed trepanation on the left parietal bone. Photograph by Valerie Andrushko.

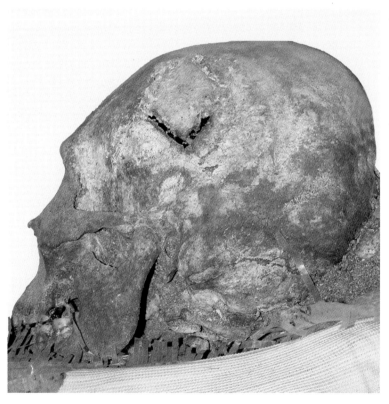

Figure 7.15
Kanamarca skull in the field laboratory before cleaning, with the removed bone fragment in place. Photograph by Valerie Andrushko.

Peru. Of the 162 trepanned skulls I recorded from Inca sites in the Cuzco area, there were no other examples of this technique.

The rarity of quadrilateral trepanations in the Cuzco region raises an interesting question about the partial skull, reportedly from the Yucay Valley near Cuzco, which was presented to Squier in 1865 by María Ana Centeno de Romainville. Was this simply a curiosity brought back in Inca times from a tomb in the central highlands, or did it belong to someone living in the Yucay Valley who was operated on by a central highlands trepanner? According to Susan Niles, who has done extensive ethnohistoric work on the Yucay Valley, at the time of the Spanish conquest this region had a diverse population that included not only natives of the Cuzco area, but also thousands of Inca subjects (*mitimaes*) brought there from different parts of the empire to work on the royal estate of the Inca ruler Huayna Capac (Niles 1999:126). Niles notes that most of these immigrants were either from Collasuyu (the southern quarter of the empire) or from Chinchaysuyu (to the north), and that some identified themselves as being natives of the central highlands (Niles 1999:131). Thus, it is possible that central highlanders transplanted by the Inca brought their trepanation skills and techniques (rectangular incisions) along with them to the Yucay Valley. Unfortunately, the lack of any archaeological documentation for either the Squier skull or the Museo Inka skull makes it difficult to contextualize these two anomalous specimens.

Archaeological excavations conducted at the site of Kanamarca in 2004 encountered the first documented case of a rectangular trepanation from the Cuzco region (Figures 7.14 and 7.15). Kanamarca is an Inca site located 148 kilometers southeast of Cuzco. Excavations in 2004–2005 uncovered thirty-eight burials, including that of an adult woman with a rectangular trepanation on the left side of the skull (Andrushko 2007; Verano and Andrushko 2008). This is also the first documented case from Peru in which the portion of bone removed during the trepanation procedure was replaced in its original location following surgery. It is unclear whether the bone was replaced while the patient was still alive or after death, since there is no evidence of bone reaction around the margins of the opening. Most importantly, the Kanamarca burial is the first archaeologically documented case of a rectangular trepanation performed in the Cuzco region, and provides support for the argument that the two other cases of rectangular trepanations are indeed from the Cuzco region as well.

Drilling and Cutting

Although Quevedo does not mention these skulls in his publications, the Museo Inka has in its collection three, possibly four, examples of trepanation by drilling and cutting, one of the rarest forms of trepanation in South America. One of these skulls is from Ollantaytambo (Llanos 1936:140); the others do not have site designations, but are identified as coming from the Cuzco area.

The drilling and cutting method was a rarely practiced and time-consuming method of making openings into the skull, as it required the drilling of multiple holes and the subsequent cutting of the bone between them. While powered drills used in modern craniotomies cut through bone quickly, a hand-powered drill, possibly used with sand or some other abrasive, would probably take considerable time to bore through the vault bones.

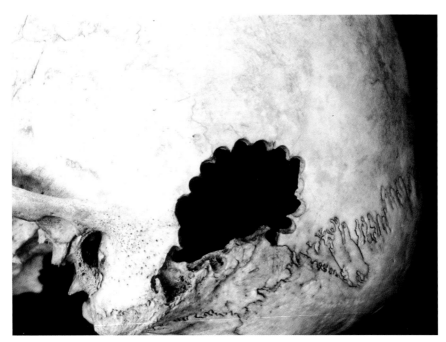

Drilling carried with it an increased risk of accidentally penetrating the dura mater, adding to its problematic nature. This may explain why trepanations done by this method are so rarely seen in Peru or elsewhere in the world. In fact, it is generally stated in the trepanation literature that no examples of successfully healed trepanations by this method have ever been found. Two possible exceptions can be found in the Museo Inka collection, although bone healing makes the original details of the openings ambiguous.

Figure 7.16 shows a classic example of trepanation by drilling and cutting, with no sign of bone reaction, suggesting that the patient died during or shortly after the procedure. The location chosen for the trepanation (above the left mastoid process) may be significant. It is similar to two examples from Paracas of trepanations placed above the mastoid process. An eroded area (lytic defect) at the inferior margin of the trepanation and pitting of the mastoid process suggest that, as in the cases from Paracas, the opening may have been made in an attempt to treat an infection or wound to the mastoid area. The attempt was unsuccessful.

Figure 7.17, an adolescent male, has two trepanations on the posterior aspect of the skull. The first, located on the occipital bone, shows extensive and irregular bone reaction (osteoclastic activity) around its margins, suggesting that the wound had become infected. This trepanation may have been executed by the drilling and cutting method, but lytic destruction of bone around the margins has removed any direct evidence. The second trepanation, which may have been meant to relieve symptoms associated with the first, clearly was executed by the drilling and cutting method. No evidence of bone reaction is seen around the margins of this second intervention, indicating that it was not successful.

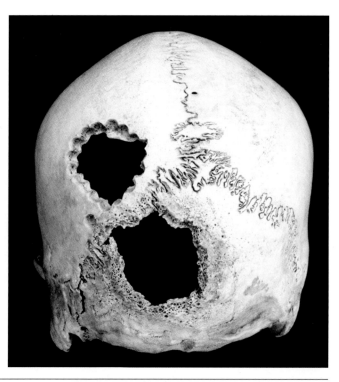

Figure 7.17
Adolescent male with
two trepanations, one
with pronounced bone
reaction (infection?) on
the occipital bone and
the other, on the parietal,
showing no signs of
healing. Museo Inka 2589.

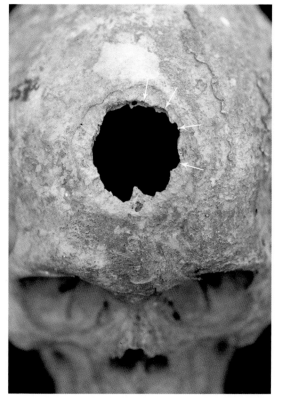

Figure 7.18
An adult male with a
trepanation on the frontal
bone with what appear
to be crescent-shaped
marks from drilled holes
(arrows). Museo Inka
2572/MO-H 332.

An adult male skull from the Cuzco area also has two trepanations, both of which show extensive healing. Of particular interest is the opening on the frontal bone (Figure 7.18), which shows scalloped margins that may preserve portions of drill holes. If so, this is a rare case that shows healing while preserving evidence of the drilling and cutting method.

OLLANTAYTAMBO

The largest sample of trepanned skulls from the southern highlands comes from the site of Ollantaytambo, located in the Urubamba River Valley, seventy kilometers northwest of Cuzco. A royal estate of the Inca emperor Pachacuti, Ollantaytambo was a carefully laid out Inca town with associated ceremonial and funerary precincts, extensive terraced fields, and hilltop forts (Hemming and Ranney 1982; Protzen 1993). Small burial structures (chullpas) and funerary caves are found across the river from the town, in the areas from which rock was quarried to build Ollantaytambo (Protzen 1993:146–147). Although Ollantaytambo has been explored and mapped by various researchers, beginning with Hiram Bingham in 1915, only limited excavations have been conducted there.

In 1936, Luis Llanos excavated in the ceremonial and funerary precincts above the town and recovered human skeletal remains from a number of tombs. Unfortunately, all of the tombs had been looted. Llanos reported finding three trepanned skulls, two of which I was able to locate in the Museo Inka's collections. The majority of the Ollantaytambo skulls in the museum's collections appear to have been accessioned at a later date, based on their catalog numbers, and I am uncertain from where at the site they originated. Presumably they were collected from both the funerary precinct above the town as well as from the burial structures near the quarries.

Today the Museo Inka has sixty-two trepanned skulls from Ollantaytambo. This is an important collection because it constitutes the largest sample of trepanned skulls from a single archaeological site in Peru (Paracas comes in a close second). It is distinguished as well by the number of skulls with multiple trepanations: fifteen skulls have two trepanations, four have three, and two have four. Counting all of the multiple openings, a total of eighty-two trepanations are present on the sixty-two skulls. Most of these (75.3 percent) show long-term healing, nearly double the survival rate of Paracas and substantially better than that of the central highlands.

Demography

With the exception of three adolescents and one child, all of the trepanned skulls from Ollantaytambo are from adults. Although it is possible that some healed trepanations observed in adult skulls represent surgeries received as children, this seems unlikely. Twenty adults in the Ollantaytambo sample have a trepanation with only short-term or no healing, indicating that the patients died shortly after the procedures. If children were operated on with any frequency, one would expect to see a similar number of unsuccessful trepanations, given that the risk of infection, bleeding, or brain trauma should be comparable in children and adults.

The cranium of the single trepanned child from Ollantaytambo lacks the bones of the face, so its age at death can only be estimated based on the size and thickness of the vault bones. It has a single trepanation over the sagittal suture, just posterior to the bregma, which shows only short-term healing (Figure 7.19a). As noted previously, this is a risky place for a trepanation due to the possibility of tearing the sagittal sinus. But there is some evidence of bone reaction following the procedure, indicating that catastrophic hemorrhage was not the cause of death. Examining the margins of the opening, we can see that some portions are quite irregular, while others (particularly the right margin) are smoothly beveled (Figure 7.19b). Perhaps the trepanation was located on the edge of a preexisting depressed fracture, penetrating wound, or localized scalp infection.

While the sex of the child and one of the adolescents could not be assessed by visual criteria, sex could be assigned to the other two adolescents and to the adult skulls based on standard criteria, such as general size and robusticity of muscle markings (Buikstra and Ubelaker 1994; Walker 2008). The Ollantaytambo sample is interesting in this regard. Most other collections of trepanned skulls from Peru as well as from Neolithic Europe show a marked sex bias of males over females. Ollantaytambo, in contrast, shows a male to female sex ratio that is nearly fifty-fifty. In my analysis of the collection, I classified twenty-nine skulls as female and thirty as male. Why so many females in this sample? As I discuss below, the generally low frequency of skull fractures at Ollantaytambo combined with the infrequent association of skull fracture and trepanation suggests that trepanations may have been done for reasons other than acute head injury.

The Ollantaytambo skulls presumably represent the population living in the nearby town in Inca times, although little is known about the specific contexts from which these remains were collected. The burial structures and crevices around Ollantaytambo were looted long ago, and today human bones can only be seen on the surface of a few of them (Llanos 1936:130–148; Protzen 1993:146–147). Examination of the Ollantaytambo skulls, however, suggests that this was an ethnically homogeneous population, at least in terms of head modification. I found only two intentionally modified skulls in the collection, one male and one female. This contrasts with many other Cuzco-area burial sites, where a significant proportion of skulls were culturally modified (Andrushko 2007; MacCurdy 1923). It also contrasts strongly with some sites nearby Ollantaytambo such as Tambobamba (below), where all individuals had culturally modified skulls. Perhaps the two outliers at Ollantaytambo married into the local population or were natives of some other area assigned to work there. The Inca reportedly brought laborers from the Lake Titicaca region to build Ollantaytambo (Hemming and Ranney 1982:109–110), and some of them may have died there. The annular form of cranial modification seen in these two skulls is a form commonly found among the Aymara of the Lake Titicaca area (Andrushko 2007), although it occurs in other Peruvian highland regions as well (Verano 2003b). One of the two unusually shaped skulls from Ollantaytambo, the adult female, has a large healed lesion on the frontal bone that could be a superficial trepanation by scraping, but it may simply be a healed injury (Figure 7.20). It is not typical of circular trepanations seen in other crania at Ollantaytambo. The second deformed skull, an adult male, has a minor healed injury but is not trepanned.

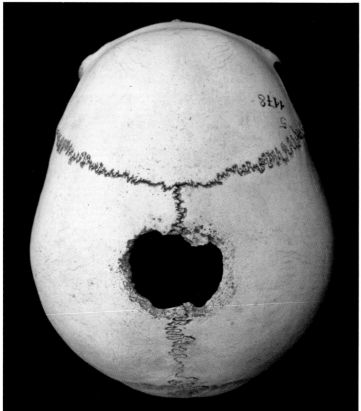

a

Figure 7.19
(a) Child from Ollantaytambo with a trepanation (38 × 47 mm) displaying short-term healing; and (b) detail of the trepanation, showing variation in the smoothness and regularity of the margins. Museo Inka MO-H 303, 5/1178.

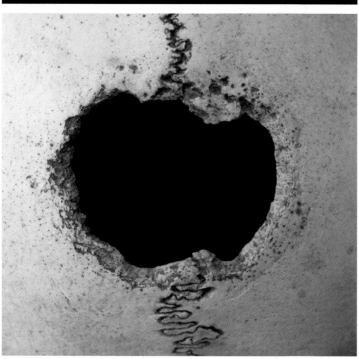

b

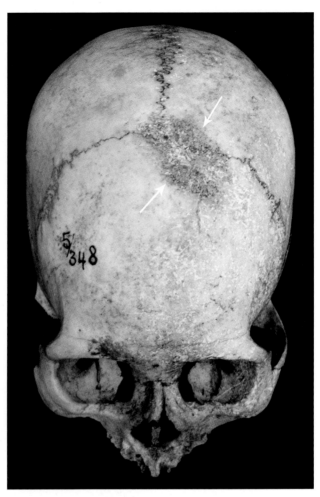

Figure 7.20
Adult female cranium from Ollantaytambo with an oval-shaped healed lesion (30 × 44 mm) on the frontal bone (arrows). Museo Inka 5/348, 18.

Skull Fractures and Trepanation

Skull fractures, whether healed or unhealed, are relatively rare in the Ollantaytambo sample (see, for example, Figure 7.21). Depressed fractures or penetrating wounds are seen in only thirteen of the sixty-one trepanned skulls (21 percent). Most of these (nine of thirteen) are old healed injuries, two of which show short-term survival and two that show no bone response. Fractures are found in various locations, although the most common sites are on the left side of the head and the face.

Only seven of eighty-two trepanations (9 percent) provide evidence that skull fractures probably motivated surgery. Most trepanations (91 percent) appear not to have treated trauma, although some skulls have large portions of the skull vault removed, making it possible (as is the case in other Peruvian samples) that a small depressed fracture or penetrating wound was excised during the procedure. The crania shown in Figures 7.22 and 7.23 are good examples of this situation. Severe injuries to the skull did occur, however, and three cases in which trepanations attempted to treat fractures are particularly evocative.

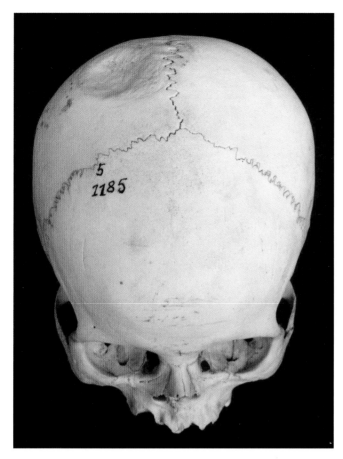

Figure 7.21
Young adult female from Ollantaytambo with a large, healed, depressed fracture of the right parietal bone. Museo Inka 5/1185.

The skull of a young adult male has a large penetrating wound of the frontal bone with a radiating fracture extending laterally across the right superciliary arch, and another fracture coursing across the orbital roof, through the right maxilla, and across the skull base (Figure 7.24). The defect in the frontal bone shows scraping around its margins, indicating that an attempt was made to treat the wound. Presumably, fragments of bone displaced by the impact would have been removed from the wound as well. There is no bone reaction around the margins of the wound or along the radiating fractures, which indicates that the patient did not survive for long. This is not surprising, given the severity of the injury.

The cranium of a young adult female has a total of four trepanations. Three are well healed, but the fourth shows no evidence of bone reaction (Figure 7.25). There is a partially healed oval-shaped fracture of the left temporal bone just above the zygomatic arch that may have been the motivation for the three trepanations located close to it. The pair closer to the back of the skull, both healed, may represent a single trepanation procedure, given their similar size, shape, and degree of healing. The third trepanation visible directly above the fracture shows no bone reaction, indicating that the patient died during or soon after the operation. Perhaps the two healed openings were surgeries done at the time of the injury, and the third represents a later, unsuccessful attempt to treat subsequent complaints.

Figure 7. 22 Adult female from Ollantaytambo with a large unhealed trepanation (98 × 70 mm) on the left parietal bone. A linear fracture extending from the anterior margin of the defect (arrow) may be a perimortem fracture, but it is not unequivocal. Museo Inka 5/1169.

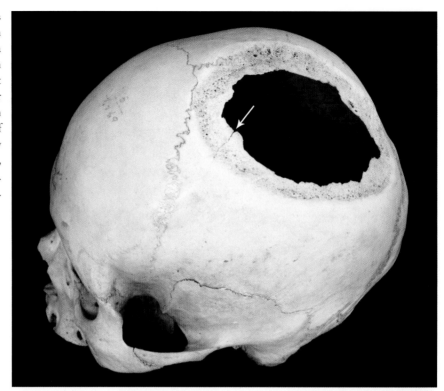

Figure 7.23 Adult male from Ollantaytambo with a large, oval-shaped, scraped trepanation (55 × 103 mm) with two openings through the inner table of the skull. There is no evidence of healing and no visible indication of why the trepanation was done. Museo Inka 5/1196.

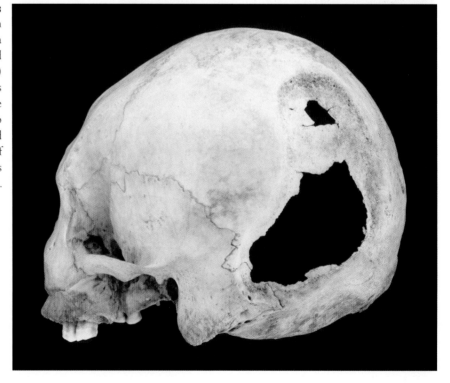

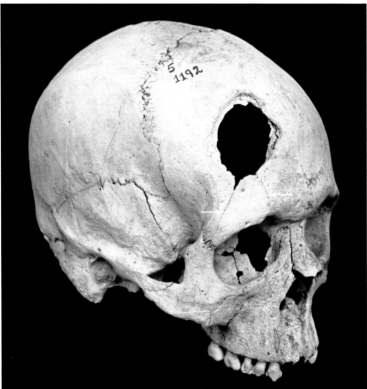

a

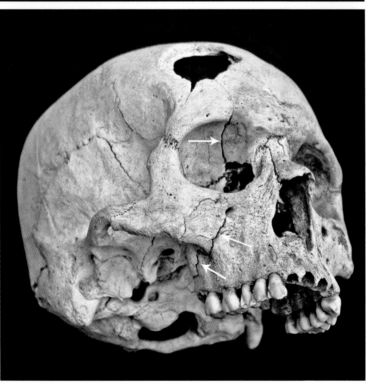

b

Figure 7.24
(a) Young adult male
from Ollantaytambo with
a depressed fracture or
penetrating wound on
the frontal bone with a
radiating fracture extending
across the right superciliary
arch (arrows). (b) Another
fracture travels across the
roof of the right orbit and
down across the right
maxilla (arrows). Museo
Inka 5/1192.

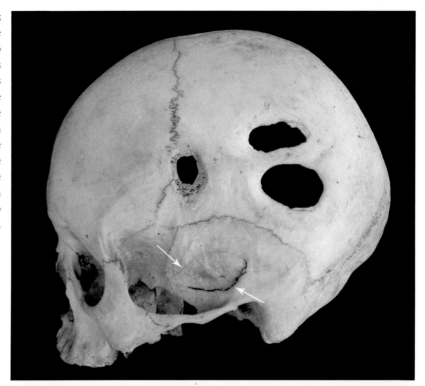

Figure 7.25
Young adult female from Ollantaytambo with four trepanations (three visible in this photo). The three openings may be associated with an oval-shaped fracture of the temporal bone located just above the zygomatic arch (arrows). Museo Inka 5/1176.

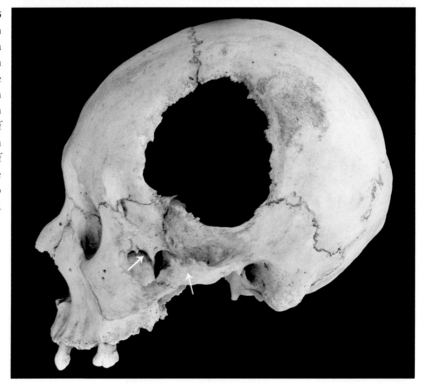

Figure 7.26
Adult male from Ollantaytambo with a large healed trepanation (70 × 60 mm) of the left temporal region associated with healed fractures of the zygomatic arch and greater wing of the sphenoid bone (arrows). Museo Inka 5/1168.

An adult male cranium presents an impressive case of a large, healed trepanation in the left temporal fossa (Figure 7.26). This area would have been both a difficult and dangerous area to trepan due to the need to cut through the temporal muscle and arteries to reach the bone, and because middle meningeal arteries lie just under the temporal bone, increasing the risk of heavy bleeding. One additional complication in this case was what appears to have been a blow to the left side of the head. The zygomatic arch has healed fractures of multiple bones, and spicules of bone extend downward from the greater wing of the sphenoid bone, suggesting earlier fractures as well. Presumably the trepanation was performed to treat an injury to the squamous portion of the temporal bone. In this case, the patient survived.

Ambiguous Cases

Even in a sample like that from Ollantaytambo, where trepanation was common, there are cases in which healed openings in the skull might be attributed to other causes. An example is an adult male cranium with an oval defect on the midline of the skull, partially occluded by bony spicules (Figure 7.27). This may represent a scraped trepanation, or it might simply be a depressed skull fracture with some of the bone fragments resorbed or sloughed off during healing. Its regular shape, and the fact that circular and oval trepanations were the dominant technique at Ollantaytambo, suggests that this might in fact be a healed trepanation.

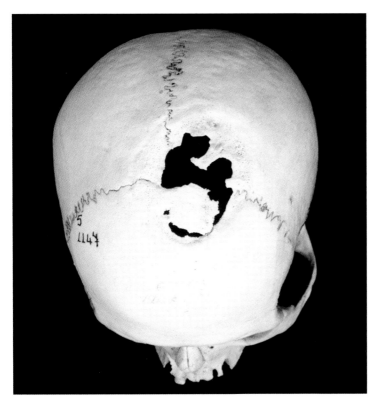

Figure 7.27
Adult male from Ollantaytambo with a healed oval-shaped lesion on the top of the skull. Probable trepanation by scraping. Museo Inka 5/1147.

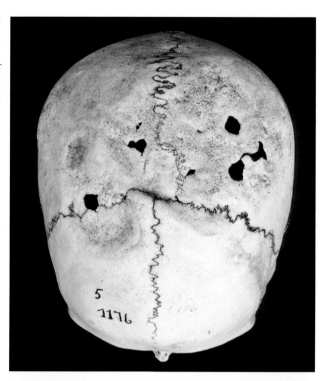

Figure 7.28
Adult female from
Ollantaytambo with
a large healed area of
inflammation with multiple
defects through the inner
table. Museo Inka 5/1176.

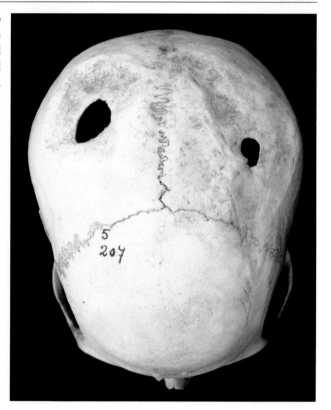

Figure 7.29
Old adult female from
Ollantaytambo with healed
defects on the parietal
bones. Museo Inka 5/207.

The cranium in Figure 7.28 is more problematic. It shows a large healed area of inflammation of the skull vault with multiple defects through the inner table. This case appears to be a scalp infection that eventually healed. While it may have been treated by scraping of the outer table, the healing would have removed any evidence of scrape marks. The only hints of possible human intervention are the beveled edges on the anterior margins of the inflamed area, which show a regularity that might reflect scraping of the bone.

Another ambiguous case is the cranium of an older adult female that has two healed defects, one on each parietal bone (Figure 7.29). The position of these holes and the surrounding thinned areas suggests biparietal thinning, in which the parietal bones grow thinner with advanced age, sometimes producing defects that penetrate the bone (see Chapter 3). In this skull, however, there is thickening of the bone (sclerosis) around the openings, and the defect on the left side is located more anteriorly than that on the right, which makes trepanation a possible diagnosis as well.

Multiple and Paired Trepanations

Multiple trepanations are common at Ollantaytambo. The most impressive example is the cranium of an adult male with four large trepanations, all well healed (Figure 7.30). According to Quevedo (1943a:117), it was collected from the Cueva de Hamppatuyoc, a cave near Ollantaytambo. The four trepanations are oval to circular in form and similar in size, ranging from thirty to forty-five millimeters in maximum diameter. The skull has no visible healed injuries, and all four openings show extensive healing, indicating long-term survival following the procedures.

Some Ollantaytambo crania with multiple trepanations show different degrees of healing across the defects, indicating that they were made at different times. Multiple holes made at the same time suggest that the trepanner was searching for something—perhaps for a blood clot or some other indication of injury or disease. An example is a young adult male with three trepanations (Figure 7.31). One, located on the left parietal bone, is a circular, well-healed opening. At some later point, a trepanner made two more openings—one behind the other—along the sagittal suture. Fresh cuts and grooves on and around the margins of these later openings indicate that this was an unsuccessful surgical procedure. Neither trepanation shows any evidence of bone response. The only visible indication of why these two openings might have been made is a series of small erosive defects on the left parietal and frontal bones that seem to mark inflammation of the bone surface, possibly from a scalp infection or injury. Perhaps there was suspicion of intracranial bleeding, since the skull was not simply scraped but cut through to expose the dura.

Another young adult male from Ollantaytambo has four trepanations (Figure 7.32). Three show extensive healing, but the final one (at far right in the photograph) shows no bone reaction at all, indicating that the patient died during or shortly after surgery. There are no fractures or other indications of why these trepanations were done. Perhaps they represent an attempt to treat recurrent headaches or some other neurological symptom. The failure of the fourth trepanation, given its similar size and location relative to the others, is puzzling.

An older adult male (Figure 7.33) has three healed trepanations aligned obliquely across the skull. One of the more intriguing skulls in the Ollantaytambo sample, it presents

Figure 7.30
Adult male with
four well-healed
trepanations:
(a) superior view;
and (b) lateral view.
From the Cueva
de Hamppatuyoc,
near Ollantaytambo.
Museo Inka 2580.

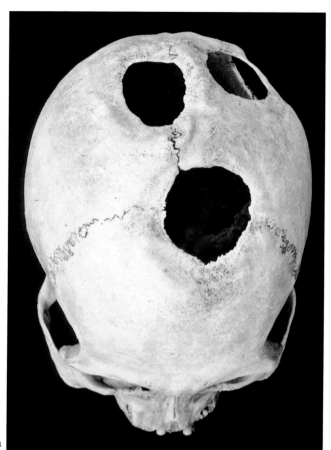

a

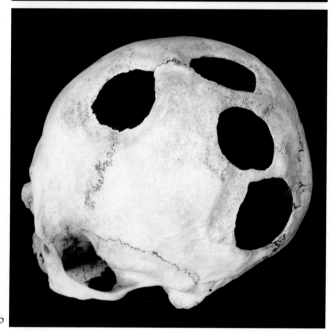

b

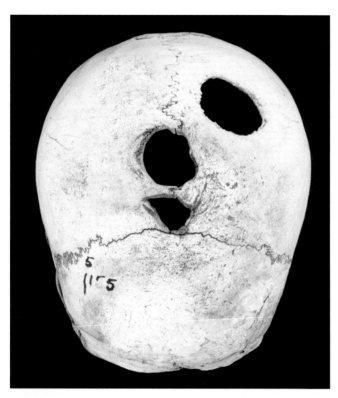

Figure 7.31
Young adult male
from Ollantaytambo
with a well-healed
trepanation on the
left parietal bone
and two unhealed
trepanations along
the sagittal suture.
Museo Inka 5/1155.

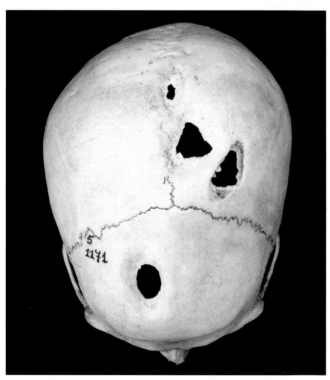

Figure 7.32
Young adult male
from Ollantaytambo
with three healed
trepanations and
one (at far right)
with no signs of
healing. Museo
Inka 5/1171.

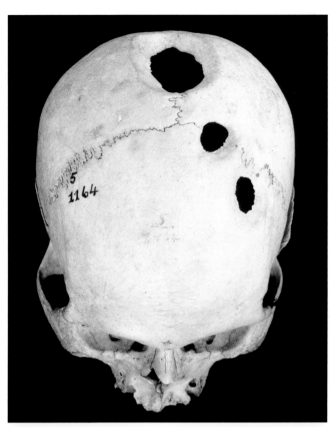

Figure 7.33
Old adult
male from
Ollantaytambo
with three healed
trepanations.
Museo Inka 5/1164.

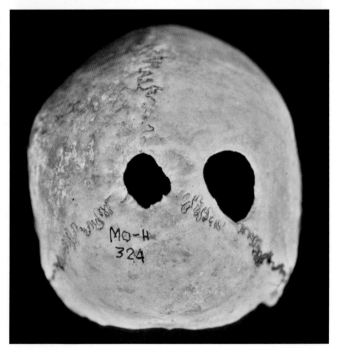

Figure 7.34
Adult male
with two healed
trepanations along
the sagittal suture.
Museo Inka 5/1167.

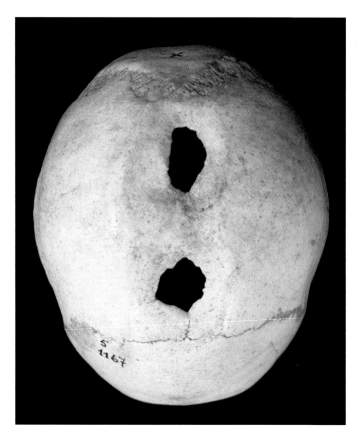

Figure 7.35
Adult female
with two healed
trepanations side
by side on the rear
of the skull. Museo
Inka 5/1197.

a linear alignment resembling craters left by an aerial bombing run. All three openings are well healed, so it is not possible to say whether they were done simultaneously or at different times. Again, there is no indication of the reason for the trepanations.

Figure 7.28 (described above in the context of trauma), Figure 7.34, and Figure 7.35 are special cases of skulls with two openings that may be paired trepanations. There are similar examples from other southern highland sites, some of which are unhealed and thus clearly represent single procedures (these will be described below). In the three examples from Ollantaytambo, the trepanation pairs are all healed, but their adjacent locations, as well as their similar size and shape, suggest that they may have been done at the same time. These paired openings might indicate a search for something specific, or perhaps there was some symbolism involved in the placement of two (or perhaps three) openings.

OTHER CUZCO-AREA SITES WITH TREPANNED SKULLS
Pachar

Pachar is located five kilometers southeast of Ollantaytambo. The Museo Inka has a single trepanned cranium from the site of Pachar. It is an adult male showing pronounced annular cranial modification and a healed depressed injury above the right orbit (Figure 7.36a).

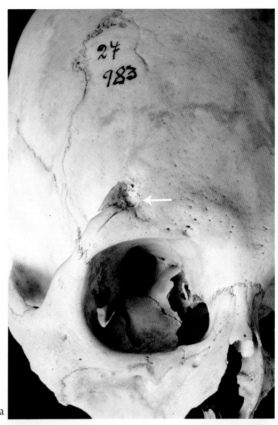

Figure 7.36
(a) Adult male from Pachar with a healed fracture from a blow above the right orbit (arrow). (b) Left lateral view of the cranium, with massive blunt force trauma and evidence of cutting around the lower posterior margin of the broken out area. Museo Inka 27/983.

a

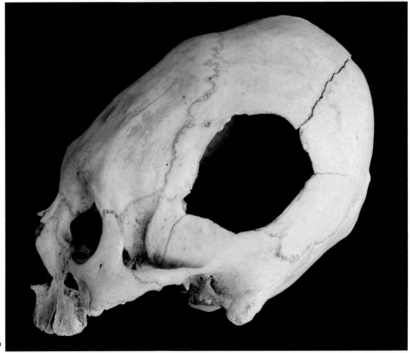

b

The small, circular shape of the injury suggests that it was created by a star-headed mace. While this trauma healed well, a later injury to the vault was substantially more serious. A major blunt force injury to the left parietal area produced radiating fractures that coursed anteriorly across the temporal fossa and posterolaterally across the left and right parietal bones (Figure 7.36b). Evidence of surgical intervention is visible on the lower posterior margin of the defect, where the edge shows a clean cut. There is no evidence of survival.

Alturas de Tambobamba

Tambobamba is located about sixty kilometers southwest of Cuzco. The ancient settlement was one of a series of way stations, or *tambos*, along the Inca road system. The Museo Inka has six trepanned skulls, two adult females and four adult males, from the Alturas de Tambobamba. All show pronounced annular cranial modification and have between one and three well-healed trepanations each (Figure 7.37). The trepanations are oval to circular in shape and relatively small in size, with diameters ranging between fifteen and thirty-five millimeters. None are associated with skull fractures, except for one possible case, in which two trepanations are placed near a small, healed, depressed fracture. In the other skulls there is no clear reason for the trepanations.

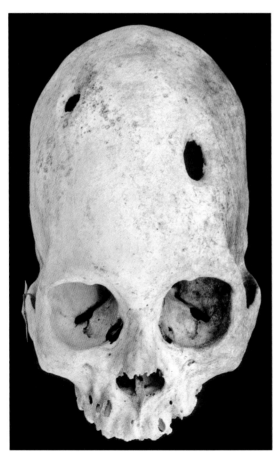

Figure 7.37
Adult male from Alturas de Tambobamba with annular cranial modification and three healed trepanations (the third is located on the left parietal bone and is not visible in this photograph). Museo Inka 3594.

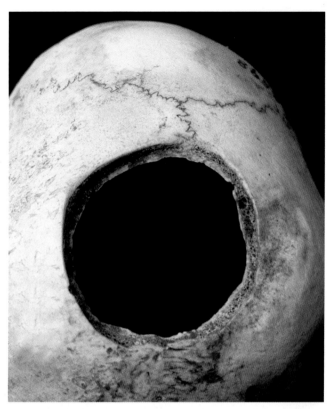

Figure 7.38
Adult male from Acomayo with a large unhealed trepanation (63 × 65 mm). Just to the right of the trepanation is a healed depressed fracture. Museo Inka 2598.

Acomayo

Acomayo lies about fifty kilometers southeast of Cuzco. The Museo Inka has three trepanned skulls that were collected there in 1934, and the Museo Nacional de Antropología, Arqueología, y Historia del Perú has a trepanned skull that was donated to the museum in 1951. All four skulls come from adult males. Two have annular cranial modification; two are unmodified. Each has a single trepanation made by the circular grooving method, and all openings are of nearly the same size, approximately sixty millimeters in diameter. Based on this small sample, the success rate (50 percent) was not particularly good: two openings show long-term healing, but the other two show no bone reaction, indicating that death occurred during or shortly after the surgery. The reason for trepanning is not obvious in any case. Although three skulls have healed depressed fractures (Figure 7.38), no perimortem injuries can be observed.

Sacsahuaman

Sacsahuaman was an impressive fortress and ceremonial complex constructed by the Inca above the city of Cuzco (Gasparini and Margolies 1980; Hemming and Ranney 1982). It was badly damaged during the early colonial period, when stones were removed to build Cuzco's churches and other buildings. Scientific study of the ruins has been sporadic and limited in scale. The first systematic attempt to conserve the architecture and conduct archaeological excavations was in the 1930s (Julien 2004). A number of Inca burials were

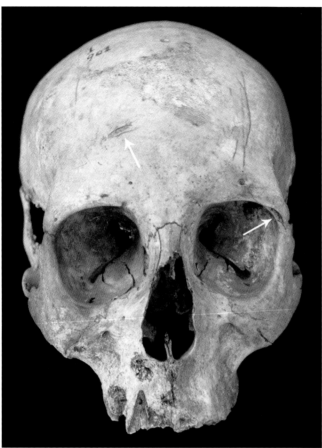

a

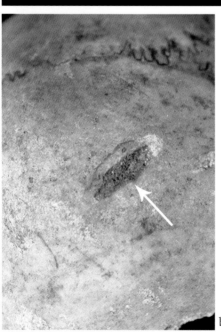

b

Figure 7.39
(a) Frontal view of an adult cranium from Sacsahuaman with two sharp force injuries: one in the forehead area and one over the left eye orbit (arrows); and (b) close-up of a sharp force grazing wound on the left parietal bone. Museo Inka 1/901.

found during these excavations, some of which I was able to examine in 1992 and 2002. These include one skull with perimortem sharp-edge trauma that was not trepanned, and three skulls with multiple healed and unhealed fractures and trepanations. Perhaps reflecting the fortress function of Sacsahuaman, all skulls are male and all have injuries. Figure 7.39 is a particularly interesting case because it shows sharp force injuries unlike the typical wounds produced by native Andean weapons, and may document injuries inflicted by a Spanish sword. Two of the wounds are located on the skull vault, and one penetrating wound grazed the outer edge of the left eye socket. The three trepanned crania from Sacsahuaman, on the other hand, are not remarkable; the trepanations are circular to oval in form, similar to those found at other sites in the Cuzco region. One of the crania is of interest because it has a well-healed trepanation associated with a fracture of the temporal bone (Figure 7.40), a dangerous area for fractures due to the risk of tearing the meningeal arteries and a rare location for trepanations.

More recent excavations conducted at a cemetery in the northwest corner of Sacsahuaman in 1999 produced the skeletal remains of an additional forty-three individuals (Andrushko et al. 2006). Interestingly, for those burials that could be sexed, most (twenty-nine of forty-one) were females and only twelve were adult males. Trepanation was not observed in any of these individuals, which, along with the very different sex distribution, suggests that the skulls from the 1930s excavations may represent quite distinct burial contexts and social groups from those more recently excavated.

Figure 7.40
Adult male from Sacsahuaman with two healed trepanations. The trepanation on the left temple is associated with a skull fracture (arrow). Museo Inka 1/327.

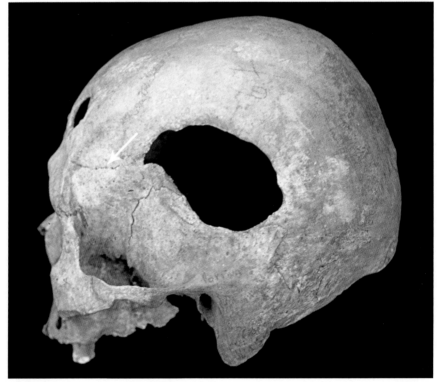

Chokepukio

Chokepukio is an archaeological site located in the Lucre Basin, approximately thirty kilometers southeast of Cuzco. It has a long history of occupation, dating as far back as 400 BC and extending through the Late Horizon Period. In recent years, Chokepukio has been the focus of multiple seasons of excavation directed by Gordon McEwan (McEwan et al. 2002). A total of eighty-nine Inca-period burials have been recovered at the site, including five individuals with trepanations (Andrushko et al. 2006; Andrushko and Verano 2008). Three of the trepanations are clearly associated with skull fractures. Two of the three appear to be unsuccessful attempts to treat victims with severe head wounds (Figures 7.41 and 7.42), while the third shows evidence of long-term healing. Two other individuals have trepanations (one healed, one with no healing) without any indication of why the procedure was initiated. All trepanations at Chokepukio are of the southern highlands circular cutting form, except one, which appears to reflect scraping.

Although a small sample, the Chokepukio skulls are important because they are among the few trepanations from the southern highlands that have been found in intact burials excavated under controlled conditions. It is hoped that additional burials with trepanations will be found in future archaeological excavations in the Cuzco area.

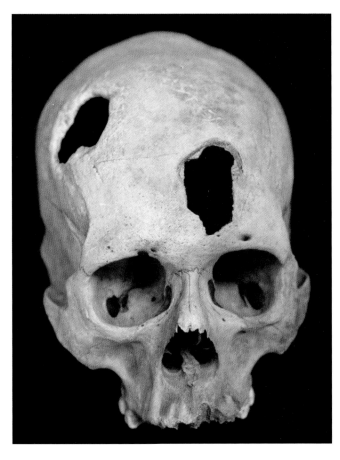

Figure 7.41
Adult male from Chokepukio with two trepanations. The one located on the right parietal bone is well healed. The one on the frontal bone is associated with a skull fracture and shows no healing. Cut marks can be seen across the frontal bone and to the right side of the opening. Photograph courtesy of Gordon McEwan.

Pikillacta

Two trepanned skulls have also been found at the Middle Horizon Period–site of Pikillacta, also in the Lucre Valley. One is held at the Museo Inka, and the other was excavated by McEwan and described in his 1987 publication (McEwan 1987:appendix 2). The Museo Inka skull was acquired in 1949. It has a single, healed, circular opening. The skull found by McEwan has three openings, all showing extensive healing. These two skulls come from a site that was built and abandoned during the Middle Horizon Period (ca. AD 600–900), and they are important evidence that trepanation was practiced in the Cuzco area before Inca times.

Unprovenanced Skulls from the Cuzco Region

In addition to skulls from known sites described above, the Museo Inka also has fifty-three trepanned skulls identified as coming from the Cuzco area but lacking more specific information. Like the Tello collection from the central highlands, these skulls probably were gathered by university and museum archaeologists from burial structures and caves in the Cuzco area during the early twentieth century. While of unknown antiquity and provenance, they are similar in technique to trepanned skulls from known Inca sites, and

Figure 7.42
Adult male from Chokepukio with a large unhealed trepanation (45 × 50 mm) on the right parietal bone, associated with a skull fracture. A linear fracture extends out from the right margin of the defect to the squamosal suture, which has separated as well. Photograph courtesy of Gordon McEwan.

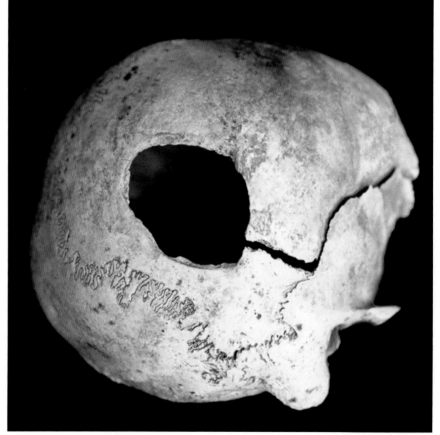

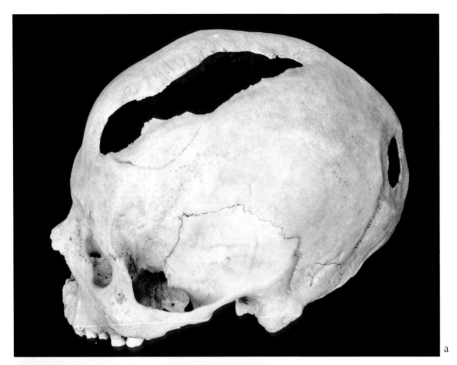

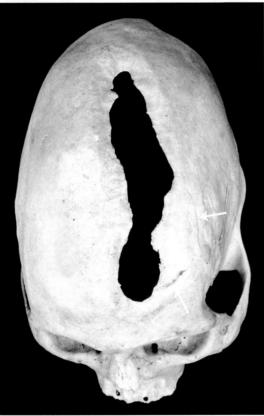

Figure 7.43
(a) Left lateral view of an adult male with two healed trepanations. The larger trepanation, which extends along the sagittal suture, is 117 mm in length. It appears to be associated with a healed linear fracture (arrow). (b) Superior view, with healed fracture indicated by arrows. Museo Inka 2579.

thus have some value as comparative specimens. In addition, twenty-three (43 percent) have healed or unhealed skull fractures, and there are several examples of trepanations associated with these injuries. The sample shows a strong bias toward men, consisting of thirty-eight males, twelve females, and three individuals of uncertain sex. Twenty-seven of the skulls show no cranial modification, while twelve present an annular form. Some of the more interesting crania will be described below.

The skull of a young adult male with two healed trepanations is included in Sergio Quevedo's 1943 survey of trepanation in the Cuzco region (Quevedo 1943b:202, cat. no. 2579). Quevedo describes it as an example of an unusual trepanation, more linear than circular in form. Indeed, the trepanation on the top of the skull has the appearance of a long irregular gash, which begins at the frontal bone and follows the sagittal suture posteriorly (Figure 7.43). Despite its risky placement directly over the sagittal sinus, the operation was a success, judging from the extensive healing of its margins. Although not noted by Quevedo, one can see a healed linear fracture, semicircular in shape, to the left of the trepanation. Perhaps this fracture was the motivation for trepanning. A second, more classically "Inca" trepanation (by circular grooving) is also present on the back of the skull (visible in Figure 7.43a). This opening also is well healed.

The Museo Inka has three crania that are good examples of unsuccessful attempts to treat acute skull fractures. The cranium in Figure 7.44 has a circular trepanation placed over an irregular area of necrotic bone that has several small fractures radiating outward from the defect. There is a larger area of subperiosteal new bone apposition over the temple,

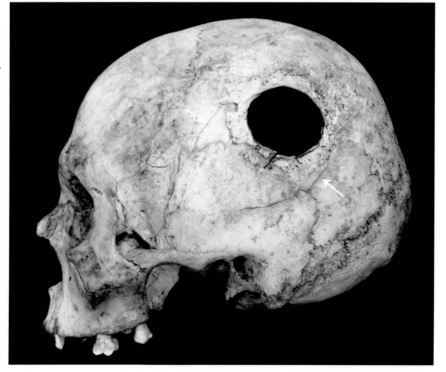

Figure 7.44
Adult male with a trepanation (30 × 35 mm) placed over a skull fracture and area of necrotic bone. Multiple fracture lines radiate outward from the circular trepanation (arrows). Museo Inka 2569.

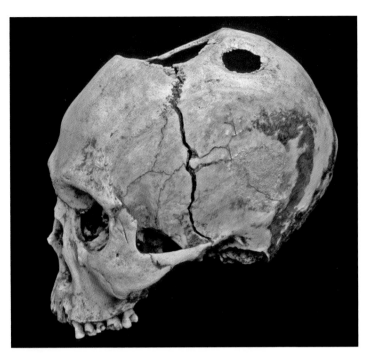

Figure 7.45
Adult male with
two trepanations,
one healed and
one unhealed. The
larger unhealed
trepanation appears
to have been placed
over the impact
point of a major
blunt force injury
that sent radiating
fractures down
both sides of the
skull. No evidence
of healing. Museo
Inka s/n (no catalog
number).

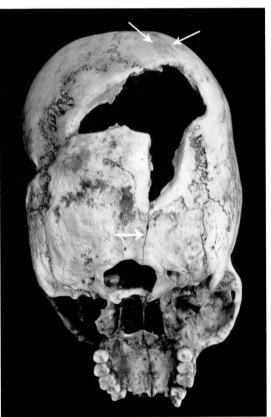

Figure 7.46
Adult male with a large
irregular trepanation of the
back of the skull, associated
with a circular impact
fracture above (arrows
above) and a radiating
fracture below (arrow
below). Museo Inka s/n
(no catalog number).

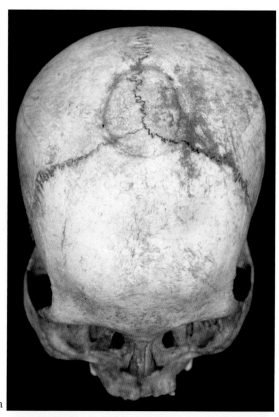

Figure 7.47
(a) Superior view of an adult female with a trepanation that was begun but never completed; and (b) close-up of incomplete trepanation. Museo Inka MO-H 246, s/n 150, 2632.

a

b

marking the spread of an infection. There is no evidence of healing, indicating that the patient probably succumbed during or shortly after the surgical intervention. The cranium in Figure 7.45 has two trepanations—one healed and one unhealed. The larger opening shows major fractures radiating out from its margins, the largest of which extends down the temporal bone through the temporomandibular joint. The third example (Figure 7.46) has a large irregular opening on the back of the skull. There are two clues as to why the trepanation was placed here: a small, circular impact fracture above the trepanation, and a linear fracture extending from the bottom of the trepanation to the foramen magnum. There is no evidence of healing, indicating that the intervention was not successful.

Figure 7.47 shows a rare example of an adult female from the Cuzco area with an incomplete trepanation. The top of the skull has a 35 × 45 millimeter oval area where the outer table of the skull was grooved with a sharp instrument. Two small openings into the diploic space are visible on the lateral margins of the groove. Interestingly, the bone shows smoothing of the margins of the groove and obliteration of the cut marks, indicating survival. Why the trepanation was begun but then aborted is unknown. There is no fracture or other indication of the purpose of this partial intervention.

SOUTHERN HIGHLANDS: POOLED SAMPLE

Combining the skulls from Ollantaytambo and the other sites described above with the unprovenanced Cuzco-area skulls, our database contains 160 trepanned skulls from the southern highlands. Many of these have multiple trepanations, resulting in a total of 226 openings. The following data are derived from this pooled regional sample, which permits a general overview of trepanation techniques, locations, and success rates, and allows examination of the association between skull fractures and trepanation for the southern highlands as a whole.

Techniques

The most commonly practiced trepanation techniques in the southern highlands are circular or oval cutting (55 percent) and scraping (45 percent). Only three examples of trepanation by linear cutting are known from the Cuzco area: Squier's skull (see Chapter 2, Figure 2.4), an unprovenanced cranium in the Museo Inka collections (see Figure 7.13), and the adult female burial from Kanamarca (see Figure 7.14). Only two examples of trepanation by the drilling and cutting method were found in the Museo Inka collections (see Figures 7.16 and 7.17). Other than these unusual cases, trepanation techniques in the southern highlands are consistent and demonstrate impressive success rates.

Locations

Figures 7.48 and 7.49 present data on the locations of trepanations and skull fractures in the pooled southern highlands sample. The fracture data includes both healed and unhealed fractures. Most trepanations (33 percent) were placed on the left side of the skull (primarily on the left parietal bone), followed by the frontal bone (24 percent), right vault (19 percent), and mid-vault (13 percent). The occipital region was the least common location

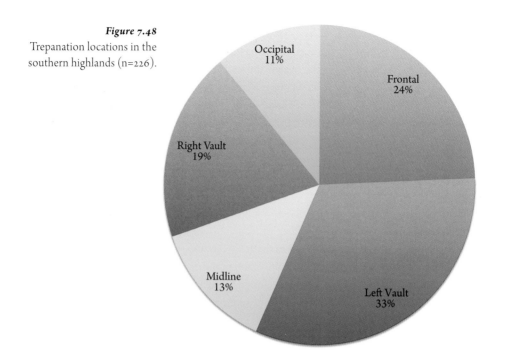

Figure 7.48
Trepanation locations in the
southern highlands (n=226).

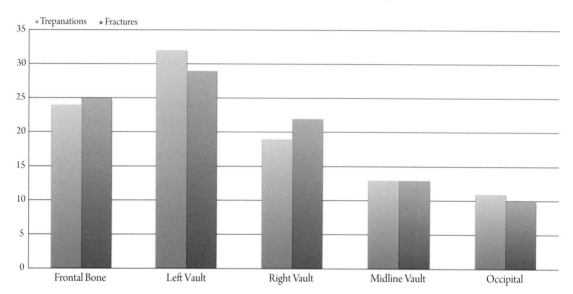

Figure 7.49 Comparison of trepanation and skull fracture locations in the southern
highlands (%).

for trepanning (11 percent). Skull fracture locations are quite similar, with the highest frequency on the left vault (29 percent), followed by the frontal (25 percent) and right vault (22 percent). These frequencies are similar to observations in the south coast and central highland Peruvian samples, although in the southern highlands more trepanations are found on the left side of the skull than on the frontal bone. The frequency with which sutures were affected (36.6 percent) and the rarity of trepanations executed in the temporal fossa (8.7 percent) and nuchal region of the occipital bone (1.9 percent) is also similar to that of the south coast and central highland samples.

The motivations for trepanning in the southern highlands are not always clear, as most trepanations are not associated with visible skull fractures. Trepanations executed for reasons other than acute head injury, such as posttraumatic headache or other symptoms, might be located anywhere on the skull, and in examples of multiple trepanations, openings are often spread across different areas of the skull (see, for example, Figures 7.2, 7.30, 7.32, and 7.33). Nevertheless, the overall correspondence between skull fracture and trepanation location in the southern highlands is similar to that of other geographic regions, confirming that particular regions of the skull faced an increased risk of injury—and thus an increased frequency of trepanation.

Success Rate

The success rate for southern highlands trepanations is impressive. Of 226 trepanations, 166 (73.5 percent) show extensive healing, indicating long-term survival of the patient; twenty-three trepanations (10.2 percent) show short-term survival; and thirty-seven (16.4 percent) show no bone reaction, indicating that the patient died during or shortly after surgery. The 73.5 percent success rate is more impressive still when one considers trepanations associated with visible skull fractures. Of the sixty trepanations that showed short-term or no healing, seventeen (28 percent) had skull fractures that were probably the reason for surgery. Many of these showed extensive radiating fractures, indicative of a severe head injury that might have been fatal even without trepanation (see Figures 7.36, 7.44, and 7.45). Large trepanations that removed substantial portions of the cranial vault likely represent attempts to treat head trauma as well, although no evidence remains. Were it possible to recognize and exclude the obviously "hopeless" cases of severe head injury, the overall survival rate would certainly exceed 73.5 percent.

Individuals with multiple trepanations are informative as well, because we can examine whether going back for a second or third (or seventh) trepanation was advisable. Of the thirty-two skulls with two trepanations, twenty-five (78.1 percent) show healing of the second opening. Six of the eight individuals with three trepanations (75 percent) had a successful third procedure. And the most notable repeat patients, two with four trepanations each, one with five, and one with seven, all survived. An impressive feat by any measure. The British Museum of Natural History owns the Andean record holder for number of healed trepanations: a cranium from the Cuzco region with seven healed openings (Figure 7.50 and 7.51). This case, and the others with four and five healed openings, suggests that returning to an experienced Cuzco trepanner incurred relatively little risk, provided that one did not have a severe head injury with a poor prognosis.

Figure 7.50
Photograph of a cast
(oblique superior view)
of the British Museum
of Natural History skull
from Cuzco, showing
five of the seven
trepanations. National
Museum of Natural
History, Smithsonian
Institution, 381898 (cast of
BMNH catalog number
1956.10.10.1).

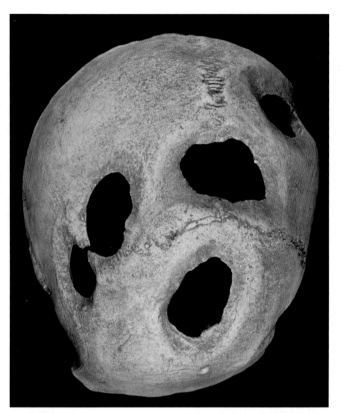

Figure 7.51
Drawing of the British
Museum of Natural
History skull from Cuzco,
showing all seven healed
trepanations. Redrawn after
Oakley et al. 1959:fig. 4.

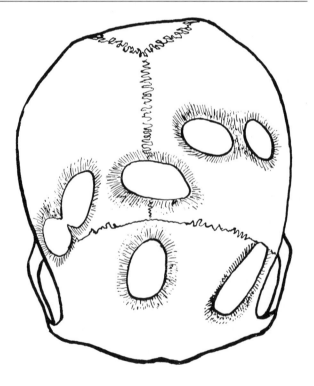

HOLES IN THE HEAD

NEW DISCOVERIES OF TREPANNED CRANIA FROM THE CUZCO REGION

Recent research by Valerie Andrushko (Andrushko 2007; Andrushko and Verano 2008) has revealed new data on trepanned skulls from the Cuzco region. This new material has not been entered into our trepanation database, so it is described separately here. It has been recovered from archaeological excavations at six Inca sites, one in the city of Cuzco and five located 4.5 to 147.5 kilometers from the Inca capital, and includes sixty-six individuals with a total of 109 trepanations. These new samples are significant because the crania come from well-documented archaeological excavations, and there is a sufficient comparative sample of non-trepanned individuals from the same sites to permit calculation of the frequency of trepanation in each sample. Thus, the issue of collection bias, which plagues nearly all other trepanation samples, is avoided.

Of 411 individual crania from the six sites, Andrushko found that sixty-six (16.1 percent) were trepanned at least once. Trepanation prevalence varied by site from a low of 4.8 percent to a high of 35.6 percent. All but one of the trepanations were done using the circular grooving or scraping techniques. The most impressive case is a cranium with seven perforations of the left and right parietal bones (Figure 7.52). In terms of the number of openings, this skull ties that of the British Museum of Natural History cranium (see Figures 7.50

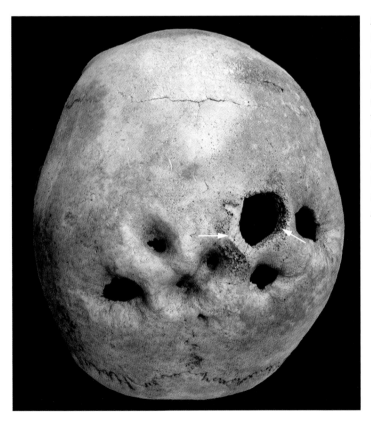

Figure 7.52
Cranium from the site of Qotakalli with seven openings on the left and right parietals. Six show extensive healing; one was in the early stages of healing at the time of death, as indicated by active bone remodeling (arrows). Photograph courtesy of Valerie Andrushko.

and 7.51), although in this case, the concentration of openings in a single area suggests that some may have been made during a single operation rather than on seven different occasions. An outlier in terms of trepanation technique is the cranium from Kanamarca with a trepanation by linear cutting (described above and illustrated in Figures 7.14 and 7.15).

Of the fifty-four trepanned adults whose sex could be determined, males were significantly more likely to be trepanned than females (thirty-five males compared to nineteen females; a male-to-female sex ratio of 1.84 to 1). Similar to our larger pooled data set from the Cuzco region, children were rarely trepanned. A single child of seven to eight years of age at death is among this sample of sixty-six trepanned individuals. Comparing other age groups, it is notable that unhealed trepanations are found primarily in adolescents and young adults, while older adults tend to have well-healed trepanations. This suggests that surgery was most often done on adolescents and young adults. A greater risk of head injury from violent encounters may explain this: twenty-nine of the sixty-six trepanned individuals (44 percent) have healed or perimortem skull trauma, and in seven cases trepanations are directly associated with perimortem fractures.

Geographic and Temporal Distribution

As part of her dissertation research, Andrushko examined skeletal remains from five other Cuzco sites that had Inca and pre-Inca occupations: Sacsahuaman, Kusicancha, Machu Picchu, Wata, and Qhataqasapatallacta. With the exception of a few examples from Sacsahuaman (see discussion above), trepanned skulls were not found at these sites. We do not know why trepanation was practiced at some sites in the Cuzco region and not at others. Perhaps there was a greater need for such procedures at certain places and times, such as during periods of warfare, when head injuries would have been more common (Andrushko and Torres 2011). Or perhaps there were some trepanners known for exceptional skill, who developed local traditions and trained apprentices in the surgical arts. Don Brothwell, drawing on earlier work by Stuart Piggott (1940), noted that concentrations of trepanned skulls were found in some regions of Europe during Neolithic times, and he proposed that there may have existed special "centers of surgical activity" (Brothwell 1994). Certainly there are regional concentrations in Peru as well (south coast, central highlands, and northern highlands). The Cuzco region seems to show local variation in the practice, with trepanners both in the center and periphery of the Inca heartland.

Only a small number of southern highland trepanned skulls come from secure pre-Inca contexts. While a few trepanned skulls from Cuzco periphery sites date to the Late Intermediate Period (ca. AD 1000–1300), most are associated with the Inca occupation of these sites. A few trepanned skulls have been found at the Middle Horizon site of Pikillacta (ca. AD 600–900) in the Lucre Valley south of Cuzco (see discussion above), but overall, the evidence suggests that trepanation emerged relatively late in the Cuzco region, coincident with the rise and expansion of the Inca Empire in the mid- to late fourteenth century.

Success Rate

Of 109 trepanations in Andrushko's study, eighty-nine (82 percent) show extensive healing, a success rate slightly higher than our larger pooled southern highlands sample. Clearly, trepanners in the Cuzco region achieved a level of skill superior to those in other regions and time periods. This may reflect both technique and experience. The scraping and circular grooving methods seem to have had a higher success rate than the linear cutting and drilling methods, and the low mortality rate suggests that Inca trepanners had developed a high level of skill.

OLD AND NEW DATA FROM SOUTHERN HIGHLAND SITES

Although we are confident that we have located and recorded all large collections of southern highlands trepanned skulls, many museums in Peru, the United States, and Europe have single specimens or small collections, typically assembled in the late nineteenth and early twentieth centuries. Examples can be found in private collections in Peru as well. In most cases, these skulls are of unknown provenance and date, and thus are of limited research potential, but their collectors and collection history are of interest. One example is a collection of trepanned crania made by Max Uhle in 1905.

Uhle, often called the father of Peruvian archaeology because of his important early fieldwork in coastal Peru, visited Cuzco in 1905 as part of an exploration of archaeological sites in the southern highlands. He visited a number of cemeteries and burial caves in the area surrounding Cuzco, all of which had been looted, but many of which had skeletal material exposed on the surface. He collected crania from cemeteries on the road from Cuzco to Pisac between Cochahuasi and Huancalli; from burial caves at Sauma, about a kilometer north of Chinchaypuquio; and from a burial cave at Colmay, about seven kilometers northwest of Chinchaypuquio. Uhle's collection included seventeen crania with trepanations. Apparently, he never analyzed or published this material, as there is no mention of it by MacCurdy or later scholars who studied trepanation in the Cuzco region. John Rowe published a summary of Uhle's visit to Cuzco, noting the sites he visited and the limited information available on his travels and activities (Rowe and Uhle 1954:11). The crania Uhle collected from Cuzco and other parts of Peru are now in the collection of the Phoebe A. Hearst Museum of Anthropology at the University of California, Berkeley, where I recently had the opportunity to study them.

The trepanned skulls collected by Uhle are typical examples of southern highland trepanation technique. All were done by circular grooving, scraping, or oval cutting (Figure 7.53). Most have single trepanations, but four individuals have two (e.g., Figure 7.54), and three individuals have three (e.g., Figure 7.55), for a total of twenty-nine trepanations. The success rate for these trepanations is impressive: twenty-four of the twenty-nine openings (92 percent) show long-term healing, while only two were unsuccessful. Four are associated with visible skull fracture, but in the other cases there is no evidence of the purpose of the trepanations. As can be judged from cranial size and morphology, males outnumber females by about two to one in this sample. Like the trepanned skulls described by MacCurdy, there is heterogeneity in skull shape in the Uhle collection. Most crania show annular oblique (circumferential) deformation, but a few are unmodified. Unfortunately, Uhle did not report finding grave goods or other indicators of cultural affiliation that might

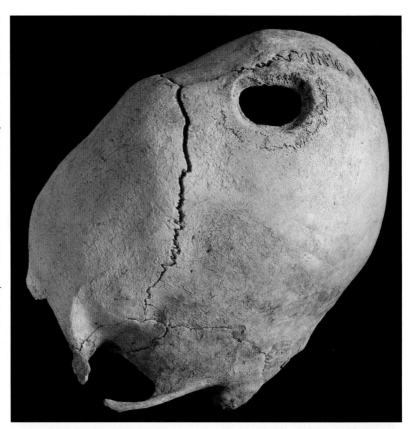

Figure 7.53
Trepanation by the circular grooving technique in an adult female with annular cranial deformation. A halo of necrotic bone and an irregular line of osteoclastic activity can be seen surrounding around the opening, indicating short-term survival only. From Colmay, Cuzco, collected by Max Uhle. Catalog number 12-3228, courtesy of the Phoebe A. Hearst Museum of Anthropology and the Regents of the University of California.

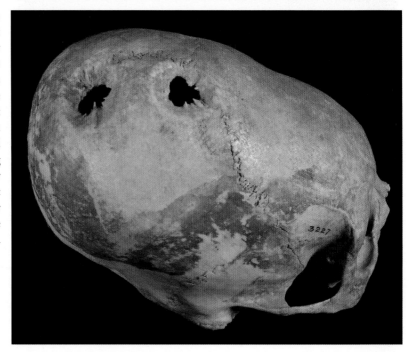

Figure 7.54
Cranium of an adult female with annular cranial deformation. Two well-healed trepanations by the scraping technique are present on the right parietal bone. From Colmay, Cuzco, collected by Max Uhle. Catalog number 12-3227, courtesy of the Phoebe A. Hearst Museum of Anthropology and the Regents of the University of California.

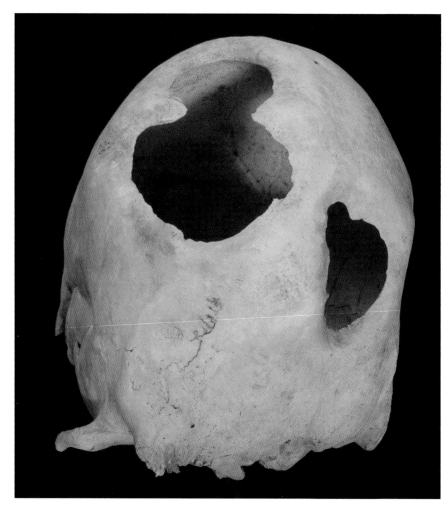

Figure 7.55
Partial cranium
(oblique posterior view)
of an old adult female
with annular cranial
deformation. There
appear to be three well-
healed trepanations
(two seem to be
separate openings that
intersect one another,
while the other is an
isolated opening). All
three were made using
the circular grooving
or scraping technique.
From Colmay, Cuzco,
collected by Max
Uhle. Catalog number,
12-3235, courtesy
of the Phoebe A.
Hearst Museum of
Anthropology and
the Regents of the
University of California.

allow approximate dating of this material, but the surgical technique and high rate of success are consistent with Inca trepanation, and Uhle noted that the Colmay burial cave was located near Inca architecture.

New Data from the Department of Apurimac

As part of her dissertation research, bioarchaeologist Danielle Kurin recently conducted excavations at four Late Intermediate Period (ca. AD 1080–1280) funerary caves in the provinces of Andahuaylas and Chincheros, located in the Department of Apurimac, about 160 kilometers west of Cuzco (Kurin 2012, 2013). Skeletal remains recovered from these caves include 256 crania, thirty-two of which (12.5 percent) are trepanned. Some have multiple trepanations, reflecting a total of forty-five separate procedures.

Scraping is the most common trepanation method, seen in 58 percent of cases. Drilling and cutting is the second most common method (24 percent), followed by circular grooving (20 percent). A single example of linear cutting was found on an isolated parietal fragment. Kurin interprets this as postmortem experimentation rather than trepanation of a living patient, because the cuts were made on the *internal* rather than the external surface of the bone (Kurin 2013:488, fig. 5; see below). Of the forty-five trepanations Kurin recorded, 66.6 percent show either partial or long-term healing. Most successful were trepanations by scraping (all of which show at least partial healing), followed by circular grooving (55.6 percent success rate). Drilling and cutting was nearly always unsuccessful, with one exception that shows short-term survival. Most trepanations are found on the left parietal bone, similar to my own data on central and southern highlands trepanations.

Kurin found that more than half the crania had skull fractures, either near the site of trepanations or on other parts of the cranium, suggesting an association between the two. However, only in about 25 percent of the cases is the trepanation directly associated with or adjacent to the fracture. Three crania do not show fractures but have openings placed in areas of healed bone inflammation (osteitis), indicating another possible motive for the procedure. None of these individuals survived, however, indicating that the attempt at treatment was not successful.

Only adult crania at Kurin's Andahuaylas sites have trepanations; crania of fifty-two children were examined for trepanations, but none were found. Trepanation is significantly more frequent in adult males than in adult females. Kurin tested for an association between individuals with and without cranial modification (both are found at Andahuaylas sites) and trepanation, but did not find a statistically significant difference in frequency.

Figure 7.56
A cranium of an adult male from the site of Natividad (Department of Apurimac), which has a total of ninety-three partial and complete drill holes on the right frontal and parietal bones. Photograph courtesy of Danielle Kurin and Wiley Periodicals, Inc.

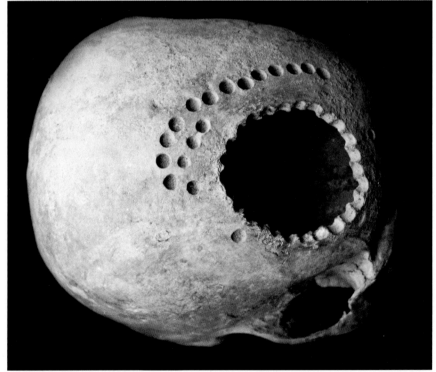

Kurin's most unusual discovery is evidence on two crania (as well as on the parietal bone fragment mentioned above) of apparent postmortem experimentation. Each of the crania has a large number of drilled holes that create openings typical of the drilling and cutting method. There are additional features such as a linear groove formed by an overlapping series of incomplete drilled holes in one cranium and linear sequences of discrete holes through the outer table in the other (Figure 7.56). The parietal fragment mentioned previously has linear cuts through the inner table of the bone. Kurin argues convincingly that all three of these cases are postmortem experiments on crania rather than trepanations on living patients. Polishing of the posterior and basilar portions of one cranium, indicating extensive handling, provides additional support for postmortem manipulation. Interestingly, each of the two complete crania had a well-healed trepanation by the scraping method.

The idea of Peruvian trepanners experimenting on cadavers has been proposed by some scholars and discounted by others, including myself (see Chapter 4). Until Kurin's recent discoveries, convincing evidence of such experimentation has been lacking. Of course, one can only speculate on the motives for drilling holes in skulls after death. Does it reflect the training of apprentices in trepanation techniques, or are these simply marks of a trepanner idly passing time with his or her tools? Kurin makes other intriguing observations on possible treatments associated with trepanations in her Andahuaylas sites, such as cutting of the hair around trepanation sites, a possible cranioplasty, and evidence of the application of poultices to surgical wounds.

These new discoveries from Andahuaylas are important. They are the first trepanned skulls from the southern highlands of Peru to be directly radiocarbon dated, confirming that skull surgery was practiced in this region prior to the rise of the Inca Empire, and show experimentation with multiple techniques. The sample also provides important evidence of postmortem experimentation. The context for these discoveries is not without ambiguity, however. The Andahuaylas burial caves, like most in the Andes, contain commingled skeletal remains. The caves have been disturbed over the centuries by visitors, both human and non-human, resulting in damage to and removal of both skeletal material and associated grave goods. As a result, crania must be analyzed as isolated elements. Despite these taphonomic challenges, this new material is an important contribution to our knowledge of trepanation practices in the southern highlands of Peru.

TREPANATION IN THE BOLIVIAN ALTIPLANO

Trepanation was practiced in late prehistoric times not only in the southern highlands of Peru, but also in the Altiplano (Andean plateau) of southern highland Peru and Bolivia. This region is defined by its high altitude, averaging about 3,750 meters (12,300 feet), and an ecological zone characterized by grasslands, salt flats, and volcanic mountains. It possesses the world's highest navigable lake, Lake Titicaca (at an altitude of 3,800 meters), which defines a portion of the border between modern Peru and Bolivia. Just south of Lake Titicaca are the ruins of the monumental center of Tiwanaku, which rose to dominate the region from around AD 500 to 1100 (Janusek 2007).

Although Lake Titicaca and the ruins of Tiwanaku were described by European explorers during the mid-sixteenth century (Cieza de León 1941 [1553]), the first archaeological investigations did not occur until the late nineteenth century (Stübel and Uhle 1892). Important among these early investigations was fieldwork conducted in 1895 by Adolf Bandelier on Lake Titicaca's Island of the Sun and at various sites along the margin of the lake, as well as south of the capital of La Paz (Bandelier 1904, 1910). Bandelier excavated a large number of burials, and he reported collecting nearly 1,200 crania from Bolivian mortuary contexts, including sixty-five crania he identified as having trepanations (Bandelier 1904). Most of the crania came from chullpas near the town of Sica Sica, located about 115 kilometers south of La Paz, while others were found in excavations on the lake margin, on the Island of the Sun, on the flanks of Illimani, and on the eastern slope of the cordillera near Pelechuco and Charassani (Bandelier 1904; Chapin and Bandelier 1961).

With the exception of Bandelier's early publications, very little has been written on ancient trepanation in Bolivia. Several general overviews of the history of Bolivian neurosurgery have been published (Alvarado Reyes 2004; Dabdoub and Dabdoub 2013), but these provide only short summaries of prehistoric trepanation. Although they include photographs of trepanned skulls, their geographic origin, antiquity, or current location are not indicated. Bandelier sent his collection of Bolivian trepanned skulls to the American Museum of Natural History, which had funded his research. There they were "investigated and arranged by Dr. Aleš Hrdlička" (Bandelier 1904:440). Apparently, Hrdlička did not publish the collection, and it has has been largely unstudied since then, with the exception of a recent publication by Christina Torres-Rouff, which examines Bandelier's skeletal collection from the Island of the Sun. Although the focus of her article is not trepanation, Torres-Rouff includes a photo of a trepanned skull from Kea Kollu Chico (an adult female with an unhealed trepanation) and reports frequency data on skull fractures, trepanation, cranial deformation, and skeletal health indicators in comparative samples from the Tama Tam and Kupa Pukio chullpas (Torres-Rouff 2013).

In 1993, I had the opportunity to visit the museum and examine their trepanation collection, which includes Bandelier's Bolivian material and a small sample of trepanned skulls from the southern highlands of Peru, including the famous Squier skull that is described in Chapter 2. During my visit, I recorded and photographed thirteen trepanned crania from the Bandelier collection. One was excavated from the hillside site of Kea Kollo Chico on the Island of the Sun, and the others were from the Tama Tam chullpa and other sites near Sica Sica, and from Chujun Paki (near Huata) and Cachilaya (on the southeastern shore of Lake Titicaca). Eleven of the crania have a single trepanation, while two from the Tama Tam chullpa have multiple openings. The trepanations on eleven of the crania show long-term healing, while one shows none and one shows short-term healing, indicating a success rate of 84.6 percent. Although the sample is small, it indicates a survival rate superior to that of the central highlands of Peru and similar to that of the southern highlands. Trepanation techniques also resemble those of the southern highlands: circular grooving and cutting and scraping (Figures 7.57 and 7.58). The motive for trepanning is not clear in most individuals, but there are three unequivocal cases (Figures 7.58, 7.59, and 7.60) and one possible case (Figure 7.61) of significant skull fractures with

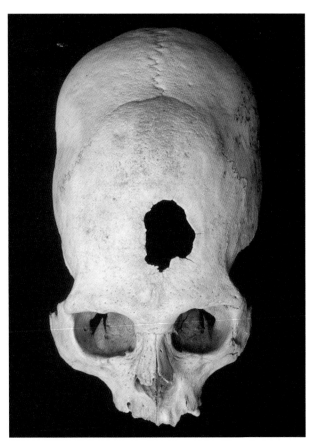

Figure 7.57
Cranium of an adult male from Cachilaya, Lake Titicaca, with a well-healed trepanation on the frontal bone created using the scraping method. Bandelier collection B-3063 © 2015, Division of Anthropology, American Museum of Natural History.

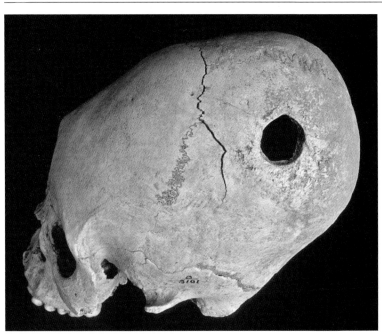

Figure 7.58
Cranium of an adult female from Lluchuni-Amaya with a trepanation by circular grooving that shows partial healing. The cranium also shows probable perimortem blunt force trauma (separation of the coronal suture and a radiating fracture extending inferiorly from it). The fracture may have been the motivation for trepanning in this case. Bandelier collection B-3101 © 2015, Division of Anthropology, American Museum of Natural History.

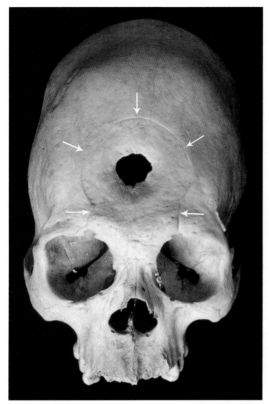 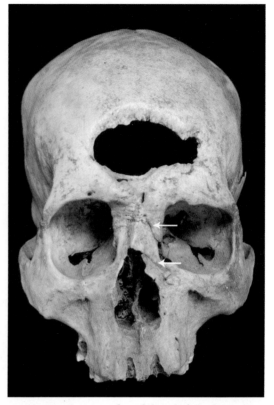

Figure 7.59 Cranium of an adult male from the Tama Tam chullpa, near Sica Sica, showing a large, circular, depressed fracture of the forehead region, with radiating fractures extending inferiorly across both superciliary arches (arrows). A circular trepanation, presumably by scraping, is located at the center of the depressed fracture. Both the trepanation and the fractures are healed, indicating survival. Bandelier collection 99/3106 © 2015, Division of Anthropology, American Museum of Natural History.

Figure 7.60 Cranium of an adult male from the Churkoni Group chullpa, Sica Sica region. This individual appears to have received a major blow to the forehead, which fractured the frontal bone and sent radiating fractures down through the left nasal bone and nasal process of the left maxilla (arrows). A trepanation was done on the frontal bone adjacent to the fractured area. It shows long-term healing, indicating that the operation was successful. Bandelier collection 99/3347 © 2015, Division of Anthropology, American Museum of Natural History.

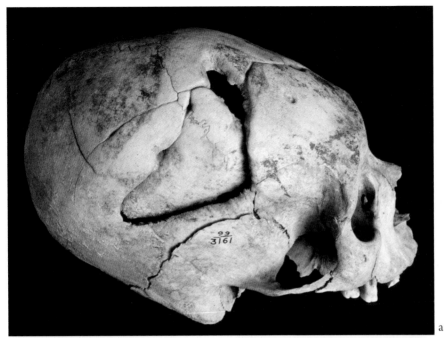

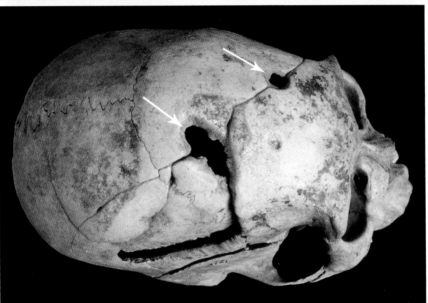

Figure 7.61 (a) Lateral view; and (b) superior view of the cranium of an adult male from the Tama Tam chullpa, near Sica Sica, with massive trauma to the skull and two possible trepanations. Extensive healing makes it unclear whether the two openings indicated by arrows are trepanations or penetrating wounds. The extensive fracturing of the right side of the vault, with the displacement of a large triangular piece of bone, is more consistent with blunt force trauma than with radiating fractures from penetrating wounds. It is remarkable that this individual survived. Bandelier collection 99/3161 © 2015, Division of Anthropology, American Museum of Natural History.

associated trepanations. Notably, although these fractures were severe, three out of four show long-term healing.

Dating and Context

Bandelier's crania from chullpas near Sica Sica appear to date to the Altiplano Period (ca. AD 1100–1400) (Torres-Rouff 2013), whereas the trepanned crania from Kea Kollo Chico may be substantially earlier, as the cemetery in which they were found dates to the Middle (ca. 1300–500 BC) or Upper Formative Period (ca. 500 BC–AD 500). These early dates come from recent fieldwork on the Island of the Sun directed by Charles Stanish and Brian Bauer (Stanish and Bauer 2004). If Bandelier's crania indeed date to the Middle Formative Period, they would be contemporary with or even earlier than the Paracas cavernas tombs. If they date to the Upper Formative Period, they are probably later. Dating of the osteological material remains problematic, due to the lack of detailed information on the graves Bandelier excavated from Kea Kollo Chico.

Until the past few years, the only published example of a trepanned skull from an early context in the Altiplano was a trepanned cranium found in 1970 in a tomb on the eastern slopes of the Cordillera Real in the province of Bautista Saavedra, east of Lake Titicaca (Wassén and Bondeson 1972). Uncalibrated radiocarbon dates for the tomb indicate that it dates from AD 400 to 800. The cranium, which has three openings, appears to have been a funerary offering, along with medicinal plants, snuffing paraphernalia, and other objects associated with the burial of a "medicine-man" (Wassén and Bondeson 1972).

Three trepanned skulls have been found recently in archaeological excavations at sites on the Copacabana Peninsula near the southern end of Lake Titicaca. Sara Juengst and Sergio Chávez (2015) report that ceramics date two of these crania to the Early Horizon Period (800 BC–AD 100 and 400 BC–AD 100) and one to the Late Intermediate Period (AD 1000–1200). One cranium has two well-healed trepanations by linear cutting, one has an incomplete linear cutting trepanation placed at the margin of a depressed skull fracture, and the third has a well-healed opening that Juengst interprets as having been made with the drilling and cutting method, although the degree of healing makes it hard to distinguish from a scraping trepanation. The diversity of trepanation methods in these crania is interesting, as are the early dates for two of them, confirming that trepanation was practiced in the Altiplano substantially earlier than the Late Intermediate Period.

A Tradition Continuing into the Historic Period

While conducting fieldwork in Bolivia in 1895, Bandelier was told that trepanation was still performed in rural areas by traditional healers (Bandelier 1904). Informants on the peninsula of Huata told him that traditional Aymara healers made openings in skulls by incision and scraping, using simple tools such as pocket knives and chisels. Although these were secondary accounts, Bandelier inquired further and found a woman from Huata who had suffered a skull fracture in the temporal region and had been trepanned. The operation reportedly was executed by a well-known traditional surgeon by the name of Paloma using a pocket knife. The woman told Bandelier that the operation was painful, but that the wound had healed without complications. Paloma apparently was widely known and came to the attention of several medical school professors in La Paz, who, having heard about the simple tools he used, presented him with a set of surgical instruments as a gift. Reportedly, he never used them, preferring his own (Bandelier 1904:443).

Bandelier heard other accounts of trepanations conducted in rural areas of Bolivia as well as in southern highland Peru. A local healer near Cuzco apparently trepanned a man who had suffered a skull fracture during the 1850s. Bandelier sought more information from his Aymara field workers, showing them trepanned skulls from the excavations and asking their opinion, but they claimed not to know of the practice and were reluctant to speak about it. The Aymara woman with the healed trepanation resisted further inquiries. Bandelier noted that "she disappeared as soon as possible and avoided us studiously thereafter" (Bandelier 1904:442).

Accounts like these confirm that trepanation continued to be practiced in remote areas of the Andes into the modern historical period. In fact, scattered reports of trepanation in Bolivia continued into the twentieth century. Perhaps this is not surprising, given that modern medical facilities and doctors were unavailable in rural areas of Bolivia until after agrarian reform in 1953, making native healers and herbalists the only option for the indigenous poor of this region (Bastien 1987). Winifred Brooke (in Oakley et al. 1959), who visited the Baptist Mission at Huatahata, Lake Titicaca, in 1950, was told by a local nurse of an Aymara "medicine man" who performed trepanations on local patients:

> The nurse told me that when she first came to Huatahata two or three years earlier, the medicine man trepanned the head of another young man there and she saw him doing the operation. He first made both the patient and himself drunk, no doubt on *chicha*, the common Bolivian drink. He did the operation with a rusty nail and a stone (used I believe as a hammer). He did not put back the piece of bone he removed, but later on the skin healed over the hole (Oakley et al. 1959:93).

As recently as 1976, Bastien was told of a patient who was diagnosed with an intracranial tumor by doctors in La Paz, but could not afford to have it removed surgically. He instead sought out a local herbalist who trepanned him with a knife and removed the tumor with his fingers. The patient, who lived near Tiwanaku, reportedly recovered from the operation (Bastien 1987:17).

Reports such as these suggest that in rural areas of highland Peru and Bolivia, trepanation remained an accepted method for treating head injuries for centuries following European contact. The accounts differ in details, but they are consistent in reporting that surgeries were done with simple tools by practitioners known for their expertise in treating head wounds.

Ethnographic Parallels and Modern Experimentation

A skull which has been operated upon seldom by itself tells why the operation
was undertaken.

—T. Dale Stewart (1958:480)

AS T. DALE STEWART NOTES WITH A HINT OF IRONY, A TREPANNED SKULL
rarely reveals the specific motives behind its surgical defect. Without clear evidence of a
fracture or infection, one can in most cases only speculate as to the reasons for trepanning
a particular skull. As reviewed at the end of Chapter 7, there are scattered accounts of traditional cranial surgery in highland Peru and Bolivia continuing into the mid-twentieth
century. These provide some information on motives and surgical technique, but they
are few in number and are largely secondhand accounts. However, more extensive ethnographic reports of trepanning have come from other parts of the world, and these
provide an important comparative perspective on trepanation in Andean South America.
Also, beginning with Paul Broca's trepanations on human cadavers and dogs in the 1870s,
a number of scientists experimented with stone and metal tools in an attempt to replicate ancient trepanation techniques. These experiments culminated in two controversial mid-twentieth-century surgeries in Peru that were performed on living patients
with Inca copper and bronze tools borrowed from archaeological museums. Later, an
unusual modern experimentation with self-trepanation emerged in the 1960s in Europe
and North America.

Ethnohistoric and modern eyewitness accounts of traditional cranial surgery in the
South Pacific and in North and East Africa provide useful comparative models for understanding ancient Peruvian trepanation. They document independent traditions of skull
surgery performed with simple tools to treat acute head injury and its complications
with a high rate of success. The accounts are consistent in emphasizing that trepanation
was conceptualized by its practitioners as a practical approach to treating head injury
and headache.

THE SOUTH PACIFIC

In the late eighteenth and early nineteenth century, a number of explorers and anthropologists reported that trepanation was practiced on various islands in the South Pacific. These reports were often secondhand, but they provide information on the reasons for performing skull surgery (most commonly for skull fractures caused by sling stones or clubs) and the tools with which it was done (simple implements made of chipped stone, shark teeth, seashell, and bamboo). Summaries of these early accounts are found in Crump (1901), Handy (1923), Wölfel (1925), Ford (1937), Heyerdahl (1952), and Martin (1995, 2003). Describing trepanation in Melanesia, Edward Ford noted: "The operation was undertaken for the immediate treatment of traumatic cranial injuries, and in certain areas its performance was extended to the treatment of severe headache and other ailments, and as a prophylactic measure, in children, against the occurrence of such affections in subsequent life" (Ford 1937:477).

One of the most detailed descriptions of South Pacific trepanation was written by Richard Parkinson, who in the mid-1800s was the first European settler on the Island of New Britain, off the north coast of New Guinea. He wrote a book about his experiences there, *Dreissig Jahre in der Sdsee* (*Thirty Years in the South Seas*), which was published in 1907 in Stuttgart. Passages from this book have been translated into English by Graham Martin (1995), and I quote from them below. Based on firsthand observations of trepanation by the Tolai, Parkinson wrote:

> The surgical knowledge of the natives undoubtedly reaches its high point in the treatment of skull fractures caused by stones from slingshots. If a native is knocked out by a slingshot the unconscious combatant is immediately dragged from the scene of the fight and taken to a wise man skilled in the care of these wounds. This expert then decides the nature of the wound. . . . If the slingstone has depressed the temple then he declares the wound mortal at once and no operation is undertaken. If on the contrary the frontal bone (the forehead) is knocked in, he proceeds immediately to trepanation. His instruments are the simplest imaginable, a fragment of obsidian, a sharp shark's tooth, or a sharpened mussel shell.
>
> Then with one of the previously described instruments the operator makes a long cut obliquely over the bruise down to the bone of the skull. Two assistants pull the scalp flaps slowly and carefully apart . . . till the whole fracture can be seen. The next task is the removal of the bony splinters. With a sharpened bit of coconut shell the individual fragments of bone are carefully raised till the brain is visible . . . the next stage of the operation begins when the operator smooths the edges of the hole . . . so that all sharp corners are removed till the hole is round or elliptical. Once these things have been done, the actual operation is finished and the operator takes the necessary steps to encourage healing of the wound.

After the scalp flaps were pulled back into place, the wound was washed with green coconut water and covered with a woven fiber mat. Only then did Parkinson observe a ritual designed to ensure that the wound would heal and the patient survive:

Now he [the operator] has to do what his patients believe to be the only effective measure, namely various magical procedures that are the only things which will produce real healing. In this case they have two especially healing substances, called *mailan* and *aurur*, which must be blown into the air, hung around the patient's neck, or fixed somewhere else on the body. Without these substances the operation is not completed, and in the opinion of the natives could not have a favourable course. Whether it is the result of the surgical skill of the operator, or the result of the magic mixture, it is certain that the operation is usually very successful (Martin 1995:257–258).

Parkinson based this last statement on the reported success rate of Tolai surgeons, one of whom recalled that he had done thirty-one surgeries, with a loss of only eight patients—a success rate of 75 percent (Martin 1995). This is comparable to the best trepanners of ancient Peru.

In addition to the testimony of eyewitness and secondary accounts of trepanation, there are also examples of South Pacific trepanned skulls that were sent by Parkinson and others to museums in Europe. Though such skills are few in number and most lack detailed information on dating and context, museums in Germany, France, and England have examples from both Melanesia and Polynesia (Margetts 1967; Martin 1995; Stewart 1958; Wölfel 1925). One of them is that of a young adult male from Banks Island, Melanesia, who was trepanned by a native healer in 1901 for a severe skull fracture from a sling stone. The operation was unsuccessful, and the man died two hours later (Crump 1901). At some point following his death his skull was collected, and it later ended up in a museum collection in London. In 1993, G. C. Stevens and Jennifer Wakely did an innovative study of the skull using scanning electron microscopy to characterize the cut marks around the trepanation opening. They compared them to experimental cuts they made with metal, stone, and mollusk shell tools on laboratory bone samples and found the best match with cuts made with mollusk shell. Although Crump did not describe the tool that was used in this this operation, the experimental results lend support to ethnographic accounts that shell was one of the materials used to trepan in Melanesia (Stevens and Wakely 1993).

Unfortunately, it is not known how, why, or when trepanation originated in the South Pacific. One of the more imaginative hypotheses was proposed by Thor Heyerdahl, who argued in his book *American Indians in the Pacific* that trepanation was introduced from Peru: "We have ample evidence to suggest that the Peruvians brought trepanning and its associates down-wind into the Pacific at an early period when Polynesia was still virgin land. . . . Some islands . . . present sufficient evidence to show that the trepanation bridge formerly spanned the whole water from the coast of Peru to the islands in Melanesia" (1952:665). Heyerdahl's theory of South American voyagers and diffusion of such practices as trepanation is provocative, but it has not found support from archaeological, linguistic, ethnobotanical, or genetic data. It is more likely that trepanation evolved independently in the South Pacific, as it did in other parts of the world, as a practical treatment for head wounds. It could easily have spread by contact between the Pacific Islands, particularly those in what is now French Polynesia, where there is known to have been extensive maritime travel and trade. But there are large gaps in the distribution of trepanation across Oceania, making it unlikely that the practice was invented in a single location and then spread by diffusion (Littleton and Frifelt 2006; Martin 1995). Whatever its origins, trepanation disappeared from the South Pacific by the end of the nineteenth century amid cultural disruption from warfare, colonization, and epidemics (Martin 1995).

NORTH AFRICA

In the late nineteenth and early twentieth centuries, scientific expeditions to Algeria, Morocco, Libya, and Sudan documented the practice of trepanation among the Uareg and Kabyle Berbers, the Tibu, and the Chaouïa (Rawlings and Rossitch 1994). Evidence gathered by these expeditions includes ethnographic accounts of surgeries, physical examination of individuals with healed trepanations, tools used for trepanning, and bone plugs removed from patients (Hilton-Simpson 1922; Oakley et al. 1959). A. Roger Akester reported the following observations he made in Tibesti:

> During the Cambridge Tibesti Expedition, 1957, a party composed of members of Cambridge University and of the 10th Armoured Division in Tripoli penetrated the region of extinct volcanoes which rise abruptly from the flat wilderness of the Sahara Desert. After leaving the great crater of Emi Koussi, the rim of which forms the higest peak in the Sahara (11,150 feet), our biologists spent two weeks in the village of Yibbi Bou, where we set up a clinic for the local people, the Tibu . . . and their camels. We came across a most remarkable case of trephining while we were there. A Tibu, with two huge scars in his scalp . . . had been operated on seven years previously. He carried in his pocket two battered sardine tins telescoped together to form a box in which he kept two fragments of his own skull. These fragments fitted the scars on his head perfectly (Akester, in Oakley et al. 1959:94–95).

Interviews with various North African trepanners and their patients reveal some common features of skull surgery in the region. Trepanations were done for skull fractures and headaches caused by head injuries (Hilton-Simpson 1922; Rawlings and Rossitch 1994). Surgeons studiously avoided penetrating the dura mater to avoid infection. According to M. W. Hilton-Simpson (1922), they also avoided the cranial sutures, as these were thought to record the destiny of the patient written by the hand of Allah. Wounds were not sutured, but were dressed with sheep's butter, resin, herbs, and honey. Tools used in trepanning included pocket knives, metal probes and picks, simple saws, and, in some cases, hand drills. Hilton-Simpson (1922) has written the most detailed description of the various tools used in the early twentieth century by Shawiya surgeons of the Aures Massif, Algeria, and includes photographs of many of them in his publication (Figure 8.1). Scarification of the head and trepanation appear to have ancient roots in North Africa. Herodotus claimed that cauterization of the scalp was practiced in Libya, and trepanned skulls predating the Roman Empire have been found in Algeria (Margetts 1967; Stewart 1958).

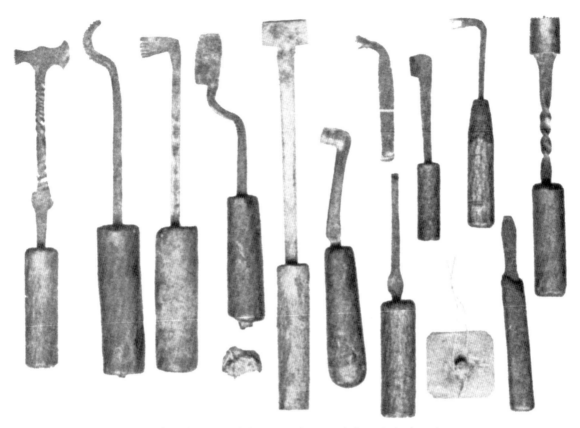

Figure 8.1 Trepanning tools of the Shawiya, including saws, elevators, drills, and a lead weight (square object, lower right), which was wrapped in cloth and temporarily placed over a trepanation opening to keep the brain from extruding after surgery. The drill at the far right is a crown trepan that was reportedly made by a local jeweler. Modified after Hilton-Simpson 1922:pl. 5.

EAST AFRICA

While the North African accounts are interesting, much more detailed and extensive reports of trepanation come from East Africa. The Kisii of highland southwestern Kenya and, to a lesser extent, the Tende of Tanzania have been observed, photographed, and filmed performing cranial surgery. While the antiquity of trepanation in East Africa is unknown, it was clearly practiced in the late nineteenth century, based on reports by doctors, police, and magistrates in British and German colonial documents (Margetts 1967). It was not until 1958, however, that the practice came to the attention of the scientific community through publications by Grounds (1958), Coxon (1962), and Margetts (1967). Since then, many reports have been published on Kisii trepanation, including firsthand observations by medical doctors, interviews, photographs, and videotapes, as well as surveys of methods, indications for surgery, survival rates, and complications. As a result, Kisii trepanation is arguably the most thoroughly documented traditional surgery anywhere in the world.

Edward Lambert Margetts, a Canadian psychiatrist, was one of the first Western physicians to describe the practice of trepanation among the Kisii. Margetts spent eight years in Nairobi in the 1950s treating patients and serving as director of the Mathari Mental Hospital. During this time, he became interested in non-Western healing traditions, including trepanation. In a 1967 publication, he described three patients who had been trepanned successfully by Kisii "head surgeons" (*omobari omotwe*) for headaches following head injuries. The most impressive case Margetts observed was that of a man who had hit his head on a door lintel and suffered from chronic headaches. Five years after the injury, he sought out an omobari, who performed a trepanation, followed by more operations over the next seven or eight years. When the man removed his hat, Margetts was amazed to see how much of his skull vault appeared to have been removed (Figure 8.2). Radiographs confirm that a significant portion of the vault was removed by the surgeries (Figure 8.3). Margetts subsequently met the omobari who had done the trepanations. He was a man of about seventy years of age, who said that he had been trepanning patients since he was in his twenties, exclusively for headaches following trauma. He had been taught the skill by his father, and he used a curved scraping tool to cut through bone. He could not remember the total number of patients he had trepanned, but guessed that it must have been in the hundreds, and he claimed never to have lost a patient (Margetts 1967).

During his years in Nairobi, Margetts obtained a set of Kisii trepanation tools (Figure 8.4) and the skullcap of a patient who apparently had died shortly after a trepanation (Figure 8.5). The tools are very similar to trepanning kits that have been described and photographed by other investigators (Furnas et al. 1985; Grounds 1958; Meschig 1983); they are for the most part handmade from scrap metal. The skullcap shows an unhealed trepanation with visible scrape marks. Although presumably done with a metal tool, it is quite similar in form and scrape marks to trepanations from Paracas (compare with Figure 5.15).

A number of Kisii trepanation procedures have been observed and photographed since the 1950s. In 1997, Michael Mueller, a science writer, was traveling in Kenya and had the opportunity to witness a trepanation. The patient was a woman with a history of headaches and dizziness that persisted for five years after a fall in which she struck her head on the ground. Despite multiple visits to the local hospital, her symptoms were not relieved, and her family decided to consult with a local omobari. He examined her and decided that a trepanation was indicated. The operation was performed one morning outside of her house, with the patient sitting on a chair and supported from behind by her husband. A basin full of fragrant leaves was held under her head during the operation to mask the smell of blood and to keep her calm. The omobari was assisted by his son, who was apprenticing with him. The son first shaved the woman's head and washed it with a banana-based soap while the omobari sterilized his tools in a pot of boiling water. The surgeon then examined her head and asked where the headache was most severe (Figure 8.6). Satisfied that he had located the appropriate place, he made a cross-shaped incision in the scalp. Assistants then retracted the scalp flaps to expose the bone. The surgeon noted bleeding from two locations on the cranium, which he scraped with a hacksaw blade until the bleeding stopped (Figure 8.7). He considered this sufficient to cure the patient's symptoms, so he did not

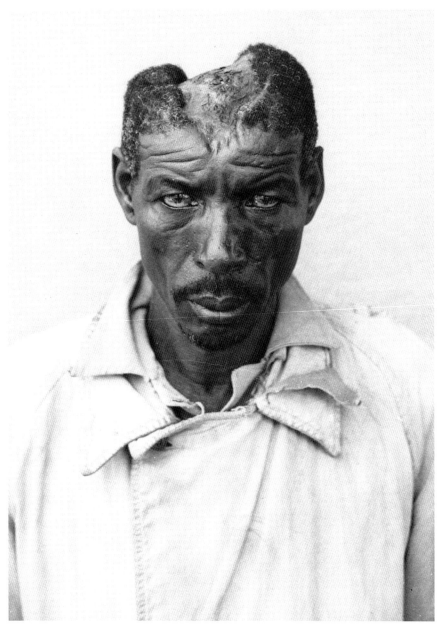

Figure 8.2 Kisii man of about fifty years of age who had multiple trepanations to treat recurring headaches following a blow to the head. Photograph by Edward Margetts, courtesy of the San Diego Museum of Man.

Figure 8.3
Anterior-posterior
radiograph (a), and lateral
radiograph (b) of the Kisii man's
head, showing the large area of
missing bone at the top of the
skull. Photographs by Edward
Margetts, courtesy of the San
Diego Museum of Man.

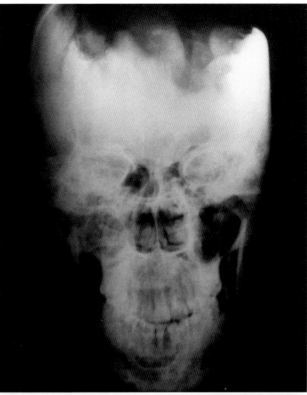

a

b

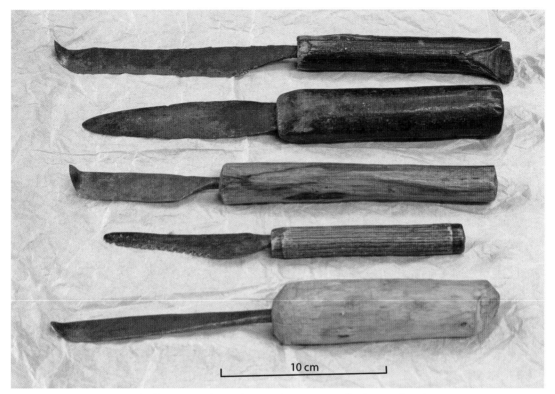

Figure 8.4 Trepanation tools of a Kisii omobari. There are three scrapers (with curved tips), a saw, and a knife. Collected by Dr. Grijendra Kumar Sood in 1956 and presented to Edward Margetts. Photograph courtesy of the San Diego Museum of Man.

penetrate further. The wound was then irrigated with banana sap and the flaps closed and held in place by a cloth bandage. The patient was led back to her house, and instructions were given for her care and diet. As is the custom, the omobari returned on several occasions to check on the woman's recovery (Mueller and Finch 1994).

While other eyewitness accounts and several films of Kisii trepanations exist, the most extensive survey of cranial surgery was conducted in the 1980s by a joint American and Kenyan team (Furnas et al. 1985). Plastic surgeon David Furnas and colleagues from the University of Nairobi, St. Joseph Hospital in Kilgoris, and the Kisii District Hospital conducted interviews with eight omobari, filmed several procedures, and saw more than one hundred patients. They found that women slightly outnumbered men and that adults outnumbered children in trepanation frequencies. Including simpler procedures such as scalp incision and scraping of the cranium, they calculated that as many as 5 percent of Kisii had been treated surgically. The team estimated that as many as five hundred to eight hundred procedures were done per year, by perhaps one hundred omobari. These are surprising numbers, given that in 1958, Grounds had estimated that only twenty to thirty Kisii omobari were still practicing trepanation. Both figures, however, are only estimates, as omobari are not officially registered with the Kenyan government or health services. Technically,

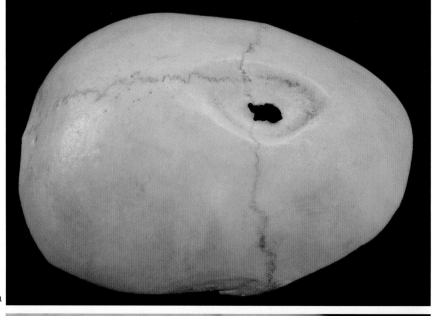

a

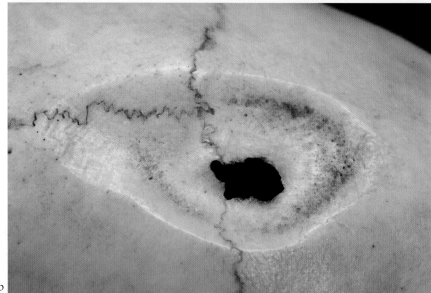

b

Figure 8.5 (a) A trepanned skull cap from Kisii General District Hospital, South Nyanza, Kenya. Although its origin is unknown, the form of the trepanation and technique (scraping) is typical of traditional Kisii surgery. It shows no evidence of healing. (b) Close-up of the trepanation, showing scrape marks. Margetts collection; photographs courtesy of the San Diego Museum of Man.

Kisii trepanation is illegal in Kenya, but authorities have long looked the other way. They only investigate if a death occurs (Furnas et al. 1985; Grounds 1958).

Furnas and his colleagues saw a number of patients who had been trepanned multiple times. Typically, these were cases in which symptoms persisted after the initial trepanation. Only three fatal complications were identified during their study: two deaths from meningitis and one from tetanus. Two patients with excessive bleeding were taken to hospitals, where they were given blood and recovered.

The eight omobari interviewed by Furnas and his colleagues were older men: all but one were over fifty years of age. All had learned their skills through a period of apprenticeship with a relative or a master omobari. When asked why they trepanned, they were consistent in saying that it was for treating acute head trauma or for headache, dizziness, drowsiness, or epilepsy attributed to earlier head injury. Surgical tools and techniques were

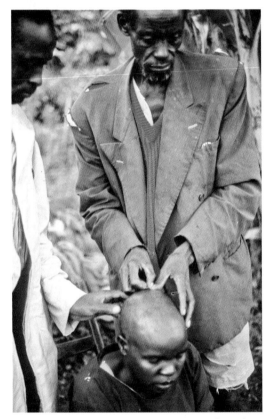

Figure 8.6 The omobari and his apprentice (at left) examine a patient's head to determine where to operate. Photograph, 1977, courtesy of Michael Mueller.

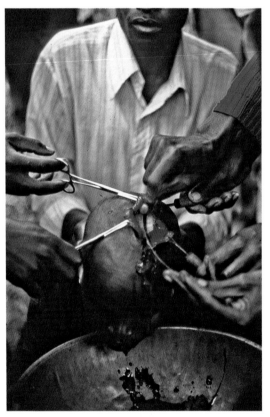

Figure 8.7 The patient's scalp has been retracted and the omobari is using the curved blade of a hacksaw to scrape areas of bone where he detected bleeding. Both traditional Kisii tools (on the right) and two modern hemostats (on the left) are used to retract the scalp flaps. The hemostats were reportedly a gift from a Dutch physician. Photograph, 1977, courtesy of Michael Mueller.

similar to those reported by observers in the 1950s, with some additions (also reported by Mueller and Finch 1994). For example, some omobari have acquired drugs such as procaine (a local anesthetic, used to numb the scalp) and penicillin (to avoid infection), and a few have been given gifts of modern surgical tools such as hemostats, which they use to retract scalp flaps (visible in Figure 8.7).

From their study, Furnas and his colleagues conclude that Kisii trepanation is a successful surgical procedure with a low rate of complications and a high degree of satisfaction as reported by patients. They note, however, that the traditional Kisii omobari is becoming an endangered species. Practitioners lament that few young people today are interested in learning their skills, and they are concerned that the practice may disappear in the near future. Nevertheless, demand for the services of omobari will probably remain high. Although recent decades have seen great progress in neurosurgical training and medical facilities in Kenya (Qureshi and Oluoch-Olunya 2010), at the time of Furnas's survey, Kenya had only four registered neurosurgeons to serve a population of over sixteen million (Dar 1985). But apparently the final chapter on East African trepanation has yet to be written. Furnas returned to Kenya in 1993 to investigate reports that the Marakwet, a group that inhabits the former Rift Valley Province, also practices trepanation, a fact that was largely unknown until recently (Mueller and Finch 1994).

MODERN EXPERIMENTATION WITH ANCIENT TOOLS

Once the scientific community generally accepted that trepanation was practiced in ancient times, questions naturally arose about what tools and techniques were used by ancient skull surgeons. Paul Broca was a pioneer in this area, performing experimental trepanations on human skulls using chipped flint and glass tools. The objective of his initial experiments was to see how quickly openings could be made in the skulls of children and adults. Broca found that he could quickly trepan the relatively thin cranial bone of a child's skull (in as little as four minutes), while it took considerably longer to scrape through the vault bone on an adult (about fifty minutes, counting time out to rest his hand). Although his experiments on human skulls used cadavers, Broca also trepanned several living dogs to demonstrate that he could safely make openings in their skulls without damaging the dura or brain (Clower and Finger 2001). Other experiments using Neolithic stone tools on human cadavers were done by Just Marie Lucas-Champonnière, T. Wilson Parry, and L. Capitan in attempts to reconstruct the specific manner in which openings were made in European Neolithic skulls (Lastres and Cabieses 1960; Lucas-Championnière 1912; Ruffer 1918).

In Peru, Julio Tello and Francisco Graña and his colleagues did experimental trepanations on human cadavers, using prehistoric metal and stone tools (Graña et al. 1954; Tello 1913). Experiments on the dead, however, were not sufficient for some surgeons, who wanted to demonstrate that Inca bronze and copper tools could be used to trepan a living patient. Two independent experiments, done by different surgical teams, were performed in hospitals in Cuzco and Lima in 1944 and 1953. Although they received largely positive reports in Peruvian newspapers at the time (Anónimo 1945; Graña et al. 1954; Quevedo 1970), these surgeries were viewed by some medical professionals as an unnecessary exercise, given that prior experiments on cadavers had demonstrated the ability to make openings in the skull with similar tools, and ancient Peruvian skulls provided direct evidence that trepanations were performed successfully (Lastres and Cabieses 1960:146; Stewart 1958:475). Certainly, such experiments would be highly controversial if attempted today.

The 1944 Surgery in Cuzco

The first experiment on a living patient using Inca tools was performed at the Hospital "Antonio Lorena" in Cuzco on September 8, 1944, by Dr. Manuel Callo Zevallos, assisted by Drs. Sergio Quevedo and Carlos Aragón Saravia. The most detailed report of this surgery appeared the following day in Cuzco's daily newspaper *El Sol*, in a story entitled "Una soprendente trepanación del cráneo realizada en el Hospital de Belén utilizando, únicamente, instrumental incaico suministrado por el Museo local" (A surpising trepanation of the skull performed in the Hospital of Belén using exclusively Inca instruments supplied by the local Museum). A shorter report in English was published subsequently in *El Palacio* (Anónimo 1945). The full text of the *El Sol* article can be found in volume one of Juan Lastres's *Historia de la medicina peruana* (1951:194–195) and in Graña's publication (Graña et al. 1954:45–46), which also includes what is apparently the only published photograph of the procedure (Graña et al. 1954:fig. 27). The most detailed account of the surgery and the events leading up to it did not appear until more than twenty-five years later in a lengthy article by Sergio Quevedo (Quevedo 1970). The following account is drawn largely from this source.

Prior to the surgery, Quevedo performed experiments on cadavers with Inca tools lent to him by the director of the Museo Arqueológico de la Universidad Nacional San Antonio de Abad. These experiments proved useful in testing the tools' utility in making cranial openings. Quevedo found that the crescent-shaped tumi knife, frequently claimed to be the principal tool the Incas used to trepan, was of no use in cutting through bone, although it was effective for incising the scalp and scraping away the periosteum. Quevedo experimented with other tools, including a small chisel-like bronze tool (*cincel*) that he struck with a small metal bar. Unfortunately, he found that the cincel tended to slide and bounce off the smooth surface of the skull vault rather than cut into the bone. After some reflection he came up with a simple solution: he used an obsidian knife to score the bone, creating a groove that allowed the chisel to be gently hammered without bouncing or sliding. He found this to be the most satisfactory way of cutting a piece of bone out of the skull.

Having tested his tools, Quevedo was now ready to do the experiment on a living patient. An opportunity soon presented itself in the form of a twenty-two-year-old woman, a native of Calca who had been struck on the head by a falling tree. She had not received medical treatment at the time of the accident, and although she had no obvious neurological deficit, she suffered from occasional convulsions. It was decided that a craniotomy was appropriate. The surgical team was assembled, and tools from the archaeology museum were brought to the hospital and sterilized. After preparing the patient, local anesthesia was applied by injection of the scalp. A rubber tube was wrapped tightly around the head to control bleeding. The principal surgeon, Dr. Callo, informed the patient of the special nature of this surgical procedure and assured her that a complete set of modern surgical tools had been assembled and would be employed in case any problem arose, no matter how "small" (Quevedo 1970:59). Using the tumi, obsidian knife, and chisel, a piece of bone was removed and the borders of the opening were smoothed. A thin piece of sterilized plastic was placed over the opening and the scalp retracted and sutured with an Inca bronze needle. According to the report in *El Sol*, the operation was completed in fifty-five minutes and was followed by a good postoperative recovery.

Unfortunately, although it did not receive notice in the press, the patient's long-term recovery was not the success that had been hoped for. According to Quevedo (1970:69–70), several days after surgery she suffered convulsions and a developed a high fever. Despite treatment with medications available at the time, she died of pneumonia. The initial enthusiasm surrounding this medical experiment was short-lived. Would the outcome have been different had modern surgical tools been used? One can only speculate at this point, but no further surgical experiments with Inca tools were done, at least not in Cuzco.

Surprisingly, even though they knew of this first experiment and of the loss of the patient to postoperative complications, a second group of surgeons performed a nearly identical procedure in a Lima hospital nine years later.

The 1953 Surgery in Lima

On September 10, 1953, surgeons Francisco Graña and Esteban Rocca performed a craniotomy in a Lima hospital using ancient stone and metal tools loaned by the Museo de Antropología, Arqueología, y Historia del Perú. Like Quevedo, the surgeons had practiced with the tools previously on cadavers, assuring themselves that they could use them to make openings into the skull. They experimented first with obsidian knives, finding that they did not function well as drills (obsidian being brittle), but that bifacially chipped obsidian knives easily made linear cuts that allowed for the removal of a rectangular piece of bone. In a second experiment on a cadaver they decided to use only metal tools, cutting the scalp with a tumi knife and then using a chisel and bronze bar (in the same manner as the Cuzco surgery) to cut out a circular piece of bone. In a third experiment, the chisel and bar were used to cut out an oval piece of bone. Satisfied that they had mastered the technique, they chose a patient for the experiment: a young adult male who had suffered a blow to the left side of the head that had produced a subdural hematoma.

The surgery was done under general anesthesia. As in the Cuzco case, a rubber tube was tied firmly around the head to control bleeding. An incision was made in the scalp with a tumi knife, and the chisel and bar were used to cut out a circular piece of bone. The dura, when exposed, showed a bluish color marking the location of the subdural hematoma. The dura was cut with the chisel and the blood aspirated. Suturing and treating of the wound was then performed using standard surgical methods and materials. According to the surgeons, the patient made a full recovery (Graña et al. 1954:263–286).

The Cuzco and Lima surgical experiments, while publicized as "successful," were controversial. The first patient died shortly after her surgery, and details of the postoperative life of the second patient were not reported. It is not clear from published accounts whether either patient gave formal consent for these experiments, or how aware they were of what was being done to them. Most surprising, perhaps, is that these trepanation experiments were done twice, using nearly identical tools and procedures.

Self-Trepanation

> You fancy getting the trepanning done?
> —John Lennon, to Paul and Linda McCartney
> 1986 interview of McCartney in
> *Musician* magazine (Colton 1998)

Reports of self-trepanation—intentionally drilling a hole in one's own skull—first appeared in the 1960s. These were not experiments using archaeological tools, nor were they attempts to replicate ancient surgical techniques. The preferred tools were electric drills of various types; none were specifically designed for cranial surgery. The objective of the procedure was to make a small opening in the skull that was believed to increase blood circulation to the brain and enhance consciousness.

The recognized founder of the self-trepanation movement is Bart Hughes, who as a medical student at Amsterdam University experimented with various means of enhancing consciousness. At some point, Hughes became convinced that consciousness was influenced by the volume of blood in the brain, a phenomenon he called "brainblood-volume." Reasoning that the upright posture of humans was starving the brain of blood, compounded by the fact that the adult braincase was effectively a sealed box, Hughes hypothesized that creating an opening in the cranium would increase blood flow to the brain and, as a result, enhance consciousness (Colton 1998). In 1965, he tested his hypothesis by drilling a small hole through his frontal bone. Hughes reported that the operation lasted about forty-five minutes, although the cleanup of his apartment walls and ceiling took much longer (Turner 2007). Convinced that trepanation had improved his state of mind, Hughes began promoting the idea and soon attracted disciples who wanted to have their skulls drilled as well. Because the medical community did not consider "elective" trepanation a justifiable surgical procedure, self-trepanning was the simplest option. In 1966, a friend and disciple of Hughes, Joseph Mellen, attempted to trepan himself with an antique hand trephine, but without success. He later succeeded using an electric drill, assisted by Amanda Feilding, who in 1970 would trepan her own skull with an dental drill. Bart Hughes was photographed trepanning himself (Turner 2007), but Amanda Feilding went a step further and produced a film of her operation, called *Heartbeat in the Brain*, excerpts of which were included in a documentary program *A Hole in the Head*, produced by Mad Dog Films for The Learning Channel in 1998.

In 1972, Peter Halvorson, an American traveling in Holland, was inspired by Bart Hughes and trepanned himself as well. Hughes would gradually withdraw from the public spotlight, apparently tired of giving interviews, but both Amanda Feilding and Peter Halvorson worked to promote trepanation as a means of achieving enhanced consciousness. Through the Beckley Foundation in England, which she founded in 1998, Feilding continues to support drug policy reform and medical research on consciousness and brain function. Included in her foundation's research agenda is investigation into the benefits of trepanation for cerebral circulation (Beckley Foundation 2010).

In 1998, Peter Halvorson founded the International Trepanation Advocacy Group (ITAG), which promotes trepanation in a more direct way. In 2000, ITAG sought out volunteers for elective trepanations and contracted with a medical facility in Mexico to perform the procedures. According to ITAG's website, fifteen volunteers were trepanned and then examined by magnetic resonance imaging to test for changes in blood flow following the procedure. The results were inconclusive, and the experiment was discontinued. Nevertheless, ITAG continues to promote trepanation, and has collaborated with the Beckley Foundation on clinical research exploring the effects of craniotomy on blood and cerebrospinal fluid circulation (Moskalenko 2009; Moskalenko et al. 2008).

Not surprisingly, the international medical community views elective trepanation with great skepticism and is particularly concerned about the dangers involved in self-trepanation (Gump 2010). Despite such warnings, an internet search for "trepanation" will be rewarded with a number of self-trepanation testimonials, often illustrated with photographs. Fortunately, there have been relatively few reported cases of individuals incurring serious health risks by attempting to trepan themselves (Wadley et al. 1997). Neither the Beckley Foundation nor ITAG recommend self-trepanation, given the obvious risks involved with drilling into one's own skull. But there have been some lapses. In 2001, Peter Halvorson pled guilty to practicing medicine without a license after being filmed on a television news show operating on a woman with a hand trephine. The judge in the case sentenced Halvorson to three years' probation and a five hundred dollar fine, and ordered that he undergo a psychiatric evaluation (Associated Press 2001).

Although the efforts of Bart Hughes, Amanda Feilding, and Peter Halvorson have yet to produce a large following, they are sincere in their belief that trepanation is a route to increased consciousness, clarity of thinking, and happiness. I had the opportunity at a trepanation conference in April 2000 to dine with Amanda and her husband, Lord Jamie Neidpath (both trepanned), and Amanda and I have continued to correspond since. At our dinner and since that time she has expressed the hope that I can find evidence in ancient Peruvian skulls of trepanation undertaken to enhance consciousness. I told her that, unfortunately, determining such motives from dry skulls alone would be most difficult, and that the only reason for trepanning that I had been able to infer from bone evidence was the treatment of skull fractures. As indicated above, ethnographic accounts of traditional surgeons in the South Pacific and in East and North Africa are consistent in reporting that trepanation was and is done for practical medical reasons. Whether modern trepanning produces positive changes in mood and consciousness is a personal matter perhaps best left to those who have experienced such changes.

9 ANCIENT TREPANATION FROM THE PERSPECTIVE OF MODERN NEUROSURGERY

DAVID KUSHNER and
ANNE R. TITELBAUM[1]

FROM THE PERSPECTIVE OF MODERN NEUROSURGERY, THE SUCCESS OF prehistoric trepanation in Peru is impressive, considering the potential risks of cranial surgery and the many possible postsurgical and perioperative complications related to brain injury and other medical conditions. As noted elsewhere in this volume, the precise reasons for prehistoric surgeries remain unclear, although there does appear to be an association of trepanation with evidence of cranial trauma. It seems plausible that traumatic brain injury was the primary reason for most trepanations and was probably the main reason that this procedure was developed. However, trepanation was also performed on individuals whose skulls show no clear evidence of trauma, suggesting that the procedure was also performed for other reasons.

In a modern clinical setting, traumatic brain injury is a leading reason for neurosurgical intervention. Other conditions that necessitate cranial surgery include those that involve significant brain swelling, such as large ischemic strokes or disorders that result in intracranial mass lesions like brain tumors or abscesses. The modern neurosurgical interventions that are most closely related to trepanations include craniotomy, decompressive craniectomy, and burr-hole procedures. Each of these interventions carries risk of intraoperative and postoperative complications that may include infection and mortality even with all the advantages of modern medicine.

Modern neurosurgery transitioned into a distinct profession during the first quarter of the twentieth century, following the important developments of an understanding of cerebral localization, antiseptic and aseptic techniques, improvements in anesthesia, and technological advances such as diagnostic imagery (for a comprehensive history, see Greenblatt et al. 1997). Since its inception as a profession, neurosurgical research has continued to hone the understanding of brain anatomy, physiology, and internal medicine, while also improving surgical outcomes through better surgical tools, techniques,

1 The authors are grateful to Dr. Robert Quencer, M.D., professor and chair of the department of radiology, and Dr. Jose Romano, M.D., professor of neurology, both of the University of Miami Miller School of Medicine, for providing the CT scans used to illustrate this chapter.

preoperative considerations, general anesthesia, intraoperative monitoring of vital functions, postoperative monitoring, skilled nursing, intensive care, intracranial pressure monitoring, mechanical ventilation, antibiotics and pharmaceuticals, neuroimaging, delivery of fluids and nutrition, knowledge of possible postsurgical complications, and the availability and strategy of inpatient and outpatient rehabilitation. The aim of this chapter is to examine the similarities and the many differences of trepanation and modern neurosurgery, which ultimately underscore the astonishing success of this procedure in prehistoric Peru.

REASONS FOR TREPANATION AND DECOMPRESSIVE NEUROSURGERY/PATHOPHYSIOLOGY

Emergency alleviation of pressure on the brain caused by potentially life-threatening and quality-of-life-threatening intracranial mass lesions was probably the primary reason for trepanation in ancient Peru, as well as being the reason for many modern neurosurgical procedures today. Enlarging intracranial mass lesions, such as tumors, abscesses, and fluid collections like hematomas, put increasing pressure on the brain, which exists in a finitely limited space within the confines of the skull. The tight intracranial space provides little room to accommodate abnormal lesions along with the normal brain anatomy. As a mass lesion expands within the intracranial space; it causes a rise in intracranial pressure that in turn puts pressure on the brain, leading to brain dysfunction that may manifest clinically with a progression of symptoms, variably including headaches, dizziness, confusion, weakness or paralysis, numbness, imbalance or incoordination, vision impairment, seizures, and loss of consciousness or coma.

Clinical deterioration from a mass lesion in the form of worsening of symptoms may occur acutely over minutes to hours, less rapidly over days to weeks, or slowly over months to years. In general, the brain swelling and intracranial bleeding that occurs in moderate to severe brain trauma will result in a rapid clinical deterioration from mass effect (the increasing pressure produced by progressively enlarging lesions) that will require emergency neurosurgical decompression interventions to prevent permanent loss of functional independence or death. Likewise, the massive brain swelling or bleeding that occurs with certain types of stroke may require emergency decompression interventions. In contrast, slowly expanding mass lesions, such as tumors or abscesses, may manifest with slowly worsening symptoms. Unchecked, mass effect can result in various brain herniation syndromes, which in turn are likely to result in permanent, severe neurological impairments or death.

Brain herniation syndrome, a cause of coma and considered a neurosurgical emergency, occurs when rising intracranial pressure from bleeding, brain swelling, or other mass lesions forces parts of the brain to be squeezed through constricted abnormal locations within or outside of the skull. Injuries involving the cerebrum are known as supratentorial lesions, as these occur above the tentorium cerebelli. There are three possible supratentorial herniation syndromes: cingulate, central, and uncal herniation. Cingulate herniation occurs when a focal mass effect shifts a brain hemisphere across the intracranial midline by pushing the cingulate gyrus under the falx cerebri. Cingulate herniation can result in secondary strokes to portions of the frontal lobe supplied by compromised anterior cerebral arteries (Figure 9.1). Central herniation occurs when diffuse supratentorial pressure on both brain hemispheres forces the diencephalon and adjacent midbrain downward through the tentorial notch. Central herniation often results in secondary injury to the thalamus and midbrain (Figure 9.2). Uncal herniation occurs when mass effect on a temporal lobe forces the uncus and hippocampal gyrus through the tentorium, compressing the midbrain and posterior cerebral artery and potentially resulting in secondary strokes in the occipital lobe.

Injuries occurring in the posterior fossa beneath the tentorium cerebelli involve the cerebellum and are known as subtentorial lesions. There are two herniation syndromes that may occur in this part of the brain: upward transtentorial or downward cerebellar herniation. Upward transtentorial herniation happens when the pressure from a posterior fossa mass lesion forces parts of the cerebellum or midbrain upward through the tentorial notch. Upward herniation causes secondary injury to parts of the cerebellum and midbrain

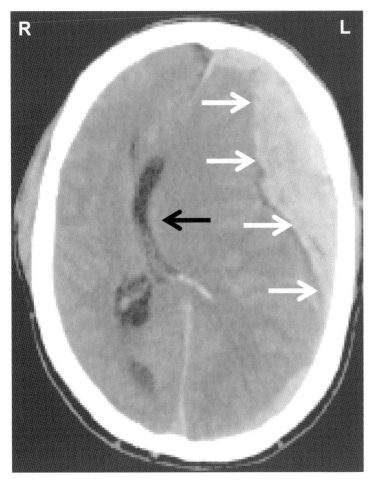

Figure 9.1
Transverse CT scan of a right hemisphere epidural hemorrhage. White arrows mark the dural edge. The black arrow indicates the direction of cingulate brain herniation across the midline due to mass effect. Image courtesy of the University of Miami Miller School of Medicine.

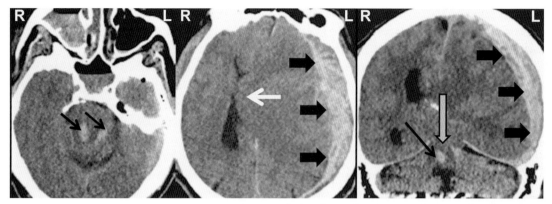

Figure 9.2 Two transverse CT scans (left and center) and a coronal CT scan (right) showing a subdural hemorrhage compressing the left cerebral hemisphere, indicated by thick black arrows. The white arrow marks a cingulate herniation with midline shift. The gray arrow marks central herniation mass effect on the brainstem. Thin black arrows point to areas of brain stem bleeding from herniation. Images courtesy of the University of Miami Miller School of Medicine.

while also causing hydrocephalus by blocking the flow of cerebrospinal fluid, further exacerbating a rise in intracranial pressure. Lastly, downward herniation of parts of the cerebellum through the foramen magnum may also occur with pressure from posterior fossa lesions. Herniation of the cerebellum will compress the medulla and upper cervical spinal cord, and is often fatal.

Emergency decompressive neurosurgical interventions, including burr-hole, craniotomy, and craniectomy procedures, are done to prevent or reverse the potentially devastating complications of brain herniation syndromes. Burr holes are small openings that are drilled into the skull usually for the purpose of draining localized epidural, subdural, or cerebrospinal fluid, or for the placement of catheters to measure intracranial pressure. A craniotomy is a large opening that is temporarily made in the skull usually with the objective of removing large mass lesions. A craniotomy surgery concludes with the skull flap being fixed back in place with the use of hardware that may include screws and clips to hold the bone in place, with the overlying scalp then closed over it (Figure 9.3). A craniectomy is a very large opening that is made in the skull either unilaterally or bilaterally (over both brain hemispheres) to accommodate massive cerebral swelling that may be caused by trauma or certain types of stroke. A craniectomy operation ends with the skull flap removed and the dura and scalp closed over the surgical area (Figure 9.4).

The Peruvian trepanations discussed in great detail in other chapters of this book varied in size and location in a way similar to modern emergency decompressive neurosurgical interventions. The concept that intracranial bleeding, brain swelling, and pressure within the skull are potentially dangerous was apparently understood by the ancient Peruvians who successfully performed trepanations, as demonstrated by the long-term survival rates. Today, we further understand that a complicated pathophysiological cascade of events may gradually unfold with rising intracranial pressure, in which normal

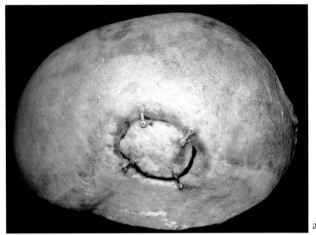

a

Figure 9.3
(a) Modern craniotomy on the left parietal of an older adult male, with hardware securing the bone plug in position. Hole: 39 × 38 mm; plug: 36.5 × 28 mm. (b) Detail showing healing of the surrounding bone. (c) Endocranial view showing its position relative to the grooves of the middle meningeal vessels. Photographs by Anne R. Titelbaum.

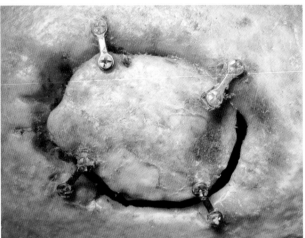

b

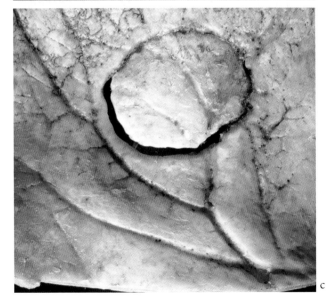

c

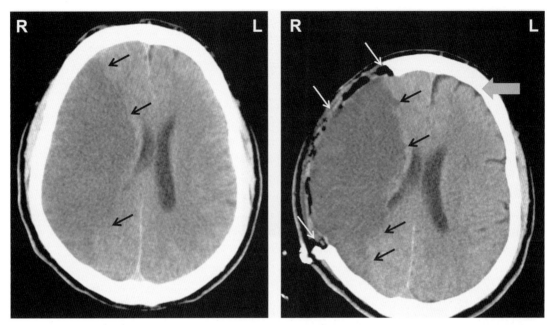

Figure 9.4 Transverse CT scans showing a significant edema, demarcated by small black arrows, due to ischemic stroke causing mass effect with midline shift (left), and the same patient following a frontal-temporal-parietal craniectomy, indicated by white arrows (right). The gray arrow points to the skull, which appears white (note the absence of bone in the area of craniectomy). This postcraniectomy image shows interval resolution of the mass effect/midline shift that was relieved by the craniectomy. Images courtesy of the University of Miami Miller School of Medicine.

blood flow to the brain, known as cerebral perfusion pressure, may become compromised, resulting in impaired oxygen and nutrient delivery to brain tissue. This blockage causes secondary brain injury, further brain swelling, and a potentially devastating uncontrollable rise in intracranial pressure that warrants a decompressive surgical intervention.

HEAD TRAUMA, TREPANATION, AND MODERN NEUROSURGERY

Relevant clinical aspects of head trauma deserve attention, as there appears to be an association of head trauma with many of the trepanations performed in ancient Peru. As previously mentioned, head trauma is also a leading reason for modern decompressive neurosurgical interventions. Blunt trauma and penetrating head injury resulting from accidents or interpersonal violence were the likely causes of prehistoric head trauma necessitating trepanations. The etiologies of modern head trauma include warfare, violence, and accidents involving motor vehicles, bicycles, pedestrians, construction, and sports. Modern penetrating trauma may result from various weapons, including bullets and shrapnel from battlefield blast injuries.

Pathologic features of head trauma that often warrant modern neurosurgical interventions and that were likely reasons for historic trepanations include skull fractures, brain contusions and swelling, intracranial bleeding, and all forms of penetrating injury. Skull fractures may result in "open" or "closed" head trauma. Any skull fracture that results in a communication between the intracranial space and the outside air constitutes an open head injury and requires neurosurgical attention (Kushner 1998). Open head trauma occurs with depressed fractures, skull fractures that are linear with overlying scalp lacerations, and those injuries that involve the potential for dural tears, including fractures of the frontal bone and other regions of the cranial vault. In closed head trauma, there is no potential for contact between the intracranial space and the environment outside the skull. Any skull fracture, open or closed, may have underlying associated pathology, such as brain contusions or bleeds. Contusions, areas of bruising, bleeding, or swelling that occur on the surface of the brain, are usually the result of blunt impacts. Symptoms of contusions vary with the location on the brain and may variably include confusion, loss of consciousness, weakness, numbness, imbalance and incoordination, and impairments of vision and perception. Large or multiple contusions can be a source of significant swelling and mass effect. Symptoms from contusions underlying skull fractures may have prompted trepanation in the past. It is quite possible that multiple trepanations for multiple contusions at various locations may have been effective in reducing dangerously elevated intracranial pressure and mass effect.

Epidural hemorrhage is a life-threatening neurosurgical emergency that frequently occurs with temporal bone fractures that tear the middle meningeal artery or vein. Other causes may include injury to dural venous sinuses or to other blood vessels. This bleeding happens between the skull and the dura mater. The large hematomas resulting from these bleeds will result in brain herniation syndromes if untreated. Emergency trepanations could have allowed for drainage and decompression of these hematomas.

Subdural hemorrhage is bleeding that occurs beneath the dura mater and usually superficial to the arachnoid mater. Such hemorrhage may be due to the tearing of bridging veins or a ruptured dural venous sinus. This type of bleeding may be rapid or slow, and is often self-limited, but may be a significant source of mass effect from the resultant hematomas or blood clots. It is conceivable that trepanations may have allowed for decompression of these bleeds either directly through lacerated dural membranes beneath depressed skull fractures, or through openings that may have been intentionally made through dura mater.

Subarachnoid hemorrhage involves bleeding into the cerebrospinal fluid-filled spaces of the brain from small blood vessels injured by trauma. Symptoms of isolated subarachnoid bleeds might include headache and confusion. In some cases, blockage of the normal flow of cerebrospinal fluid by this type of bleeding could lead to hydrocephalus, which would result in urinary incontinence and gradual worsening of gait and cognition (see below). It is unlikely that trepanations would have been useful in treating this type of bleeding due to its deep location; however, in many cases a small subarachnoid hemorrhage would be self-limiting and self-healing. Nevertheless, subarachnoid bleeding is often associated with other pathologic manifestations of trauma that may have benefited from trepanation.

Penetrating trauma may occur from different types of weapons that perforate the skull and enter the brain to various depths, usually along a linear trajectory. This form of injury causes damage to brain and vascular structures through the pathway of the perforation. Signs and symptoms will vary, depending on the injured anatomy. Also, in some cases debris from the scalp, skull, or the weapon may become lodged in the brain. Presumably, trepanation procedures may have had some success with shallow penetrating injuries, particularly for debriding foreign fragments and for decompression of the swollen brain.

Intraparenchymal hemorrhage describes bleeding and blood clot accumulation within the substance of the brain. This form of hemorrhage may occur with torn vasculature from violent trauma or from the accumulation of blood from multiple nearby areas of brain contusions. This type of bleeding is also a potential source of dangerous mass effect that requires neurosurgical attention. It is not likely that trepanation procedures would have been able to access these lesions, but trepanations may have allowed for indirect alleviation of mass effect that may have improved the possibility for at least short-term survival.

POTENTIAL COMPLICATIONS OF HEAD TRAUMA AFFECTING SURVIVAL

Long- and short-term survival after trepanation would have been affected by postsurgical complications that are still a concern today. Possible complications include infection; seizures; hydrocephalus; metabolic, physical, cognitive, emotional, or behavioral problems; and problems directly related to the neurosurgical procedure.

There are several concerns that involve the actual surgeries. First and foremost, there are some injuries that are so severe that they compromise survival despite the best surgical efforts. In some cases the timing of surgery may also affect survival, particularly if initiated too late. Some of the trepanations with no signs of bone healing may have been performed too late or been done on subjects with brain trauma so severe as to preclude survival. Additional problems include undetected perforations through the dura mater and underlying membranes that could lead to meningitis or cerebrospinal fluid leaks. Accumulation of cerebrospinal fluid beneath the dura may result in a subdural hygroma, which can cause mass effect and poor recovery. Also, recovery and survival after modern craniectomies and large trepanations may be affected by the worsening of underlying hemorrhages and contusions, development of bleeding in the opposite hemisphere, herniation of the brain through the open skull defect, and development of hydrocephalus or seizures.

Postsurgical infection continues to be a problem after neurosurgery despite the availability of numerous oral and intravenous antibiotics. The most common infections after neurosurgical procedures are pneumonia and infection of the surgical wound, which could lead to meningitis, encephalitis, subdural empyema (pus collection), or a brain abscess, all of which would probably be fatal following trepanation. Seizures commonly complicate recovery after severe brain injuries, especially in the aftermath of contusions, intracranial bleeding, or depressed skull fractures. Penetrating head trauma places individuals at a high risk for developing posttraumatic epilepsy. An investigation of veterans with penetrating head trauma found that more than 50 percent of Vietnam veterans developed epilepsy, while more than 30 percent of Iran and Iraq veterans developed an ongoing seizure disorder (Orman et al. 2012). While the reasons for the lower rate of seizures in the latter group are unclear, it may be due to advances in the treatment of brain trauma. While there are many modern anticonvulsant medications to control seizure disorders, it is unknown if seizures could have been treated following trepanation in ancient Peru. Uncontrolled seizures can have life-threatening consequences.

As noted above, hydrocephalus occurs when there is an obstruction of the normal flow of cerebrospinal fluid through the brain's ventricular system within the subarachnoid space. Posttraumatic intraventricular blood is a common cause of obstruction. Rising intracranial pressure from the expanding volume of fluid within the blocked ventricles can result in a decline in physical and cognitive functions. Obstructive hydrocephalus is easily treated by neurosurgeons with a ventricle-to-peritoneal shunt procedure that allows for the decompression of excess ventricular fluid. Left untreated, obstructive hydrocephalus can cause a steady rise in intracranial pressure that can provoke a brain herniation syndrome, which may have been another reason for short-term survival following some ancient trepanations.

There are also myriad postsurgical metabolic concerns involving the maintenance of normal homeostasis, such as proper nutrition and hydration. Swallowing is often impaired among brain injury patients, increasing the risk of aspirating foods and liquids that can cause a life-threatening pneumonia infection. Tube feedings and intravenous hydration are used today for patients with this impairment until there is a documented return of normal swallowing ability by specific tests. Dehydration, malnutrition, and aspiration pneumonia could have occurred in Peru after trepanations in individuals with moderate to severe impairments of swallowing function, resulting in only short-term survival.

Further metabolic concerns for individuals with moderate to severe brain trauma include disorders of sodium regulation. These disorders occur from mass effect injury to the hypothalamus, which plays a role in salt homeostasis. Dangerously low blood sodium levels will result in severe seizures and death if untreated with intravenous saline. On the other hand, critically elevated blood salt levels occur with the inadequate secretion of an antidiuretic hormone, which may lead to fatal dehydration and unquenchable thirst when untreated. These posttraumatic problems of salt regulation could have also contributed to some of the short-term mortalities after trepanation.

There are several important concerns that relate to posttraumatic physical impairments that may threaten survival following head trauma. Immobility, which may be caused by paralysis, weakness, or coma, puts patients at risk for the development of blood clots, pneumonia, and pressure sores. Blood clots may enter the pulmonary circulation and lead to a fatal embolism that blocks the oxygenation of red blood cells. Prevention for pulmonary embolism involves the regular use of anticoagulant medications in immobile patients, which decreases but does not fully eliminate the risk. Pneumonia may arise due to weakness in coughing and prolonged recumbency. Respiratory therapies that include aerosolized medications help to reduce the incidence of this complication. Pressure sores are areas of injured skin that result from remaining in one position too long. Such sores could lead to life-threatening sepsis (blood infections). Care strategies involving the frequent turning and repositioning of patients who are unable to move reduce the risk of bed sores, and the administration of medication may help these wounds to heal. Following trepanation, immobility would have been a significant risk for short-term survival due to pulmonary embolism, pneumonia, and infected bed sores.

Cognitive deficits from brain injury could include coma or various impairments of perception, communication, thought processes, and memory. Coma would result in immobility and short-term survival due to the aforementioned complications. In ancient Peru, coma would have likely resulted in only short-term survival due to the inability to deliver nutrition and hydration. Disorders of perception, thought processes, and memory could result in ambulatory patients wandering off, getting lost, falling, and ending up in dangerous predicaments that could lead to secondary injuries. The risk of falls, injury, and death would be significant in highland Peru due to the steep and irregular topography (Titelbaum et al. 2013). Similarly, impairments of communication that commonly occur in association with trauma affecting the left temporal lobe may prevent a patient from being able to properly express important needs. It is likely that some of these cognitive and communication impairments could have affected survival after trepanation.

Emotional and behavioral problems frequently occur after moderate to severe brain injuries. Depression can be a direct result of injury to the brain or an emotional response to pain or traumatic injuries and related loss of function (Kushner 1998). Poor motivation, loss of appetite, and suicidal ideation from depression can impact survival and recovery, as can posttraumatic restlessness, anxiety, agitation, and aggressive behavior. Today, antidepressants, anxiolytic, and antipsychotic medications are commonly used to control these symptoms and promote recovery. Posttraumatic emotional and behavioral issues may have also impaired recovery and survival after trepanation.

Headache, the most common symptom resulting from head trauma, may be the product of a posttraumatic migraine disorder, exacerbation of a preexisting headache disorder, referred pain from associated neck or cervical spine injuries, pain associated with inner ear and vascular injuries, pneumocephalus or cerebrospinal leaks from skull fractures, or chronic subdural fluid collections, some of which may be life-threatening (Kushner 1998). Frequent moderate to severe posttraumatic headaches may indicate the possibility of intracranial pathology and interfere with the performance of routine daily activities and community responsibilities, which would be problematic in both modern and prehistoric times. It is therefore conceivable that posttraumatic headache may have been a reason for some of the trepanations (see Chapter 8). It is possible that trepanners realized the potential for associated intracranial pathology or the disabling consequences of frequent severe headaches. Today, the possibility of clinical problems, such as disability resulting from posttraumatic headaches, are well known, and it is therefore important that physicians identify the specific cause of posttraumatic headaches and administer the appropriate treatment. Untreated or improperly treated posttraumatic headaches can lead to disabling consequences.

In the modern clinical setting, rehabilitation medicine provides a holistic approach to recovery after brain trauma. The goals of rehabilitation include the prevention and treatment of secondary complications, the improvement of physical function, the provision of compensatory strategies for persistent disabilities, and the reintegration into the community (Kushner 2010). Rehabilitation begins for head injury patients during the acute care hospitalization and continues afterward in inpatient and outpatient programs that involve an interdisciplinary team comprised of physicians, nurses, specialized therapists, and usually a case manager. Physical medicine and rehabilitation treatments target physical, cognitive, behavioral, emotional, occupational, communication, and swallowing disorders. The success of modern neurosurgery in terms of long-term survival and good functional outcomes is partly due to the availability of contemporary rehabilitation. It is likely that in ancient Peru, without extensive postoperative care, recovery time would have been slowed, which would have affected survival and outcomes following trepanation.

REASONS FOR TREPANATION AND MODERN CRANIAL NEUROSURGERY OTHER THAN HEAD INJURY

As noted, trepanation has been observed among crania that show no clear evidence of trauma, suggesting that the procedure was performed for reasons other than head injury. Severe, frequent, and disabling headaches not related to previous trauma may also have been a reason for some of the trepanations (see Chapter 8). Globally, 1.7–4 percent of the world's adult population has headaches on fifteen or more days every month (World Health Organization 2012). Primary headache disorders are headaches that are not due to intracranial mass lesions or other macropathology, and they account for the majority of headaches worldwide. Migraine is the most common primary headache disorder and a significant cause of disability worldwide in terms of days lost from work (World Health Organization 2012). As the prevalence of migraine is highest among women aged eighteen to forty-four, it is perhaps not surprising that head pain accounts for the third leading cause of emergency department visits among this demographic (Smitherman et al. 2013). While today there are many pharmacologic and other nonsurgical treatment options for primary headache disorders that help to prevent disability, in prehistory trepanation may have been an attempt to cure disabling primary headache disorders.

Headaches unrelated to trauma may also be a symptom of intracranial macropathology, such as mass lesions or intracranial bleeding from such causes as aneurysms or arterial-venous malformations. Usually headaches that are caused by intracranial macropathology are also accompanied by other symptoms and signs of the pathologic lesion, such as weakness, numbness, imbalance, incoordination, confusion, or impairment of vision. The associated symptoms and signs alert modern physicians to the likelihood of potentially life-threatening causes for headaches. Thus, it is also conceivable that some ancient Peruvian trepanations might have been performed to treat suspected intracranial macropathology that presented as headaches in association with other symptoms. Patients with brain tumors, abscesses, fluid collections, and certain types of strokes may benefit from modern decompressive interventions. In prehistory, it is possible that individuals with extradural or subdural pathology may have had the best outcomes following trepanation, due to the more shallow location of the lesions beneath the skull.

Survival after trepanations not related to trauma would have been affected by the timing of surgery, characteristics of the pathologic lesion, as well as many of the same potential postsurgical complications described earlier. Outcomes after modern decompressive neurosurgical procedures are affected by these same factors, but in the clinical setting there is the advantage of contemporary medicine and postsurgical rehabilitation.

COMPARISON OF TOOLS AND TECHNIQUES

The creation of a burr hole in the skull is common to the start of many prehistoric trepanations and most modern, cranial neurosurgical procedures as well. The size of modern cranial neurosurgeries varies—from simple burr holes to craniotomies, to craniectomies. Described previously, the burr hole is basically a round and usually small opening that is drilled into the skull for various purposes. Craniotomies target a larger area of the skull and may involve a region overlying multiple portions of the brain. Craniectomies involve removing most of the cranial vault unilaterally or bilaterally, depending on the reasons for the procedure. Similar to these modern procedures, trepanations varied in size in ancient Peru, from small and focal to some that were very large. Some of the largest trepanations, seen on the south coast of Peru, are proportionally comparable in size to modern craniectomies (see Chapter 5).

Noted elsewhere in this book, the methods for prehistoric trepanations include scraping, circular grooving, linear cutting, and drilling and cutting. Whereas scraping involved the progressive removal of the outer and inner tables of the skull, circular grooving and linear cutting involved incising an outline (circular, rectangular, or triangular) with the goal of removing the central plug of bone. The drilling and cutting technique involved drilling a series of holes through the skull and then cutting through the residual bone to remove the central plug. Linear incising and drilling and cutting techniques were used less frequently than the other methods, and apparently with less success, possibly due to the increased risk of perforating the dura mater.

Skull-based neurosurgery involves the initial creation of a single or multiple burr holes through the skull, which are used for drainage of underlying fluid collections (e.g., hematomas), for placement of catheters to measure intracranial pressure, or for diverting cerebrospinal fluid in cases of hydrocephalus. Also, similar to the prehistoric drilling and cutting technique, in contemporary neurosurgery multiple burr holes may be drilled to outline points along a planned craniotomy or craniectomy, which are then connected by cutting so that a large portion of skull may be removed in a craniectomy, or removed and then replaced in the case of a craniotomy. In contrast to the prehistoric drilling and cutting method, the modern method is rapid and accurate, thanks to consistently updated technology.

Tools and techniques used in ancient Peru seem to have gradually evolved over time, just as the surgical instruments and strategies of modern neurosurgery have continued to advance. The early cutting and scraping tools were most likely bifacial obsidian points and knives like those found at the Paracas burial sites still hafted to wooden handles (see Chapter 5). Trepanations done in the central highlands of Peru during the period from AD 1000 to 1400 seemed to experiment with various methods of trepanation while continuing to use sharp stone tools for linear cutting, circular grooving, scraping, and drilling and cutting (see Chapter 4). Trepanation during the time of the Inca in the southern highlands of Peru, from the mid-1400s to the mid-1500s, seems to have predominantly involved the circular or oval grooving method and a higher frequency of multiple surgeries, which may have been determined to have the best outcome (see Chapter 7). Similarly, the evolution of modern neurosurgery has occurred as a result of experimentation with various techniques and methods to determine which procedures have the best outcomes in terms of survival and quality of life.

COMPARISON OF OUTCOMES AND SUCCESS RATES

The success of modern neurosurgery in terms of survival and improvement in quality of life for patients has steadily improved since its inception as a distinct surgical specialty during the first quarter of the twentieth century. Ongoing improvements in contemporary cranial surgical outcomes have followed continued developments in the understanding of cerebral localization, progress in antiseptic and aseptic techniques, improvements in anesthesia, general medical management strategies, and pharmaceuticals, as well as technological advances involving surgical tools and diagnostic imagery. Similarly, owing to apparent experimentation with various methods and procedures, there seems to have been a steady improvement in long-term survival of trepanation patients in Peru from 400 BC to the time of the Inca.

Long-term survival rates for prehistoric trepanation are found to be almost 40 percent in Paracas and the south coast of Peru (400 to 200 BC; see Chapter 5), 55.6 percent in the central highlands (AD 1000–1400; see Chapter 4), and about 75 percent in the southern highlands around Cuzco during the time of the Inca (mid-1400s through the mid-1500s; see Chapter 7). But some of these long-term survival averages varied regionally within these three zones during each of the time periods. For example, within the southern highlands during the time of the Inca the long-term survival rate was only 50 percent at Acomayo, which is located about fifty kilometers southeast of Cuzco. Regional variation in long-term success rates may have been affected in part by the experience of the trepanners, just as modern neurosurgical success rates may be related to a surgeon's skill, training, and experience, or to patient clinical factors.

It is important to note that the success rates of the prehistoric Peruvian trepanations, and particularly those of the Inca, rival and exceed the outcomes of early head surgeries at the start of the twentieth century. Cranial neurosurgery at the end of the nineteenth century had average mortality rates of 30–50 percent, partly due to complications related to infection, uncontrolled intracranial pressure, and excessive intraoperative blood loss (Voorhees et al. 2005). Even Harvey Cushing, an academic leader and pioneer in early modern neurosurgery, had mortality rates of 48 percent for skull-based surgeries and 50 percent for brain abscesses during the period from 1896 to 1912 (Pendleton et al. 2014; Pendleton et al. 2012). One study that specifically reviewed Cushing's early neurosurgical outcomes for head trauma found a mortality rate of 80 percent within the first two weeks after surgery, leaving only 20 percent of the patients to survive long-term (Kinsman et al. 2013). It is also noteworthy that even with all the benefits of contemporary medicine, current mortality rates for craniotomies range from 3–17 percent for subarachnoid bleeds (Agency for Healthcare Research and Quality 2006) and from 2.5–5 percent for brain tumors (Long et al. 2003), and the thirty-day perioperative mortality rate from craniectomy for brain injury may be as high as 26.4 percent (Huang Yu-Ha et al. 2013). Patient factors such as age, comorbid medical conditions, and severity of the neurosurgical disease process may certainly predetermine the surgical outcome, especially in the case of emergencies. In sum, despite the lack of the advantages of modern medicine, and considering the many possible complications of cranial surgery, it is truly amazing how successful trepanation was in ancient Peru.

:::::

In summary, there are some striking similarities as well as many differences between trepanation and modern neurosurgery, which ultimately underscore the astonishing success of this procedure in ancient Peru. It seems plausible that the rationales for prehistoric surgeries were similar to the reasons for modern cranial procedures, which include head trauma and other causes of intracranial mass effect. Although the tools and techniques were different, the process of making a burr hole in the skull is a common starting point in most trepanations as well as many modern cranial surgeries. The obvious differences include the numerous advantages of modern medicine that improve the likelihood for survival and recovery while minimizing the risk for postoperative complications. Therefore, from the perspective of modern neurosurgery, the success of prehistoric trepanation in Peru in terms of long-term survival rates is impressive, considering the potential risks of cranial surgery and the many possible postsurgical and perioperative complications related to brain injury and other medical conditions.

10 RECOVERY FROM TRAUMATIC BRAIN INJURY IN PREHISTORIC PERU

J. MICHAEL WILLIAMS

ONE MAJOR PREMISE UNDERLYING THIS EXAMINATION OF CRANIAL trepanation in Pre-Columbian Peru is the understanding that most of the trepanations represent a treatment for traumatic head and brain injury. Peru is unique in that so many head injuries were sustained using blunt force weapons and then treated by trepanation. It is also clear that the majority of people who received trepanations recovered from the injury and subsequent surgical intervention, and even lived for years following the event (see Chapters 4–7). Many of these head injuries were likely sustained in warfare, and this suggests that many people would probably have been injured at once. One can imagine that following major battles the field of conflict would have been strewn with victims of head injuries, all of varying severity. These people would have been treated for their injuries and then cared for during weeks or months of recovery. Given the grievous nature of many of these wounds, the victims would not have survived without this care. The general purpose of this chapter is to describe the neurological, behavioral, and cognitive repercussions associated with traumatic head and brain injury, and to apply these observations to the situation of ancient Peru. Presumably, one result of observing and caring for these injuries was the creation of a craft of medicine that included the use of cranial trepanation.

One of the challenges of this investigation is that there are no historical records of these trepanations and only limited knowledge of medical care in Pre-Columbian Peru. All of these analyses represent an informed conjecture regarding the relationship of skulls with evidence of injury and trepanation and a model of traumatic brain injury derived from modern cases. The analysis will understandably suffer some degree of error and uncertainty in these conjectures. By carefully evaluating the osteological evidence and maintaining a conservative posture toward conclusions, it is hoped that the error in the inferences made here will be minimized.

THE MECHANICS OF TRAUMATIC HEAD AND BRAIN INJURIES

In our times, most traumatic head and brain injuries are closed head injuries sustained in automobile accidents (Thurman et al. 1999). In a closed head injury, the brain suffers trauma because of rapid movement within the skull. Most penetrating head injuries in modern times are the result of gunshot wounds. These are devastating, and most people who sustain a gunshot wound of the brain do not survive (Lewis 1976). Blunt force injuries in modern times, such as those caused by falls and objects striking the head, are probably similar to those sustained in Pre-Columbian Peru.

Virtually all of the head injuries and brain trauma sustained in Pre-Columbian Peru were caused by blunt force trauma. This included falls, injury by weapons, and falling objects striking the head. Combat injuries were primarily caused by clubs, sling stones, spears, and sharp-edged axes (Andrushko and Torres 2011; Verano and Finger 2010). The frequent use of stone weapons is an aspect of Peruvian warfare that cannot be understated. This was likely a major cause of the large number of blunt force head injuries and gave rise to an effective craft of treatment that included trepanation. Caring for a relatively large number of people with such incapacitating injuries may also have included methods of facilitating recovery and rehabilitation.

A blow to the head with a stone club involves a circumscribed application of mechanical force that is mostly absorbed by the skull. The magnitude of the force determines how the skull fractures. Minimal force produces a linear fracture across the impact area. More severe force produces a stellate fracture with linear fractures radiating outward from the center. Significant force produces a depressed fracture with triangular segments of bone breaking away and being forced below the skull's inner table. These usually cause laceration of the dura, other meninges, and brain tissue (Lewis 1976). Since a fracture indicates the absorption of considerable force by the skull, the presence of a break suggests that the brain itself has suffered a milder injury (Brooks et al. 1980). The force of the blow is absorbed by the skull and not communicated to the underlying brain tissue. Of course, this level of injury still represents the application of considerable force to the brain. The underlying principle is that the relative impact on the brain tissue will be less compared to the impact on the brain caused by a similar force that does not cause a fracture.

Some blood loss and hematoma are almost always associated with depressed skull fractures (Donovan 2005; Ganz and Arndt 2014; Miller and Jennett 1968). This varies with the location of fracture in relation to major arteries and veins. Severing an artery produces the most severe hematoma because blood is lost at arterial pressure. This produces an area of clotted blood and a mass effect that compresses the surrounding tissue. A major constraining structure is the dura. This thick, flexible layer of tissue that surrounds the brain has the resilience of a dense layer of plastic film. Hematomas below the dura and above the brain (subdural) tend to follow the shape of the brain and produce less mass effect because they are often created by a break in the venous circulation, meaning blood is lost at lower pressure (Figure 10.1). Hematomas above the dura and below the skull (epidural) tend to produce greater mass effect because they often involve arteries, which lose blood at higher pressure (Figure 10.2). Fortunately, epidural hematomas are usually easier to treat, as the surgeon has only to open the skull and drain the hematoma. Virtually all epidural hematomas are treated by opening the skull (Springer and Baker 1988). Treatment of subdural hematomas requires opening the skull and dura. In the modern era, many subdural

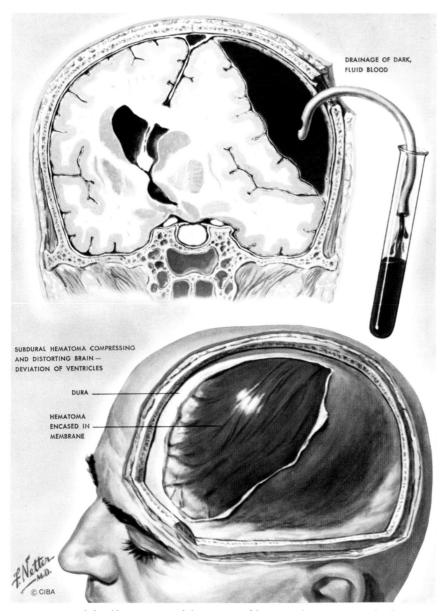

DRAINAGE OF DARK, FLUID BLOOD

SUBDURAL HEMATOMA COMPRESSING AND DISTORTING BRAIN — DEVIATION OF VENTRICLES

DURA

HEMATOMA ENCASED IN MEMBRANE

Figure 10.1 A subdural hematoma and the process of draining it by penetrating the dura mater. Illustration by Frank Netter © 2015 NetterImages.

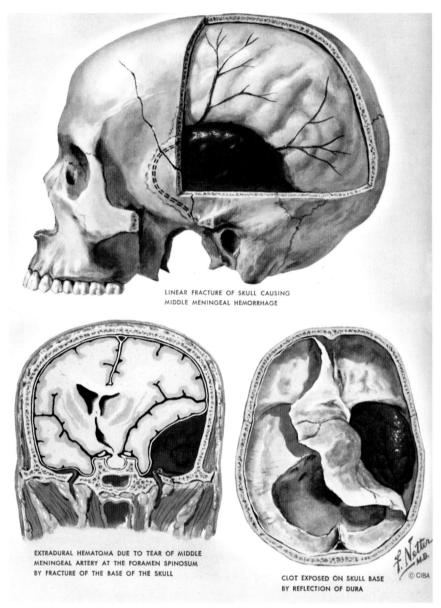

LINEAR FRACTURE OF SKULL CAUSING
MIDDLE MENINGEAL HEMORRHAGE

EXTRADURAL HEMATOMA DUE TO TEAR OF MIDDLE
MENINGEAL ARTERY AT THE FORAMEN SPINOSUM
BY FRACTURE OF THE BASE OF THE SKULL

CLOT EXPOSED ON SKULL BASE
BY REFLECTION OF DURA

Figure 10.2 Epidural hematoma as a result of a skull fracture tearing the middle meningeal artery. Illustration by Frank Netter © 2015 NetterImages.

hematomas are not treated, especially if the hematoma is not easily accessible. If the blood has not produced a mass effect, then it is allowed to stay and be reabsorbed over the course of weeks and months.

Neurons require a specific chemical environment surrounding the cell membrane in order to function. Free blood that surrounds brain tissue causes widespread disruption of this chemical balance and considerable impairment even when the neurons have not been substantially damaged or killed by the mechanical trauma or mass effect of the hematoma. The patient can still experience severe impairment or death if brain structures mediating basic life functions are compromised by the presence of blood. Patients in this situation may experience severe coma, paralysis, or delirium. They may appear to be just as disabled as the most severely injured patient. Their recovery is unique since many neurons are still viable but simply unable to function. As the hematoma resolves, patients can make dramatic recoveries. Neurons that were previously dormant are restored to normal functionality as blood leaves the brain (Patt and Brodhun 1999; Su et al. 2008). If brain tissue has been killed by mechanical forces or other deleterious pathology, then recovery is protracted and there will always be some functionality that never completely returns due to a permanent lesion (Katz et al. 2009; Luria 1963).

THE COGNITIVE AND BEHAVIORAL TOPOGRAPHY OF THE BRAIN

There are a number of obvious cognitive and behavioral manifestations of brain injury, while others are much more subtle. But even more subtle symptoms would influence the relationship of the injured person with family and friends. This section will review the basic cognitive systems in the brain and the behavioral patterns that result from lesions affecting these systems. Christopher Filley provides a more detailed description (Filley 1995).

The brain is generally divided into sensory and motor systems (Figure 10.3). The sensory systems are housed in the posterior area of the brain and the motor systems are generally in the anterior areas. For example, vision encompasses the occipital lobes, primary hearing perception is in the superior temporal lobe, and primary somatosensory perception (touch and proprioception) is located in the postcentral gyrus. Smell and taste are more primitive senses, and they have a more diffuse representation that includes the frontal lobes and the limbic system. The sensory systems are integrated in association areas that lie between the primary sensory areas. The confluence of interconnections of vision, hearing, and somatosensory perception for each hemisphere is in the parietal lobe.

The basic components of the motor systems are the primary system in the precentral gyrus, the subcortical basal ganglia, and the cerebellum. The motor systems also utilize numerous secondary motor planning and control areas in the frontal lobes. These are executed through large fiber tracts that extend down through the brain and spinal cord to moderate the activity of skeletal muscles by excitation and inhibition. The cerebellum is a structure that smoothes and coordinates these movements, especially rapid ones. The basal ganglia, lying in the white matter beneath the cortex, may be involved in driving movements and the selection of movement components.

Memory is mediated by the sensory systems and the hippocampus, a medial, subcortical structure that is part of the limbic system. Remembering new information is often compromised following traumatic brain injuries because this system is very sensitive to any disruption of function. It also takes time for memories to be consolidated, and if trauma occurs, the consolidation of new information can be lost. The duration of posttraumatic amnesia over the course of recovery is a useful predictor of later memory and cognitive outcome (Nakase-Richardson et al. 2011).

There are two major components of language: a sensory/comprehension system in the parietal and temporal lobes and a motor/expression system in the inferior frontal lobe (Bookheimer 2002). In most people, the left hemisphere mediates language. Injury of the motor language systems in the left frontal lobe causes speech impediments and other difficulties in the expression of language. Because some of the earliest cases of language disorder involved damage to these frontal areas and were widely discussed after presentations and publications by Paul Broca, this type of language disorder is named Broca's aphasia (Filley 1995). A patient's speech will be hesitant and they may be rendered essentially mute. Written language can also be compromised and may be just as hesitant, nonfluent, and impoverished as speech. Since the Pre-Columbian Peruvians had no writing system, this complication would not have been observable. Sometimes there is a residual stereotypic phrase that is uttered whenever the patient tries to speak. In Broca's most well-known case, this phrase was just the word "Tan." Sometimes the residual phrase is just a short, random collection of phonemes. But the phrase never varies, as if the system is stuck with just one utterance, no matter what the patient intends to say. One patient I encountered with Broca's aphasia could only say, "Ikabody, ikabody ama." She spoke this phrase in response to any question and sometimes in attempts at spontaneous speech. She understood the phrase to be jibberish when she said it, and would often inhibit speech because she knew that this would be the only thing that would come out when she tried. Her understanding of speech was good and she followed commands and appeared to comprehend reading material.

Soon after the discovery of Broca's aphasia, Karl Wernicke reported cases of defects in the sensory and comprehension aspects of language. This type was later named Wernicke's aphasia (Damasio and Geschwind 1984; Filley 1995). In this version of language disorder, the patient has damage to the posterior sensory systems that mediate language in the left parietal and temporal lobes (see Figure 10.3). This causes difficulty comprehending spoken and written language. Patients have trouble following commands or behaving consistently in regard to any request expressed through language. In addition, the speech of patients with Wernicke's aphasia is a garbled jumble of misplaced phonemes, as if the system for organizing language sounds were completely lost.

Spatial abilities, such as orienting the body in space, drawing figures, and manipulating objects in space, are mediated by association areas of the parietal lobes, primarily the right parietal lobe. Injury or illness that involves the right parietal lobe results in spatial disorientation. Patients will have difficulty navigating their environment, dressing (because they can no longer orient their body to the clothing), and drawing or constructing anything that incorporates a spatial arrangement. The most severe manifestation involves neglect

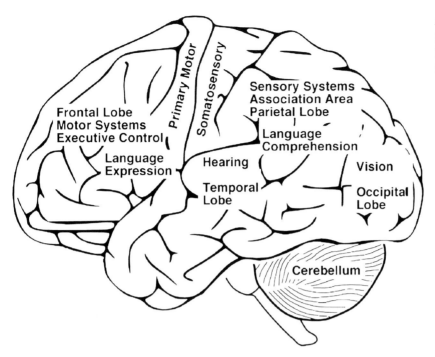

Figure 10.3
Diagram of the brain showing functional areas.

of the left side of space. Patients essentially behave as if everything on their left does not exist. They orient to the right visuospatial field as if that were the only part of the spatial environment that exists.

The final general domain of cognitive and behavioral function is executive control. The evolution of the human brain prominently includes the development of control systems in the frontal lobes. These are essentially inhibitory systems that modulate complex motor actions, emotions, language expression, memory search, and virtually every activity of the other cognitive systems (Alvarez and Emory 2006). Damage to the frontal lobes results in uninhibited social behavior, labile emotions, a concrete style of thought, and poor decision making. Most of these behavior changes are subtle and may only be noticed by friends and family who knew the patient before his or her injury.

COGNITIVE AND BEHAVIORAL RECOVERY FROM TRAUMATIC BRAIN INJURY

Most moderate and severe brain injuries are associated with a general suppression of neurological and cognitive function, causing a coma. But a coma is simply the behavioral result of inactive cortical sensory and motor systems. Coma is similar to sleep, except that sleep is an unconscious state mediated and controlled by centers in the brainstem, whereas coma is the result of brain lesion. There are two general causes of coma: damage to brainstem areas that mediate consciousness and arousal and damage to the cerebral cortex. One or both may occur in a moderate to severe brain injury. An isolated brainstem lesion produces a deep coma from which patients may not recover. If they do recover, they sometimes appear to awake from a deep sleep. Because the cortex is undamaged in this case, the patient awakens alert and competent (Katz et al. 2009; Lingsma et al. 2010).

Most trauma patients experience a combination of damage to both the brainstem and cerebral cortex and appear comatose for some interval following the injury. Coma is assessed by administering stimuli such as verbal commands and mild, harmless pain, such as rubbing the sternum or pressing the fingernails. All the accepted scales for measuring the severity of a coma incorporate these levels of response: (1) the patient responds to verbal command; (2) the patient responds to painful stimuli and does not respond to verbal command; or (3) the patient is unresponsive to any stimulus. The most shallow level of coma is associated with somnolence. In this case, the patient can converse and respond to verbal commands, but falls asleep when not interacting with others. The most severe coma is characterized by deep obtunded sleep, and the patient may have pathological breathing patterns and muscle posturing indicating the motor system is no longer controlled by the cortex (decorticate posturing). The depth and length of coma is a useful predictor of long-term recovery prospects (Williams et al. 1984).

Over weeks and months, someone with a moderate or severe brain injury will slowly recover from coma and the acute trauma. Hematomas diminish, the scalp and skull heal, brain systems that were acutely compromised by the neurochemical storm caused by the trauma resolve, and neurons rendered dysfunctional once again begin to respond and interact with each other. This is an intermediate stage of recovery in which the acute effects are resolving and the patient is emerging from coma and interacting with his or her environment. This phase is characterized by the phenomenon of posttraumatic amnesia (PTA). Since the memory system is very sensitive to disruption, patients in this phase have difficulty retaining new information. They cannot remember everyday experiences and appear amnesic (Ahmed et al. 2000). They almost always have a retrograde amnesia (RA) of a few hours that involves the loss of memories extending toward the past. For this reason, it is very common for patients to have no memory of the traumatic event that caused their injury. As the memory systems recover, the lost retrograde memories return and the patient can once again retain new experiences.

Throughout the early recovery period and emergence from coma, the patient may be agitated and impulsive. This occurs because the control and inhibition functions of the brain have been damaged by the injury. The patient may be physically uninhibited and vigorous. He or she wants to get out of bed and resist attempts to keep still and calm. Such patients are usually physically restrained and sedated, and they may be given medications that paralyze the skeletal muscles. This has a bearing on the use of trepanation on a patient who is not comatose. In modern times, patients undergoing any significant procedure are completely sedated and placed in a deep coma by anesthesia. It would be dangerous and virtually impossible to conduct a procedure such as a trepanation on an agitated patient who is not sedated. Even a comatose patient may emerge from coma and become agitated by the pain and discomfort of a trepanation. This suggests that all of the trepanations done in Pre-Columbian Peru for head injury were performed when the patient was in a deep coma or in a completely lucid state, similar to the trepanations performed by the Kisii in Africa (Furnas et al. 1985; see also Chapter 10).

In the final stage of recovery, the acute aspects of the brain injury are resolved and the patient has to cope with the neurological and cognitive impairment that remains. In general, the acute aspects of traumatic brain injury, such as hematoma and mechanical trauma, produce widespread dysfunction that has not actually destroyed neurons but that has left them unable to communicate in the systems that underlie neurological functions. Neurons are unique in this regard. Unlike other cells, their structure is only a clue to their function. Their place and network interactivity defines their functional status. The neurons that make up the visual system are structurally identical to those of the hearing system. Their unique configuration within systems subsuming vision and hearing determines their functional status. Trauma can disrupt these systems and compromise function without damaging or killing the neurons. This phase of recovery is associated with a resolution of pathology connected to functional system disruption, and the impairment that remains represents functional systems that are permanently damaged and will not recover further (Luria 1963).

The impairment associated with this residual recovery can include any functional system in the brain, including vision, motor coordination, language, spatial abilities, and memory. The manner and location in which force was applied to the brain presumably produces a higher likelihood of impairment to the systems located there. For example, modern traumatic brain injuries in car accidents involve considerable rotation forces associated with the brain movement during rapid acceleration and deceleration. This tends to permanently injure the frontal and temporal poles, due to the impact of the brain against the skull, as well as the periventricular white matter, because of the asymmetrical movement of the two hemispheres as they move back and forth during the injury (Lewis 1976). An injury in prehistoric Peru involving the direct impact of a club or sling stone probably caused greater impairment of systems near the mechanical trauma. However, widespread damage can result from the brain moving and impacting the skull on the opposite side (contrecoup injury), hematoma, and infection (Jennett and Miller 1972; Miller and Jennett 1968). For example, if the left hemisphere is struck, the person will likely have language disorder (aphasia) and weakness on the right side of the body. If the right side of the head is struck, the person will likely have spatial disorders and weakness on the left side of the body. However, if the brain moves and strikes the inner table of the left side of the skull, the patient may have both spatial disorder and aphasia. Because the visual system is in the occipital lobes, someone struck from behind may be rendered cortically blind. Someone struck in the front of the brain will have difficulty with executive control, and will probably have motor weakness and uncoordinated movements. Blunt trauma from stone weapons probably produced more localized lesions than those produced by closed head injuries in car accidents (Miller and Jennett 1968).

TWO REPRESENTATIVE CASES OF BLUNT TRAUMA TREATED WITH TREPANATION

These cases were chosen because they predate the modern use of neuroimaging and the current understanding of neuropsychology and brain functions that have been discovered since the 1940s. In the modern era, computer tomography (CT) or magnetic resonance imagining (MRI) scans are routine for new trauma cases. In this way, the surgeon can quickly view the areas of skull fracture, hematoma, or other lesions. Although the physicians involved in these cases had a much more developed model of brain anatomy and neuropathology than did practitioners in ancient Peru, they were still deriving their treatment approach and making inferences based on observations of the patient's behavior. Both of these cases also involved making openings in the skull. Although the modern surgical tools were more efficient, the placement of the opening, the release of underlying hematoma, and the resulting recovery presumably involved the same set of observations made by practitioners in Pre-Columbian Peru.

These two cases do not include the repair of a depressed skull fracture. Given the archeological evidence, many trepanations were probably conducted to simply repair or remove broken bones. There are a few Peruvian skulls that show incomplete trepanations surrounding a depressed fracture (see Chapter 4). These cases illustrate that the Peruvian method almost exclusively involved cutting around the area of broken bone. Modern repair of open depressed fractures aims to lift and repair the broken skull areas. Closed fractures are often left without repair and simply monitored for hematoma and infection (Donovan 2005; Ganz and Arndt 2014).

Thomas Oliver (1888) presents a case successfully treated using trepanation that also includes observations that could have been made by practitioners in ancient Peru. Oliver's patient was a sixteen-year-old boy who fell, striking the right side of his head, during a game of tug-of-war. He was unconscious for a brief time and awoke apparently uninjured, passing the next ten days with no symptoms. Then:

> One morning, after getting out of bed and whilst in the act of dressing himself, he had his first convulsive seizure. It was extremely sudden in its onset, without any prodromata, and was accompanied by unconsciousness. He was put to bed, and on regaining consciousness complained of pain in the right side of his head. From that day he suffered from several fits daily—each series, more severe than the preceding—and followed by an alteration in his disposition; moroseness and sullenness replacing a character previously noticed for its liveliness.
>
> An aura was now felt before nearly all the fits, particularly those that became severe, and were accompanied by unconsciousness. He thought he saw a cat, the picture of which was still present in his mind, even after all his motor disturbance had subsided, and while yet in the transitional stage from coma to complete consciousness.
>
> It was noticed that in many of the severe fits the left arm and leg were much more convulsed than the right, and that as regards precedence, they were the first to be affected, the two sides of the face suffering equally. In addition, not only were the left arm and leg frequently the seat of marked paresis, which lasted for several days after the fit; but occasionally they were the subjects of choreiform movements over which he had no control, and which at times passed over to the right arm and leg, but were never of the same extensive range as on the left side where they originated. Frequently, after a severe fit, the stage of stupor was very protracted;

for two or three days the patient would be speechless and deaf, able to take liquid food when brought to him, but never asking for it. On regaining consciousness, and whilst yet deaf, he always at first made known his wants to us in writing.

I suggested trephining as the only likely method of dealing successfully with the fits. My surgical colleagues saw the case with me, and agreed as to the advisability of the operation, recommending, however, the application of the trephine over the painful spot, rather than upon that part of the skull lying upon those portions of the brain now recognised as concerned with the initiation of the movements of the arms and legs—I mean the ascending frontal and parietal convolutions. The painful spot, as I have already mentioned, lay anterior and somewhat inferior to these two convolutions. The operation was performed by Dr. Hume, under antiseptic precautions. A piece of bone, the size of a shilling, was without difficulty removed. The bone was quite healthy, and was easily lifted from its bed, being in no way adherent to the underlying membranes. The dura mater was healthy, in no way thickened. As the dura mater was healthy it was debated for a few seconds as to the advisability of opening it. By degrees, however, it was noticed that the dura mater was becoming tense, and shortly after this membrane was shot out through the opening beyond the level of the bone, the tension now being very great. Accordingly a crucial incision was made into it, and in a few seconds there escaped from the wound several teaspoonsful of serum, containing a few flakes of lymph. The arachnoid and pia mater seemed healthy, as did also the surface of the brain and the small blood vessels which lay upon it.

A very small drainage-tube was inserted, the cut ends of the dura mater were drawn together with delicate catgut, the skin flaps were gently drawn together, a sponge applied, and the ordinary antiseptic dressings placed over all. That evening the dressings were found to be soaking, and on removal a few teaspoonsful of serous fluid were squeezed out of the sponge. More than two ounces of serous fluid escaped that day. The dressings were renewed, and never afterwards required to be changed on account of the escape of fluid. The patient had one or two minor fits on coming out of the chloroform and also for two or three days after the operation, but after this they became separated from each other by the interval of a day, then two days, a week, a fortnight, and so on, until no fit occurred during a period of six months. The wound had healed kindly and quickly, without even the least rise of temperature. The patient having long left the infirmary, feeling quite well, no longer having any localised pain in his head, followed for a time the occupation of a telegraph boy, but lately became the cash boy in a confined counting house.

Trephining, as a method of treating epilepsy, is only applicable to those cases where there is the history of an injury to the head followed by localising symptoms or by convulsions, either unilateral or more pronounced on one side of the body than the other, or where an injury to the head has been followed by a depressed fracture or separation of a portion of the inner table of the skull. Relief comes either from the operation acting as a strong counter-irritant lasting all through the period of healing, or from the reduction of tension consequent upon the escape of pent-up serum. It is several months since this paper was written and read, but the last account that I had of this patient from his mother was that he was still keeping free from fits (Oliver 1888).

This case illustrates many of the features of a blunt head injury with a prominent subdural hematoma that likely included blood at venous pressure. The delay of symptoms for ten days suggests that the blood mass was slowly building. A blood clot developing at arterial pressure produces acute effects. During the chronic phase, the hematoma develops into a mass of serous fluid (Wintzen 1980). Seizures are very common, since the cortex is involved and irritated (Temkin et al. 1991). The vision of the cat is a classic manifestation of the seizure prodromal sign or aura. Although most seizure patients have a prodromal aura, visual hallucinations such as the cat are unusual. The patient also recovered quickly. After the mass and irritating effects of the hematoma were reduced, the patient appeared to respond and recover. He did not appear to have residual impairment a few months after the injury. It is important to keep in mind that this patient likely did not have a large brain lesion with tissue damage caused by mechanical trauma. The tissue was rendered dysfunctional because the blood and other fluid produced an environment in which the neurons could not function. When the blood and fluids were drained by the trepanation, the neuronal systems returned to their pre-injury status. It is important to keep in mind that many patients would not have such a positive outcome and might only recover to a point of residual impairment that might include the loss of language, memory disorder, movement disorders, and other cognitive impairments described previously. The seizure disorder may also persist indefinitely, creating considerable adjustment problems during the remainder of the patient's life.

The second case features language disorder as the prominent symptom (Cope 1914). The case also illustrates the manifestation and recovery of coma:

E. B., aged 14, was brought to the Bolingbroke Hospital about eight o'clock on the evening of August 14, 1913, with the history that she had fallen down a flight of six steps and struck the back part and left side of her head against the step or ground. The accident had occurred three hours previously; during the intervening time she had been semiconscious and had vomited frequently. Up to the time of the accident she had been a lively and intelligent girl in full possession of her faculties. When admitted the patient's temperature was normal, pulse 76, respirations 16 per minute. She lay with eyes closed, but when approached opened them and said, "Don't hurt me, daddy," and repeated the word "daddy" frequently during the initial examination. She had no recollection of the accident, and with difficulty recalled her actions prior to the injury. At the same time she continually relapsed into a more drowsy condition; her eyeballs kept rolling upwards. There was an abrasion and a very small scalp wound behind the left ear. There were no signs of fracture of the skull base, and no paralysis of cranial or peripheral nerves. The pupils were of normal size and reacted to light; the knee-jerks were elicited and the plantar reflex was normal. Her condition did not improve; she remained in an irritable state, curled up on her right side in bed, and resented any interference. Vomiting occurred several times. She spoke no word spontaneously, but apparently heard what was said to her. At first her condition was taken to be that of simple concussion and cerebral irritation, and I was not asked to see her. Gradually, however, her pulse became slower until it was about 50 per minute, whilst her mental condition remained anomalous, in that she seemed fully conscious yet did not utter a word. On August 19, when I saw her first, the condition was much as described above. There was no paralysis, but I could not elicit the knee-jerks; there was some photophobia; the pupils were equal, slightly dilated, and reacted to light normally. Ophthalmoscopic examination showed congestion of the retinal vessels and blurring of the edges of the disks. On the next day (August 20) the aphasic condition was more fully investigated by my house surgeon (Mr. O. R. L. Wilson), to whom I am indebted for these notes. The only word she could be got to utter spontaneously was the nick-name of her sister, and this name, "Doodles," she repeated throughout the examination. She gave plenty of indication that she understood words spoken to her, but could not answer any question intelligibly, a jumbled mutter of unintelligible sounds being all that she could attempt. She was unable to repeat words spoken to her. She did not understand written questions or commands, though it was clear she saw them. She was able to write spontaneously, but her writing was not intelligible. She copied capital letters correctly, but came hopelessly to grief when attempting to copy ordinary handwriting. She was unable to write from dictation, nor could she name objects seen. Reading aloud from printed or written matter was not in her power, and she was unable even to pick out objects of which the name was given to her by speaking.

She readily understood pantomimic gestures, and imitated them. From the above examination it was evident that there was some serious lesion in the higher centres for understanding both printed and spoken words, but especially affecting the visual higher centres. On August 21 operation was undertaken. A horseshoe-shaped flap was made with its base above the left ear. The trephine was placed so that the centre pin was 2 in., or a little more, above the external auditory meatus. No clot was found outside the dura, which was tense, bulging, and non-pulsatile. When the dura was incised a small amount of dark blood was found underneath. By carefully searching in every direction under the dura by means of a flat metal instrument a considerable amount of old black blood clot was discovered in a direction towards the occipital lobe. This clot escaped under considerable tension—it almost leapt out—and altogether several drachms came away. Some more bone was removed in a backward direction and the spaces between the bone and dura and the brain and dura were carefully searched, but no more clot was found. The cerebral cortex was also explored by needle and knife, but no subcortical hemorrhage was found. The dura was sewn up with thread and the skin flap replaced and sutured with silkworm gut without drainage. The pulse at the end of the operation was 100; at the beginning it had been 50 to the minute. Recovery of speech after the operation was exceedingly quick. The next day the patient asked for some dinner, and in general showed a marvellous improvement. Within a week practically all her disabilities were removed, and instead of the stolid, non-comprehending countenance was the intelligent, mobile face, readily smiling and appreciating every remark made to her (Cope 1914).

Most case reports like this understandably report positive outcomes. But many patients have permanent impairments of cognition and neurological functions; some never emerge from coma. Most cases follow the general pattern described previously, in which the patient emerges from coma and recovers to a pattern of impairment consistent with the brain areas that have been permanently damaged. Unfortunately for the course and progress of recovery, neurons do not reproduce in the adult human brain. We have only a finite number that is established soon after birth. Their interconnections grow and then attenuate over the course of development. The adult brain networks are sculpted by experience and further development (Stiles 2012). If an adult acquires a brain lesion from trauma or illness, this process of development cannot be repeated and even further brain growth will have little influence on function. The recovered patient must live with the impairment that remains after the acute effects of brain injury have resolved (Corbetta 2012).

SPECULATIONS ON A CASE FROM PERU

Focus on an archaeological case of trepanation may clarify the possible observations made by Peruvian medical practitioners. The case chosen for this analysis is represented by a skull from the southern highlands (Figure 10.4). This man sustained a large skull fracture involving the temporal bone as a result of severe blunt force trauma. This is one of the worst locations for such an injury because of the proximity to the temporalis muscle and blood vessels that spread across the skull and brain surface from inferior to superior areas. The temporalis muscle on the left side of the head must have been essentially obliterated by the trauma. One can imagine the blood loss and pain associated with this blow, and a coma would have been a merciful result of an injury this severe. Indeed, lying in a deep comatose state would have been necessary in order for the Peruvian practitioner to treat this injury using two large trepanations, one that encompasses the fracture in the left temporal bone and another trepanation in the left frontal area. The fracture itself must have been reasonably large, and the trepanation was done by the scraping method to clear the entire area of fracture. All that remains is a linear fracture radiating away from the opening and toward the front of the skull (see Figure 10.4b). The frontal trepanation does not have a contiguous fracture. There may have been a depressed fracture in this location that was removed by the trepanation, or this trepanation may have been done as a treatment for hematoma, pain, seizures, or other pathology.

This man was most likely struck with a stone club that produced a large depressed skull fracture in the area of the temporal bone and also rendered him unconscious. A short time after this, and while he was still comatose, the trepanations were executed. Although the skull appears clean now, imagine cutting away the skin and scraping through skin, muscle, connective tissue, and bone to make these large openings in the skull. This was quite a

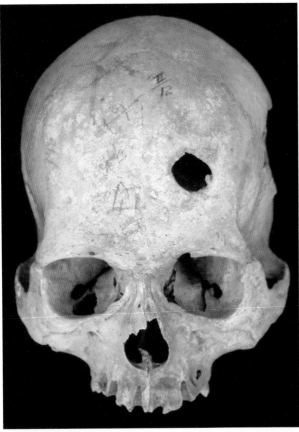

Figure 10.4
(a) Frontal view of an adult male cranium from Sacsahuaman with two healed trepanations; and (b) left lateral view with arrows marking a healed linear fracture. Museo Inka 1/327.

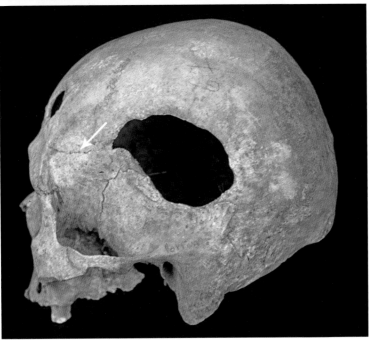

commitment to a procedure with an uncertain result. The objective of the trepanation was presumably to clear away broken bone and relieve any underlying pressure from hematoma and other swelling.

An interesting feature of such ancient Peruvian trepanations, especially those from Paracas (see Chapter 8), is their large size. The Peruvians made smaller trepanations in later time periods, but they are unique in the great number of large operations like the one depicted here. It seems that the idea was to make a trepanation that encompassed all of the affected bone, rendering a large opening. Modern surgery practice is not to operate on depressed fractures that have no hematoma and in which the bone pieces are still in place.

In the specific case at hand, the lesion and trepanation locations were directly over the language centers and motor control areas of the left hemisphere. After a period of coma, this man recovered and likely experienced global aphasia similar to the case of E. B. presented above. If the second trepanation in the frontal area treated a brain injury, then he was also weaker on the right side. These behavioral consequences would have been directly observable by his caretakers.

Both trepanations are well healed, suggesting that the patient lived for months and likely years following his injuries. He also survived and recovered from any infection that may have developed. Another obvious result of this injury was serious damage to the temporalis muscle on the left side. Moving the jaw and eating would have been extremely painful and difficult. The entire left side of his face must have been considerably swollen while he recovered. A likely set of disabling symptoms would have included aphasia, hemiplegia on the right side of the body, and chronic pain. Less likely impairments include hearing loss in the left ear, disinhibition of behavior associated with the frontal lobe injury, and memory disorder. Any cluster of these possible sequelae would have been very disabling in everyday life. This all suggests that this man was cared for and supported by his family and community while recovering from his injuries and living with disabilities.

By analysis of the available facts, it is clear that the people of ancient Peru developed a practice or craft of treating head and skull injuries using trepanation. The chapter reviewed the common sequelae of traumatic brain injury and the neurological and cognitive disabilities that ancient Peruvians would have observed and dealt with as a patient recovered from coma to the residual functional level. These include amnesia, aphasia, hemiplegia, and other apparent disabling conditions. It is clear that the most common sequelae of injury involved severe disabilities that the affected person could not have survived and dealt with alone. The family and the community were marshaled to keep the person alive during the acute phase of injury, cope with severe behavior and cognitive problems during recovery, and deal with the functional problems remaining after recovery was complete.

AS DESCRIBED IN THE VARIOUS CHAPTERS OF THIS VOLUME, EVIDENCE OF trepanation has been found in many parts of the world. While certainly not a global practice throughout human history, surveys of the literature indicate that an impressive number of both ancient and modern societies experimented with cranial surgery (Arnott et al. 2003; Campillo 2007; Germanà and Forniciari 1992; Piggott 1940). Isolated cases of "possible" trepanations also continue to be reported from new regions, although these need to be examined critically. As noted in Chapter 3, careful differential diagnosis is essential for distinguishing between genuine surgical intervention and other processes that can create holes in skulls. Some geographic regions and time periods, such as Neolithic Europe and ancient Peru, have incontrovertible evidence of trepanation based on the sheer number of crania that demonstrate a full range of unhealed, partially healed, and extensively healed openings.

EARLIEST EVIDENCE: CLAIMS AND CHALLENGES

Did trepanation first appear in Neolithic times (ca. 6000–2000 BC), or is there earlier evidence? There have been claims of trepanned crania from earlier European Epipaleolithic and Mesolithic burials possibly dating as early as 10,000 BC (Lillie 1998, 2003) and from the Epipaleolithic of North Africa (Ferembach 1962), but all of these cases are problematic. I briefly address the European crania in Chapter 3, so I will only comment on the North African cases here. Ferembach (1962) describes a cranium from Taforalt Cave (Grottes des Pigeons) in Eastern Morocco with a partially healed opening on the left parietal bone that could be a trepanation, although there is no description of tool marks that might confirm this. Another cranial fragment from the same site has a small round depression that is described as an incomplete trepanation, but in my opinion this is more likely a healed depressed fracture. The difficulty with all of these cases is that they are isolated finds, and they have healed lesions that with few exceptions have not received rigorous differential diagnosis. Personally, I remain skeptical of claims of trepanned crania predating the Neolithic Period, although some scholars are more willing to accept some of these cases (Crubézy et al. 2001).

Egypt

Ancient Egypt has produced little convincing evidence of trepanation, despite some early claims based on the incorrect diagnosis of a cranium with biparietal thinning (see Chapter 3). Trepanation might be expected to have evolved in ancient Egypt, given that head wounds from clubs and bladed weapons of war were common. The Edwin Smith Papyrus, the oldest known surgical treatise on the treatment of injuries (ca. 1500 BC) describes various types of head wounds. It recommends treatment for some (scalp lesions without skull fracture) but not for others (serious fractures with exposure of the brain); it does not discuss or recommend trepanation (Breasted 1930). There is no direct evidence of skull surgery, with the exception of a cranium dating to the Greco-Roman period with a trepanation done by cutting and drilling (Pahl 1992). A recent review of evidence from Egyptian skeletons and mummies from earlier periods in Egypt found only one example of the possible treatment of a depressed skull fracture. In this case, the authors suggest that broken fragments of bone were removed from the site of injury. However, no evidence of cutting, scraping, or drilling of the wound margins was found, so this would not be considered a trepanation (Nehrlich et al. 2003).

Greece and Rome

Only a small number of trepanned skulls have been described from ancient Greece (Agelarakis 2006; Mountrakis et al. 2011; Papagrigorakis et al. 2014) and the Roman Empire (Brothwell 1974; Rubini 2008; Tullo 2010). While this at first seems strange, given the extensive descriptions of trepanation in the medical texts of Hippocrates, Celsus, and Galen, much evidence of trepanation may have been lost due to the fact that cremation was common in both Athens and Rome (Musgrave 1990; Toynbee 1971), and identification of trepanations in cremated remains would be challenging.

China

For many years, it was believed that trepanation was not practiced in the Far East and China, although it is mentioned in classical Chinese literature (Lisowski 1967). Until recently, no published reports of trepanned skulls were available outside of China, with the exception of a 2007 article describing six possible cases from Neolithic Bronze and Iron Age sites in Shandong, Qinghai, Henan, and Heilongjiang provinces (Han and Cheng 2007). While I find several of these convincing, others may be healed fractures or cranial cysts. A few possible cases from Mongolia and southern Siberia also have been published (Bazarsad 2003; Murphy 2003). In a recent article, Xianli Lv, Zhenguang Li, and Youxiang Li argue that the sample from China is substantially larger, and note that trepanned skulls have been found at the early Neolithic sites of Liuwan, Fujia, Shanshan, and Chifeng (Lv et al. 2013). In their article, they only describe and illustrate one skull from Fujia, which indeed shows a circular defect on the right parietal bone that looks like a healed trepanation (this skull is also illustrated and described in Han and Cheng 2007). The authors provide links to online reports on other trepanned skulls, but these cases apparently have not been published, and it is difficult to believe their claim that "more trepanned skulls have been found in this region than in the rest of the world combined" (Lv et al. 2013:897). Publication of more material is clearly needed.

Mesoamerica

Besides Peru and Bolivia, the only other known center of trepanation in the New World was the Oaxaca Valley of central Mexico. Excavations directed by archaeologist Alfonso Caso in the 1930s and 1940s at the monumental site of Monte Albán recovered five skulls with trepanations (Romero 1970). Later excavations directed by Marcus Winter in 1972 and 1973 recovered five more. These burials were found in low-status residential areas outside the monumental core of the site and date to Period IIIb, about AD 40–700 (Wilkinson and Winter 1975; Winter 1989). Two distinct forms of trepanations were found: oval or circular openings made by scraping or grooving; and circular openings made with a hollow tubular drill (Figure 11.1). The latter method is particularly interesting because it is the only example of this form of trepanation known in the New World. The drill holes have vertical walls, distinct from the smaller conical holes made in the Peruvian drilling and cutting method. In fact, they are so similar to the circular bore holes made by Old World crown trephines that if examined blindly it would be difficult to distinguish the two. These drilled trepanations have been described and illustrated most extensively by Richard Wilkinson (Wilkinson 1975a, 1975b; Wilkinson and Winter 1975). Most crania with drilled trepanations show multiple openings that are quite consistent in diameter, averaging 12.8 millimeters. Wilkinson and Winter hypothesize that the drills used on these crania were adapted

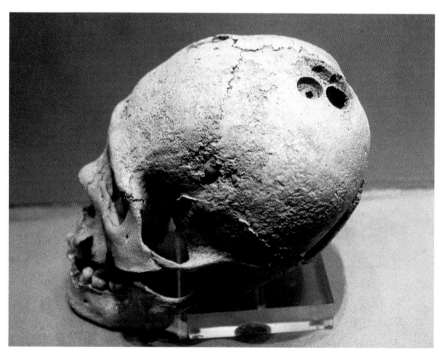

Figure 11.1
Skull from Monte Albán with multiple trepanations. The operation was unsuccessful, as there is no evidence of bone reaction. Museo de Sitio Monte Albán, Oaxaca.

from tools used to make jewelry and to drill teeth for dental incrustations. Presumably, they were made of bone or cane and used with an abrasive such as sand or crushed obsidian. Unfortunately for the patients, neither the scraping and grooving nor the drilling method was very successful. Wilkinson found some examples of short-term healing in the Monte Albán trepanned crania but no examples of long-term healing, which led him to theorize that the surgery may have been largely experimental. There are no skull fractures or any other visible indications for why these trepanations were done, so if their purpose was therapeutic, it is unclear what conditions they were meant to treat.

Since the early discoveries of 1972 and 1973, two more trepanned skulls have been found at Monte Albán (Márquez Morfín and González Licón 1992) and five have been found at other Oaxaca Valley sites (Stone and Urcid 2003). These include openings made by both the scraping and drilling methods, and they come from more diverse tomb contexts than did the original discoveries. Although seventeen trepanned crania is a relatively small sample, the crania from Monte Albán and surrounding sites represent an independent and distinctive tradition of skull surgery in the Americas.

North America

Since the early twentieth century, there have been scattered reports of American Indian crania with possible trepanations, but most of these have not survived close scrutiny (for a recent review, see Stone and Urcid 2003). While a few may indeed record experiments with treating head wounds, such as the case of an adult male cranium from northern California with a frontal lesion that was treated by scraping of the outer table with an obsidian tool (Richards 1995), others are equivocal at best. T. Dale Stewart did a thorough literature review of the North American evidence as it stood in the 1950s, and summarized it as follows:

> It is difficult to describe the feeling of dissatisfaction with the evidence and arguments which one gains in reading the individual reports and in examining the accompanying illustrations. Some of the cases undoubtedly represent old healed injuries in which there was no surgical intervention; others are fresh openings that, since they could have been made after death, do not prove the existence of surgery in the real sense. Only two or three look anything like what is often seen in Peruvian specimens (Stewart 1958:476).

Time may prove otherwise, but given the thousands of skeletons that have been excavated in the United States and Canada, it seems highly unlikely that trepanation was practiced with any frequency in North America before European contact.

GEOGRAPHIC PATTERNING IN AREAS WHERE TREPANATION WAS COMMON

Interestingly, in the two areas of the world where there is abundant evidence of cranial surgery (Neolithic Europe and ancient Peru) archaeological sites yielding trepanned skulls are not evenly scattered across the landscape. Instead, they show regional clustering.

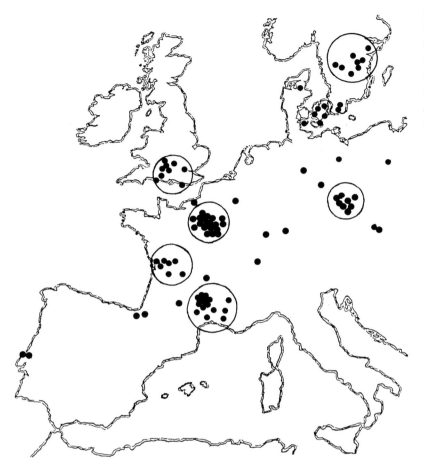

Figure 11.2
Map of Europe, showing concentrations of Neolithic trepanned skulls. After Brothwell 2003:fig. 5.

Stuart Piggott (1940) and later Don Brothwell (2003) noted this in Europe, suggesting the presence of centers of cranial surgery, from which the practice diffused to other regions (Figure 11.2). Certainly there were centers of trepanation in Peru as well (Andrushko and Verano 2008; Verano 2003a), beginning with early experimentation at Paracas and nearby sites on the south coast, followed by fluorescence in the central and southern highlands and Altiplano regions, with smaller concentrations in the northern highlands and cloud forest.

There are also clear gaps in the geographic distribution of trepanned skulls in Peru. With the exception of the Paracas Peninsula and nearby coastal valley sites, there are less than a handful of trepanned (or possibly trepanned) crania known from all of coastal Peru (Tyson and Alcauskas 1980; Uhle 1903; Verano and Delabarde 2013). All but one of these crania may date to the time of the Inca Empire, when there was extensive population movement throughout the Andean region. Trepanners or trepanned people would have moved around as well, as was probably the case with the forced resettlement of Chachapoya natives to Inca royal estates around AD 1500 (see Chapter 7). To date, no evidence of trepanation has been found in lowland Amazonia, although preservation of skeletal remains there is generally very poor.

What is perhaps more curious, given that trepanation was common throughout highland Peru and Bolivia, is that it has not been found in Chile, Argentina, or Ecuador. Even if trepanation was not an indigenous tradition in these areas, it could have been introduced with Inca expansion in the late fifteenth and early sixteenth centuries, although Inca control of these areas was quite short-lived and in many cases indirect (Malpass 1993; Von Hagen and Morris 1993). With the exception of three crania from Colombia published by Gomez (1973), no convincing examples of trepanned skulls have been reported from anywhere else in South America.

Why was trepanation so common in highland Peru? A simple argument is that this was a region with endemic warfare, where skull fractures from weapons such as sling stones and clubs were common—an ideal natural laboratory for developing treatments for head wounds. But clubs and slings were also common weapons in other parts of South America where trepanned skulls have not been found. Perhaps highland Peruvian populations had a substantially higher risk of head injury than did neighboring regions. The Hrdlička skeletal collection from the Huarochirí area (Chapter 4) and recent studies of cranial trauma in the south central highlands (Arkush and Tung 2013; Tung 2007, 2012) and Cuzco region (Andrushko and Torres 2011) confirm that head injuries were frequent in highland Peru in prehistoric times.

But skull fracture alone does not seem to tell the whole story. The frequency of multiple trepanations in Inca crania, often with openings of consistent size and with no visible association with skull fractures, suggests that some trepanations were done for other reasons. They were performed at relatively low risk to the patient, as can be judged by the number of individuals who survived multiple operations. Perhaps early success with treating head injuries encouraged trepanners to experiment with treating other symptoms, such as headaches, convulsions, or neurological changes brought on by intracranial mass lesions (Chapters 9 and 10). Whether trepanation would be of any practical value in treating non-trauma–related headaches is questioned by J. Michael Williams in Chapter 10, but experimentation may have occurred nevertheless. Kurin suggests that trepanation in ancient Peru might also have been executed for neurological disorders brought on by emotional and physical stress (Kurin 2013). While it is not possible to confirm this osteologically, it is one more potential motive for trepanning.

How did surgical knowledge spread in ancient Peru? It likely was transmitted through migration, cultural exchange between groups, and conquest, especially during the Inca Empire. Within regions where trepanation was practiced, knowledge presumably was acquired through observation and apprenticeship, similar to what has been documented ethnographically in the South Pacific and among the Kisii of East Africa (Chapter 8). And based on the data we have on the frequency of successful trepanations in ancient Peru, methods and skill improved over time.

The chapters by Kushner and Titelbaum and by Williams emphasize that the treatment and care of patients with serious head injuries does not end when an operation is completed and the wound dressed and covered. Substantial patient care would have been required over an extended period of time, particularly in cases of serious brain injuries. The recovery of normal brain function would have been variable, depending on the severity of the injury, and some patients would never fully recover. Those who suffered skull fractures needed not only a skilled surgeon but also a social network capable of providing postoperative care and support. The high survival rate of those trepanned in ancient Peru indicates that such care was provided.

Why did trepanation flourish briefly and precociously in some areas, such as the Paracas Peninsula, and then abruptly disappear? Was this simply an early experiment that gradually lost its practitioners and popularity? Did trepanation spread from Paracas up the coastal valleys into the highlands, or did it independently evolve without influence from the coast? At present, we lack archaeological evidence to answer these and many other questions about how trepanation developed and spread across time and space in Andean South America. Unfortunately, ethnohistory and written documents provide little assistance in answering these questions. There are no descriptions of trepanation by the Spanish conquistadors, priests, or chroniclers (Lastres 1951:220–223; Rowe 1946:313–314), nor is there a word for trepanation in Quechua or Aymara, the two dominant indigenous languages of highland Peru and Bolivia (Lastres and Cabieses 1960).

A lack of observations by early Spanish sources may be a reflection of the social disruption and chaos brought on by the European conquest and subsequent civil wars and epidemics. New weapons and military tactics introduced by the Spanish also changed the nature of battle wounds, with a decrease in injuries caused by slings and bashing weapons and an increase in those caused by sharp-edged swords, pikes, polearms, lances, and firearms. Even so, during the conquest of Peru, indigenous allies of the Spanish used traditional Andean weapons in battles against the Inca (Lund Valle 2009; Murphy et al. 2010).

Native religion was actively suppressed in the early colonial period, as were cultural practices such as the shaping of infants' heads—banned by the Spanish colonial government in 1585 and again in 1752 (Hoshower et al. 1995). In this environment, traditional medical practices such as trepanation may have been suppressed and executed only clandestinely. One wonders, however, why there are no accounts of trepanation until the late nineteenth and early twentieth centuries, when scattered reports appear in highland Bolivia and Peru. Was it a question of the remoteness of many highland communities, or was it suspicion of outsiders? The latter explanation is supported by Bandelier's observations on the reluctance of the Aymara to answer his inquiries (see Chapter 7).

Working with archaeological samples in the absence of written or oral history, we realize that there is much we will never know about how skull surgery evolved in ancient South America. There is room for some optimism, however. In contrast to early collections of trepanned skulls that lacked detailed information on provenance and dating, there is a growing body of new data coming out of archaeological excavations in various regions of highland Peru and Bolivia, such as those reported in Chapter 7. New discoveries of trepanned skulls are being made in controlled excavations, and some skulls now have direct radiocarbon dates. This twenty-first-century information will make it possible to refine our working chronological framework for trepanation in ancient Peru, and it can help to contextualize early collections made by Uhle, Tello, Hrdlička, and others. Radiocarbon dating of these early collections may become possible as well. The final chapter on trepanation in ancient Peru has yet to be written.

APPENDIX

Bones of the Skull, Sutures, and Selected Anatomical Landmarks

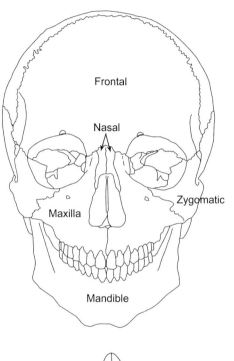

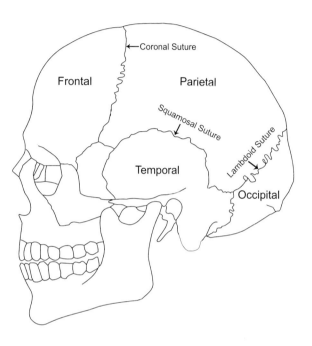

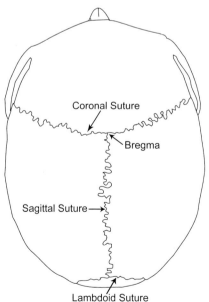

Front, left, and top views of a human skull, with selected bones, sutures, and landmarks labeled. Redrawn after Buikstra and Ubelaker 1994.

REFERENCES CITED

Adams, Francis

    1886   *The Genuine Works of Hippocrates: Translated from the Greek with a Preliminary Discourse and Annotations*, vol. 1. William Wood, New York.

Agelarakis, Anagnostis P.

    2006   Artful Surgery. *Archaeology* 59(2):26–29.

Agency for Healthcare Research and Quality (AHRQ)

    2006   Quality Indicators Website: Version 3.0. Electronic document, http://www.quality indicators.ahrq.gov, accessed June 4, 2014.

Ahmed, Saeeduddin, Rex Bierley, Javaid Sheikh, and Elaine S. Date

    2000   Post-Traumatic Amnesia after Closed Head Injury: A Review of the Literature and Some Suggestions for Further Research. *Brain Injury* 14(9):765–780.

Allison, Marvin J., and Enrique Gerszten

    1975   *Paleopathology in South American Mummies: Application of Modern Techniques.* Medical College of Virginia, Richmond.

Allison, Marvin J., and Alejandro Pezzia

    1976   Treatment of Head Wounds in Pre-Columbian and Colonial Peru. *Medical College of Virginia Quarterly* 12(2):74–79.

Alt, Kurt W., Christian Jeunesse, Carlos H. Buitrago-Téllez, Rüdiger Wächter, Eric Boës, and Sandra L. Pichler

    1997   Evidence for Stone Age Cranial Surgery. *Nature,* May 22.

Alvarado Reyes, Ramiro

    2004   Trepanaciones pre-colombinas. *Archivos bolivianos de historia de la medicina* 10(1/2):23–25.

Alvarez, Julie A., and Eugene Emory

    2006   Executive Function and the Frontal Lobes: A Meta-Analytic Review. *Neuropsychology Review* 16(1):17–42.

Andrushko, Valerie A.

    2007   The Bioarchaeology of Inca Imperialism in the Heartland: An Analysis of Prehistoric Burials from the Cuzco Region of Peru. PhD dissertation, University of California, Santa Barbara.

Andrushko, Valerie A., and Elva C. Torres

    2011   Skeletal Evidence for Inca Warfare from the Cuzco Region of Peru. *American Journal of Physical Anthropology* 146(3):361–372.

Andrushko, Valerie A., Elva C. Torres, and Viviana Bellifemine

    2006   The Burials at Sacsahuaman and Choquepukio: A Bioarchaeological Case Study of Imperialism from the Capital of the Inca Empire. *Ñawpa Pacha* 28:63–87.

Andrushko, Valerie A., and John W. Verano

    2008   Prehistoric Trepanation in the Cuzco Region of Peru: A View into an Ancient Andean Practice. *American Journal of Physical Anthropology* 137(1):4–13.

Anónimo

    1945   Peruvian Operated on with Inca Instruments. *El Palacio* 52(2):38–39.

Arkush, Elizabeth, and Tiffiny A. Tung

    2013   Patterns of War in the Andes from the Archaic to the Late Horizon: Insights from Settlement Patterns and Cranial Trauma. *Journal of Archaeological Research* 21(4):307–369.

Arnott, Robert, Stanley Finger, and C. U. M. Smith (editors)

2003 *Trepanation: Discovery, History, Theory.* Swets and Zeitlinger, Lisse.

Asenjo, Alfonso

1963 *Neurosurgical Techniques.* Charles C. Thomas, Springfield, Ill.

Associated Press

2001 Two Men Make Plea Deal for Drilling Woman's Head. *The Los Angeles Times*, March 11.

Aufderheide, Arthur C.

1985 The Enigma of Ancient Cranial Trepanation. *Minnesota Medicine* 68:119–122.

Bakay, Louis

1985 *An Early History of Craniotomy: From Antiquity to the Napoleonic Era.* Charles C. Thomas, Springfield, Ill.

Bandelier, Adolf F.

1904 Aboriginal Trephining in Bolivia. *American Anthropologist* 6(4):440–446.

1909 *The Indians and Aboriginal Ruins near Chachapoyas in Northern Peru.* United States Catholic Historical Society, New York.

1910 *The Islands of Titicaca and Koati.* The Hispanic Society of America, New York.

Barbian, Lenore T., and Paul S. Sledzik

2008 Healing Following Cranial Trauma. *Journal of Forensic Science* 53(2):263–268.

Barnes, Ethne

1994 *Developmental Defects of the Axial Skeleton in Paleopathology.* University Press of Colorado, Niwot.

2012 *Atlas of Developmental Field Anomalies of the Human Skeleton: A Paleopathology Perspective.* John Wiley and Sons, Hoboken, N.J.

Bastien, Joseph W.

1987 *Healers of the Andes: Kallawaya Herbalists and Their Medicinal Plants.* University of Utah Press, Salt Lake City.

Bazarsad, Naran

2003 Four Cases of Trepanation from Mongolia, Showing Surgical Variation. In *Trepanation: History, Discovery, Theory*, edited by Robert Arnott, Stanley Finger, and C. U. M. Smith, pp. 203–208. Swets and Zeitlinger, Lisse.

Beckley Foundation

2010 Uncovering the Significance of Trepanation. Electronic document, http://www.beckley foundation.org/2010/09/trepanation/, accessed June 4, 2014.

Bennike, Pia

2003 Ancient Trepanations and Differential Diagnoses: A Re-evaluation of Skeletal Remains from Denmark. In *Trepanation: History, Discovery, Theory*, edited by Robert Arnott, Stanley Finger, and C. U. M. Smith, pp. 95–115. Swets and Zeitlinger, Lisse.

Bookheimer, Susan

2002 Functional MRI of Language: New Approaches to Understanding the Cortical Organization of Semantic Processing. *Annual Review of Neuroscience* 25:151–188.

Breasted, James H.

1930 *The Edwin Smith Surgical Papyrus.* University of Chicago, Chicago.

Broca, Paul

1867 Cas singulier de trépanation chez les Incas. *Bulletins de la Société d'Anthropologie de Paris* 2:403–408.

Brooks, O. N., M. E. Aughton, M. R. Bond, P. Jones, and S. Rizvi

1980 Cognitive Sequelae in Relationship to Early Indices of Severity of Brain Damage after Severe Blunt Head Injury. *Journal of Neurology, Neurosurgery, and Psychiatry* 43:529–534.

Brothwell, Donald R.

1959 Notable Examples of Early Trephining. *Man* 59:95–96.

1974 Osteological Evidence of the Use of a Surgical Modiolus in a Romano-British Population: An Aspect of Primitive Technology. *Journal of Archaeological Science* 1:209–211.

1994 Ancient Trephining: Multi-Focal Evolution or Trans-World Diffusion? *Journal of Paleopathology* 6(3):129–138.

2003 The Future Direction of Research. In *Trepanation: History, Discovery, Theory*, edited by Robert Arnott, Stanley Finger, and C. U. M. Smith, pp. 365–372. Swets and Zeitlinger, Lisse.

Brown Vega, Margaret, and Nathan Craig

2009 New Experimental Data on the Distance of Sling Projectiles. *Journal of Archaeological Science* 36(6):1264–1268.

Bruesch, S. R.

1974 A Cure for Scalped Head. *Morristown Journal of Pathology* 1(1):23–26.

Buikstra, Jane E., and Douglas H. Ubelaker

1994 *Standards for Data Collection from Human Skeletal Remains*. Arkansas Archaeological Survey, Fayetteville.

Buikstra, Jane E., Donald J. Ortner, and Stephanie McBride-Schreiner

2012 Aleš Hrdlička (1869–1943): Contributions to Paleopathology. In *The Global History of Paleopathology: Pioneers and Prospects*, edited by Jane E. Buikstra and Charlotte A. Roberts, pp. 174–178. Oxford University Press, New York.

Burger, Richard L., and Lucy C. Salazar

2004 *Machu Picchu: Unveiling the Mystery of the Incas*. Yale University Press, New Haven.

Burger, Richard L., Karen L. Mohr Chávez, and Sergio J. Chávez

2000 Through the Glass Darkly: Prehispanic Obsidian Procurement and Exchange in Southern Peru and Northern Bolivia. *Journal of World Prehistory* 14(3):267–362.

Burton, Frank A.

1920 Prehistoric Trephining of the Frontal Sinus. *California State Journal of Medicine* 18:321–324.

Cabieses, Fernando

1974 *Dioses y enfermedades: La medicina en el antiguo Peru)/Gods and Disease: Medicine in Ancient Peru*. G Ediciones e Impresiones, Lima.

Campillo, Domènec

2007 *La trepanación prehistórica*. Edicions Bellaterra, Barcelona.

Carod-Artal, F. J., and C. B. Vazquez-Cabrera

2004 Paleopatología neurológica en las culturas pre-colombinas de la costa y el altiplano andino (II): Historia de las trepanaciones craneales. *Revista de neurologia* 38(9):886–894.

Carrión Cachot, Rebeca

1949 *Paracas Cultural Elements*. Corporación Nacional de Turismo, Lima.

Cederlund, C.-G., L. Andrén, and H. Olivecrona

1982 Progressive Bilateral Thinning of the Parietal Bones. *Skeletal Radiology* 8(1):29–33.

Chacon, Richard J., and Ruben G. Mendoza

2007 *Latin American Indigenous Warfare and Ritual Violence*. University of Arizona Press, Tucson.

Chapin, Heath McBain, and Adolph F. Bandelier

1961 *The Adolph Bandelier Archaeological Collection from Pelechuco and Charassani, Bolivia*. Universidad Nacional del Litoral, Facultad de Filosofía y Letras, Rosario, Argentina.

Chege, Nancy, David J. Sartoris, Rose Tyson, and Donald Resnick

1996 Imaging Evaluation of Skull Trepanation Using Radiography and CT. *International Journal of Osteoarchaeology* 6(3):249–258.

Christensen, Alexander F., and Marcus Winter

1997 Culturally Modified Skeletal Remains from the Site of Huamelulpan, Oaxaca, Mexico. *International Journal of Osteoarchaeology* 7(5):467–480.

Cieza de León, Pedro de

1941 [1553] *La crónica del Peru*. 3rd ed. Espasa-Calpe, Madrid.

Clower, W. T., and S. Finger

2001 Discovering Trepanation: The Contribution of Paul Broca. *Neurosurgery* 49(6):1417–1426.

Colton, Michael

1998 You Need It Like . . . a Hole in the Head? *The Washington Post*, May 31. Electronic document, http://www.washingtonpost.com/wp-srv/style/features/trepan.htm, accessed June 26, 2015.

Cook, Della Collins

2000 Trepanation or Trephination? The Orthography of Paleopathology. *Paleopathology Newsletter* 111:9–12.

Cope, V. Zachary

1914 Notes of a Case of Traumatic Sensory Aphasia, Treated Successfully by Trephining and Removal of Clot. *Proceedings of the Royal Society of Medicine* 7(Clin Sect):128–130.

Corbetta, Maurizio

2012 Functional Connectivity and Neurological Recovery. *Developmental Psychobiology* 54(3):239–253.

Courville, Cyril B.

1959 Cranioplasty in Prehistoric Times. *Bulletin of the Los Angeles Neurological Society* 24(1):1–8.

Coxon, Ann

1962 The Kisii Art of Trephining. *Guy's Hospital Gazette* 76:263.

Crubézy, Érik, Jaroslav Bruzek, Jean Guilaine, Eugenia Cunha, Daniel Rougé, and Jan Jelinek

2001 The Antiquity of Cranial Surgery in Europe and in the Mediterranean Basin. *Comptes rendus de l'Académie des Sciences, series IIA, Earth and Planetary Science* 332(6):417–423.

Crump, J. A.

1901 Trephining in the South Seas. *Journal of the Royal Anthropological Institute* 31:167–172.

Dabdoub, Carlos F., and Carlos B. Dabdoub

2013   The History of Neurosurgery in Bolivia and Pediatric Neurosurgery in Santa Cruz de La Sierra. *Surgical Neurology International* 4. Electronic document, http://www.ncbi.nlm.nih.gov/pmc/articles/PMC3815021/, accessed January 26, 2014.

Daggett, Richard E.

1994   The Paracas Mummy Bundles of the Great Necropolis of Wari Kayan: A History. *Andean Past* 4:53–75.

Damasio, Antonio R., and Norman Geschwind

1984   The Neural Basis of Language. *Annual Review of Neuroscience* 7:127–147.

Dar, Jawahar

1985   Perspectives in International Neurosurgery: Neurosurgery in Kenya. *Neurosurgery* 16(2):267–269.

De Divitiis, Enrico

2013   The Prehistoric Practice of Trepanation. *World Neurosurgery* 80(6):821–823.

DeLeonardis, Lisa

2005   Early Paracas Cultural Contexts: New Evidence from Callango. *Andean Past* 7:27–55.

Della Croce, Giovanni Andrea

1596   *Chirurgiae universalis opus absolutum In quo quorumcunque affectuum universo corpori humano obvenientium, & ad chirurgi curam spectantium, notio, praedictio, atque curatio perspicua methodo narrantur . . . Addita insuper est officina chirurgica, in qua nempe instrumenta omnia aliaque chirurgico convenientia suis figuris delineata expressaque cernuntur.* Robertum Meiettum, Venice.

Dement, Brittany

2012   Cranial Injury in the Central Highlands of Peru. Paper presented at the 39th Annual Meeting of the Paleopathology Association, Portland, Ore.

Di Matteo, Berardo, Vittorio Tarabella, Giuseppe Filardo, Anna Viganó, Patrizia Tomba, and Maurilio Maracacci

2013   The Renaissance and the Universal Surgeon: Giovanni Andrea Della Croce, a Master of Traumatology. *International Orthopaedics* 37(12):2523–2528.

Dobson, Jessie, and Robert Milnes Walker

1979   *Barbers and Barber-Surgeons of London: A History of the Barbers' and Barber-Surgeons' Companies.* Blackwell Scientific Publications, Oxford.

Do Carmo de Oliveira Ribeiro, Maria, Carlos U. Pereira, Ana M. C. Sallum, Paulo Ricardo S. Martins-Filho, Josimari M. DeSantana, Mariangela da Silva Nunes, and Edilene C. Horta

2013   Immediate Post-Craniotomy Headache. *Cephalalgia* 33(11):897–905.

Donovan, Daniel J.

2005   Simple Depressed Skull Fracture Causing Sagittal Sinus Stenosis and Increased Intracranial Pressure: Case Report and Review of the Literature. *Surgical Neurology* 63(4):380–384.

Doyle, Mary

1988   The Ancestor Cult and Burial Ritual in Seventeenth- and Eighteenth-Century Central Peru. PhD dissertation, University of California, Los Angeles.

Drusini, Andrea G.

1991   Skeletal Evidence of Three Pre-Columbian Coastal Peoples from Nasca, Peru. *Homo: Journal of Comparative Human Biology* 42(2):150–162.

Drusini, Andrea G., Nicola Carrara, Guiseppe Orefici, and M. Rippa Bonati

2001   Palaeodemography of the Nasca Valley: Reconstruction of the Human Ecology in the Southern Peruvian Coast. *Homo: Journal of Comparative Human Biology* 52(2):157–172.

Dwyer, Jane Powell, and Edward B. Dwyer

1975   The Paracas Cemeteries: Mortuary Patterns in a Peruvian South Coastal Tradition. In *Death and the Afterlife in Pre-Columbian America*, edited by Elizabeth P. Benson, pp. 145–161. Dumbarton Oaks Research Library and Collection, Washington, D.C.

Eaton, George Francis

1916   *The Collection of Osteological Material from Machu Picchu.* Tuttle Morehouse and Taylor, New Haven, Conn.

Ferembach, Denise

1962   *La nécropole épipaléolithique de Taforalt, Maroc Oriental, étude de squelettes humains.* Centre National de la Recherche Scientific, Rabat.

Fernando, H. R., and Stanley Finger

2003   Ephraim George Squier's Peruvian Skull and the Discovery of Cranial Trepanation. In *Trepanation: History, Discovery, Theory*, edited by Robert Arnott, Stanley Finger, and C. U. M. Smith, pp. 3–18. Swets and Zeitlinger, Lisse.

Filley, Christopher M.
   1995   *Neurobehavioral Anatomy*. University Press of
          Colorado, Niwot.

Finger, Stanley, and H. R. Fernando
   2001   E. G. Squier and the Discovery of Cranial
          Trepanation: A Landmark in the History of
          Surgery and Ancient Medicine. *Journal of the
          History of Medicine and Allied Sciences* 56:353–381.

Finger, Stanley, and W. T. Clower
   2003   On the Birth of Trepanation: The Thoughts of
          Paul Broca and Victor Horsley. In *Trepanation:
          History, Discovery, Theory*, edited by Robert
          Arnott, Stanley Finger, and C. U. M. Smith,
          pp. 19–42. Swets and Zeitlinger, Lisse.

Fletcher, Robert
   1882   *On Prehistoric Trephining and Cranial Amulets*.
          Government Printing Office, Washington, D.C.

Ford, Edward
   1937   Trephining in Melanesia. *The Medical Journal of
          Australia* 2:471–477.

Furnas, David W., M. Ashraf Sheikh, Pieter van den
Hombergh, Frank Froeling, and Issac M. Nunda
   1985   Traditional Craniotomies of the Kisii Tribe of
          Kenya. *Annals of Plastic Surgery* 15(6):538–556.

Gaither, Catherine
   2010   Osteological Report: Municipal Museum in
          Lamud. Report on file at the Municipal Museum
          of Lamud Departamento de Amazonas, Peru.

Ganz, Jeremy C., and Jurgen Arndt
   2014   A History of Depressed Skull Fractures from
          Ancient Times to 1800. *Journal of the History
          of the Neurosciences* 23(3):1–19.

Gasparini, Graziano, and Luise Margolies
   1980   *Inca Architecture*. Indiana University Press,
          Bloomington.

Gerdau-Radonić, Karina, and Alexander Herrera
   2010a Sixteen Trepanations on Eight Skulls from
          Keushu (Ancash, Peru). *American Journal of
          Physical Anthropology*, supplement 50:110–110.
   2010b Why Dig Looted Tombs? Two Examples and
          Some Answers from Keushu (Ancash Highlands,
          Peru). *Bulletins et mémoires de la société
          d'anthropologie de Paris* 22(3–4):145–156.

Germanà, Franco, and Gino Fornaciari
   1992   *Trapanazioni, craniotomie e traumi cranici in
          Italia: Dalla preistoria all'età moderna*, vol. 5.
          Giardini Editori e Stampatori, Pisa.

Goldsmith, Willliam M
   1945   Trepanation and the "Catlin Mark." *American
          Antiquity* 10(4):348–353.

Gomez, J. G.
   1973   Paleoneurosurgery in Colombia. *Journal of
          Neurosurgery* 39(5):585–588.

Gonzáles, César W. Astuhuamán, and Richard E.
Daggett
   2005   Julio César Tello Rojas: Una biografía. In
          Paracas, edited by Julio C. Tello and César
          W. Astuhuamán Gonzáles, pp. 17–51. 2nd ed.
          Universidad Alas Peruanas; Corporación
          Financiera de Desarrollo; Fondo Editorial,
          Universidad Nacional Mayor de San Marcos;
          Centro Cultural de San Marcos; Museo de
          Arqueología y Antropología, UNMSM, Lima.

González, Elena, and Rafo León (editors)
   2002   *Chachapoyas: El reino perdido*. INTEGRA AFP,
          Lima.

Goodrich, James Tait
   1997   Neurosurgery in the Ancient and Medieval
          Worlds. In *A History of Neurosurgery: In Its
          Scientific and Professional Contexts*, edited by
          Samuel H. Greenblatt, T. Forcht Dagi, and Mel
          H. Epstein, pp. 37–64. American Association of
          Neurological Surgeons, Park Ridge, Ill.

Graña, Francisco, Esteban D. Rocca, and Luis Graña
   1954   *Las trepanaciones craneanas en el Perú en la época
          pre-hispánica*. Imprenta Santa María, Lima.

Greenblatt, Samuel H., T. Forcht Dagi, and Mel H.
Epstein, eds.
   1997   *A History of Neurosurgery: In Its Scientific and
          Professional Contexts*. American Association of
          Neurological Surgeons, Park Ridge, Ill.

Gross, Charles G.
   1999   A Hole in the Head. *Neuroscientist* 5:263–269.
   2003   Trepanation from the Palaeolithic to the Internet.
          In *Trepanation: History, Discovery, Theory*, edited
          by Robert Arnott, Stanley Finger, and C. U. M.
          Smith, pp. 307–322. Swets and Zeitlinger, Lisse.

Grounds, John G.
   1958   Trephining of the Skull amongst the Kisii. *East
          African Medical Journal* 35:369.

Guillén, Sonia
   2007   Preserving the Heritage of the Chachapoya. In
          *Chachapoya Textiles: The Laguna de Los Cóndores
          Textiles in the Museo Leymebamba, Chachapoyas,
          Peru*, edited by Lena Bjerregaard, pp. 23–28.
          Museum Tusculanum Press, University of
          Copenhagen, Copenhagen.

Gump, William

2010 Modern Induced Skull Deformity in Adults. *Neurosurgical Focus* 29(6):1–4.

Han, Kangxin, and Xingcan Cheng

2007 The Archaeological Evidence of Trepanation in Early China. *Indo-Pacific Prehistory Association Bulletin* 27:22–27.

Handy, Edward Smith Craighill

1923 *The Native Culture in the Marquesas*, vol. 9. Bernice P. Bishop Museum, Honolulu.

Hemming, John, and Edward Ranney

1982 *Monuments of the Incas*. Little, Brown, Boston.

Herrera, Robinson A.

2003 *Natives, Europeans, and Africans in Sixteenth-Century Santiago de Guatemala*. University of Texas Press, Austin.

Heyerdahl, Thor

1952 *American Indians in the Pacific*. Allen and Unwin, London.

Hilton-Simpson, M. W.

1922 *Arab Medicine and Surgery: A Study of the Healing Arts in Algeria*. Oxford University Press, London.

Holck, P.

2008 Two Medieval "Trepanations"—Therapy or Swindle? *International Journal of Osteoarchaeology* 18(2):188–194.

Holliday, Diane Young

1993 Occipital Lesions: A Possible Cost of Cradleboards. *American Journal of Physical Anthropology* 90:283–290.

Horrax, Gilbert

1952 *Neurosurgery, an Historical Sketch*. American Lecture Series, no. 117. Thomas, Springfield, Ill.

Hoshower, Lisa M., Paul S. Goldstein, Ann D. Webster, and Jane E. Buikstra

1995 Artificial Cranial Deformation at the Omo M10 Site: A Tiwanaku Complex from the Moquegua Valley, Peru. *Latin American Antiquity* 6(2):145–164.

Hrdlička, Aleš

1911 Some Results of Recent Anthropological Exploration in Peru. *Smithsonian Miscellaneous Collections* 56(16):1–16.

1914 *Anthropological Work in Peru, in 1913, with Notes on the Pathology of the Ancient Peruvians, with Twenty-Six Plates*. Smithsonian Miscellaneous Collections 61, no. 18. Smithsonian Institution, Washington, D.C.

1932 Disease, Medicine, and Surgery among the American Aborigines. *Journal of the American Medical Association* 99:1661–1666.

1939 Trepanation among Prehistoric People, Especially in America. *Ciba Symposia* 1:170–177.

Huang, Yu-Hua, Tao-Chen Lee, Tsung-Han Lee, Chen-Chieh Liao, Jason Sheehan, and Aij-Lie Kwan

2013 Thirty-Day Mortality in Traumatically Brain-Injured Patients Undergoing Decompressive Craniectomy. *Journal of Neurosurgery* 118(6):1329–1335.

Ibarra Asencios, Bebel

2014 Espacio y cronología en la sierra de norte del Perú: Balance de las investigaciones arqueológicas en la provincia de Huari. In *Cien años de la arqueología de Ancash*, edited by Bebel Ibarra Asencios, pp. 11–43. Instituto de Estudios Huarinos, Huari.

International Trepanation Advocacy Group (ITAG)

2014 International Trepanation Advocacy Group (ITAG) web page. Electronic document, http://www.trepan.com/, accessed June 4, 2014.

Isbell, William H.

1997 *Mummies and Mortuary Monuments: A Postprocessual Prehistory of Central Andean Organization*. University of Texas Press, Austin.

Jackson, Ralph

1988 *Doctors and Diseases in the Roman Empire*. University of Oklahoma Press, Norman.

1990 Roman Doctors and Their Instruments: Recent Research into Ancient Practice. *Journal of Roman Archaeology* 3:5–27.

Jakobsen, Jan, J. Balslev Jorgensen, L. Kempfner Jorgensen, and Inge Schjellerup

1987 "Cazadores de cabezas" en sitios pre-inca de Chachapoyas, Amazonas. *Revista del Museo Nacional* 48:135–185. Peru.

Janusek, John Wayne

2007 *Ancient Tiwanaku: Civilization in the High Andes*. Cambridge University Press, Cambridge.

Jennett, W. Bryan, and J. D. Miller

1972 Infection After Depressed Fracture of Skull: Implications for Management of Nonmissile Injuries. *Journal of Neurosurgery* 36(3):333–339.

Jørgensen, J. B.

1988 Trepanation as a Therapeutic Measure in Ancient (Pre-Inka) Peru. *Acta Neurochirurgica* 93:3–5.

Juengst, Sara L., and Sergio J. Chávez

2015 Three Trepanned Skulls from the Copacabana Peninsula in the Titicaca Basin, Bolivia (800 BC–AD 1000). *International Journal of Paleopathology* 9:20–27.

Julien, Catherine J.

2004 Las tumbas de Sacsahuaman y el estilo cuzco-inca. Ñawpa *Pacha* 25–27:1–125.

Katz, Douglas I., et al.

2009 Natural History of Recovery from Brain Injury after Prolonged Disorders of Consciousness: Outcome of Patients Admitted to Inpatient Rehabilitation with 1–4 Year Follow-Up. *Progress in Brain Research* 177:73–88.

Kauffmann Doig, Federico, and Giancarlo Ligabue

2003 *Los Chachapoya(s): Moradores ancestrales de los andes amazónicos peruanos.* UAP, Lima.

Kaufman, M. H., D. Whitaker, and J. McTavish

1997 Differential Diagnosis of Holes in the Calvarium: Application of Modern Clinical Data to Palaeo-pathology. *Journal of Archaeological Science* 24:193–218.

Kellner, Corina Marie

2002 *Coping with Environmental and Social Challenges in Prehistoric Peru: Bioarchaeological Analyses of Nasca Populations.* PhD dissertation, University of California, Santa Barbara.

Kendall, Ann

1985 *Aspects of Inca Architecture: Description, Function, and Chronology.* British Archaeological Reports International Series, no. 242. Archaeopress, Oxford.

Kinsman, Michael, Courtney Pendleton, Alfredo Quinones-Hinojosa, and Aaron A.Cohen-Gadol

2013 Harvey Cushing's Early Experience with the Surgical Treatment of Head Trauma. *Journal of the History of the Neurosciences* 22:96–115.

Kirkup, John

2003 The Evolution of Cranial Saws and Related Instruments. In *Trepanation: History, Discovery, Theory,* edited by Robert Arnott, Stanley Finger, and C. U. M. Smith, pp. 289–304. Swets and Zeitlinger, Lisse.

Klaus, Haagen D., and Elizabeth E. Byrnes

2013 Cranial Lesions and Maxillofacial Asymmetry in an Archaeological Skeleton from Peru: A Paleopathological Case of Possible Trauma-Induced Epidermal Inclusion Cysts. *Journal of Cranio-Maxillary Diseases* 2(1):46.

Koschmieder, Klaus, and Catherine Gaither

2010 Tumbas de guerreros Chachapoya en abrigos rocosos de la provincia de Luya, Departamento de Amazonas. *Arqueología y sociedad* 22:1–30.

Künzl, Ernst, Franz Josef Hassel, and Susanna Künzl

1983 *Medizinische Instrumente aus Sepulkralfunden der Römischen Kaiserzeit.* Rheinland Verlag, Cologne.

Kurin, Danielle Shawn

2012 The Bioarchaeology of Collapse: Ethnogenesis and Ethnocide in Post-Imperial Andahuaylas, Peru (AD 900–1250). PhD dissertation, Vanderbilt University.

2013 Trepanation in South-Central Peru during the Early Late Intermediate Period (ca. AD 1000–1250). *American Journal of Physical Anthropology* 152(4):484–494.

Kushner, David

1998 Mild Traumatic Brain Injury: Toward Understanding Manifestations and Treatment. *Archives of Internal Medicine* 158:1617–1624.

2010 Principles of Neurorehabilitation. In *Neurology for the Non-Neurologist,* edited by William J. Weiner and Christopher G. Goetz, pp. 551–571. 6th ed. Lippincott, Philadelphia.

Ladino, Lady Diana, Gary Hunter, and José Francisco Téllez-Zenteno

2013 Art and Epilepsy Surgery. *Epilepsy and Behavior* 29(1):82–89.

Lastres, Juan B.

1951 *La medicina incaica.* Vol. 1 of *Historia de la medicina peruana.* Imprenta Santa Maria, Lima.

Lastres, Juan B., and Fernando Cabieses

1960 *La trepanación del cráneo en el antiguo Peru.* Universidad Nacional Mayor de San Marcos, Lima.

Lau, George F.

2011 *Andean Expressions: Art and Archaeology of the Recuay Culture.* University of Iowa Press, Iowa City.

Lewis, Anthony J.

1976 *Mechanisms of Neurological Disease.* Little, Brown, Boston.

Lillie, Malcolm C.

1998 Cranial Surgery Dates Back to Mesolithic. *Nature,* February 26.

2003 Cranial Surgery: The Epipaleolithic to Neolithic Populations of Ukraine. In *Trepanation: History, Discovery, Theory*, edited by Robert Arnott, Stanley Finger, and C. U. M. Smith, pp. 175–188. Swets and Zeitlinger, Lisse.

Lingsma, Hester F., Bob Roozenbeek, Ewout W. Steyerberg, Gordon D. Murray, and Andrew I. R. Maas
2010 Early Prognosis in Traumatic Brain Injury: From Prophecies to Predictions. *The Lancet Neurology* 9(5):543–554.

Lisowski, F. P.
1967 Prehistoric and Early Historic Trepanation. In *Diseases in Antiquity*, edited by Donald R. Brothwell and A. T. Sandison, pp. 651–672. Charles C. Thomas, Springfield, Ill.

Littleton, Judith, and Karen Frifelt
2006 Trepanations from Oman: A Case of Diffusion? *Arabian Archaeology and Epigraphy* 17(2):139–151.

Llanos, Luis A.
1936 Trabajos arqueológicos en el dep. del Cuzco bajo la dirección del D. Luis E. Valcárcel: Informe sobre Ollantaitambo de Luis A. Llanos. *Revista del Museo Nacional* 5(2), II semestre:123–156.
1941 Exploraciones arqueológicas en Quimsarumiyoc y Huaccanhuayco-Calca. *Revista del Museo Nacional* 10(2):240–262.

Lloyd, Geoffrey Ernest Richard
1975 The Hippocratic Question. *The Classical Quarterly* 25(2):171–192.

Long, Donlin M., Toby Gordon, Helen Bowman, Anthony Etzel, Gregg M. Burleyson, Simone Betchen, Ira M. Garonzik, and Henry Brem
2003 Outcome and Cost of Craniotomy Performed to Treat Tumors in Regional Academic Referral Centers. *Neurosurgery* 52(5):1056–1063.

Loring, Stephen, and Miroslav Prokopec
1994 A Most Peculiar Man: The Life and Times of Aleš Hrdlička. In *Reckoning with the Dead: The Larsen Bay Repatriation and the Smithsonian Institution*, edited by Tamara L. Bray and Thomas W. Killion, pp. 26–40. Smithsonian Institution Press, Washington, D.C.

Lothrop, Samuel Kirkland
1948 Un recuerdo del Dr. Julio C. Tello y Paracas. *Revista del Museo Nacional de Antropología y Arqueología* 2(1):53–54.

Lovell, Nancy C.
1997 Trauma Analysis in Paleopathology. *Yearbook of Physical Anthropology* 40:139–170.

Lucas-Championnière, Just Marie
1912 *Les origines de la trépanation décompressive: Trépanation néolithique, trépanation pré-colombienne, trépanation des kabyles, trépanation traditionnelle et de leur signification au point de vue de l'anthropologie zoologique par le Dr Lucas-Championnière.* G. Steinheil, Paris.

Lund Valle, Mellisa
2009 *Muerte y traumatismos en el periodo colonial temprano y su relación con los mecanismos y posibles armas causantes en el Cementerio 57AS03 de Puruchuco-Huaquerones Perú.* MA thesis, Pontificia Universidad Católica del Perú, Lima.

Luria, Alexander R.
1963 *Restoration of Function after Brain Injury.* Macmillan, New York.

Lv, Xianli, Zhenguang Li, and Youxiang Li
2013 Prehistoric Skull Trepanation in China. *World Neurosurgery* 80(6):897–899.

MacCurdy, George G.
1918 Surgery Among the Ancient Peruvians. *Art and Archaeology* 7(9):381–394.
1923 Human Skeletal Remains from the Highlands of Peru. *American Journal of Physical Anthropology* 6:217–329.

Malpass, Michael A.
1993 *Provincial Inca: Archaeological and Ethnohistorical Assessment of the Impact of the Inca State.* University of Iowa Press, Iowa City.

Margetts, Edward L.
1967 Trepanation of the Skull by the Medicine-Men of Primitive Cultures, with Particular Reference to Present-Day Native East African Practice. In *Diseases in Antiquity: A Survey of the Diseases, Injuries, and Surgery of Early Populations*, edited by Donald R. Brothwell and A. T. Sandison, pp. 673–701. Charles C. Thomas., Springfield, Ill.

Marino, Raúl, Jr., and Marco Gonzales-Portillo
2000 Preconquest Peruvian Neurosurgeons: A Study of Inca and Pre-Columbian Trephination and the Art of Medicine in Ancient Peru. *Neurosurgery* 47(4):940–50.

Márquez Morfín, Lourdes, and E. González Licón
1992 La trepanación craneana entre los antiguos zapotecos de Monte Albán. *Cuadernos sel sur* (Oaxaca) 1:25–50.

Martin, Graham
1995 Trepanation in the South Pacific. *Journal of Clinical Neuroscience* 2(3):257–264.

2003 Why Trepan? Contributions from Medical History and the South Pacific. In *Trepanation: History, Discovery, Theory*, edited by Robert Arnott, Stanley Finger, and C. U. M. Smith, pp. 323–345. Swets and Zeitlinger, Lisse.

McEwan, Gordon F.
1987 *The Middle Horizon in the Valley of Cuzco, Peru: The Impact of the Wari Occupation of Pikillacta in the Lucre Basin.* BAR, Oxford.

McEwan, Gordon F., Melissa Chatfield, and Arminda Gibaja
2002 The Archaeology of Inca Origins: Excavations at Chokepukio, Cuzco, Peru. In *Andean Archaeology I: Variations in Sociopolitical Organization,* edited by William H. Isbell and Helaine Silverman, 287–301. Kluwer Academic/Plenum Publishers, New York.

McIntyre, Loren
1975 *The Incredible Incas and Their Timeless Land.* National Geographic Society, Washington, D.C.

Meador, Kimford J., David W. Loring, and Herman F. Flanigin
1989 History of Epilepsy Surgery. *Journal of Epilepsy* 2(1):21–25.

Mendonça de Souza, Sheila M. F., Karl J. Reinhard, and Andrea Lessa
2008 Cranial Deformation as the Cause of Death for a Child from the Chillon River Valley, Peru. *Chungara, revista de antropología chilena* 40(1):41–53.

Merbs, C. F.
1989 Trauma. In *Reconstruction of Life from the Skeleton,* edited by Mehmet Yasar Iscan and Kenneth A. R. Kennedy, pp. 161–189. Alan R. Liss, New York.

Meschig, Rolf
1983 *Zur Geschicht der Trepanation unter Besonderer Berücksichtigung der Schädeloperationen bei den Kisii im Hochland Westkenias.* Triltsch Druck und Verlag, Dusseldorf.

Meyer, Mark
1979 Trephination in Pre-Columbian Peru. Unpublished honors thesis in Anthropology, Harvard College, Cambridge, Mass.

Miller, George R.
2003 Food for the Dead, Tools for the Afterlife: Zooarchaeology at Machu Picchu. In *The 1912 Yale Peruvian Scientific Expedition Collections from Machu Picchu: Human and Animal Remains,* edited by Richard L. Burger and Lucy C. Salazar, pp. 1–64. Yale University Division of Anthropology, Peabody Museum of Natural History, New Haven, Conn.

Miller, J. D., and W. Bryan Jennett
1968 Complications of Depressed Skull Fracture. *Lancet* 2:991–995.

Moodie, Roy L.
1919 Studies in Paleopathology. *The Surgical Clinics of Chicago* 3(3).

Moseley, Michael E.
1992 *The Incas and Their Ancestors: The Archaeology of Peru.* Thames and Hudson, New York.

Moskalenko, Yuri E.
2009 *Non-Invasive Evaluation of Human Brain Fluid Dynamics and Skull Biomechanics in Relation to Cognitive Functioning: A Review of Three Years of Scientific Collaboration between the Institute of Evolutionary Physiology and Biochemistry, Russian Academy of Sciences [and] the Beckley Foundation, UK.* Beckley Foundation Press, Oxford.

Moskalenko, Yuri E., S. V. Mozhaev, and G. Weinstein, et al.
2008 Effects of Cranial Trepanation on the Functioning of Cerebrovascular and Cerebrospinal Fluid Systems. *International Journal of Psychophysiology* 69(3):302–303.

Mountrakis, C., S. Georgaki, and S. K. Manolis
2011 A Trephined Late Bronze Age Skull from Peloponnesus, Greece. *Mediterranean Archaeology and Archaeometry* 11(1):1–8.

Mueller, Michael D., and Charles S. Finch III
1994 Kisii Trepanation: An Ancient Surgical Procedure in Modern-Day Kenya. *The Explorers Journal* 72:10–16.

Muñiz, Manuel Antonio, and W. J. McGee
1897 *Primitive Trephining in Peru.* Sixteenth Annual Report, Bureau of American Ethnology, Smithsonian Institution, Washington, D.C.

Murphy, Eileen M.
2003 Trepanations and Perforated Crania from Iron Age South Siberia: An Exercise in Differential Diagnosis. In *Trepanation: History, Discovery, Theory*, edited by Robert Arnott, Stanley Finger, and C. U. M. Smith, pp. 209–221. Swets and Zeitlinger, Lisse.

Murphy, Melissa S., Catherine Gaither, Elena Goycochea, John W. Verano, and Guillermo Cock
2010 Violence and Weapon-Related Trauma at Puruchuco-Huaquerones, Peru. *American Journal of Physical Anthropology* 142:636–649.

Muscutt, Keith
1998 *Warriors of the Clouds: A Lost Civilization of the Upper Amazon of Peru.* University of New Mexico Press, Albuquerque.

Musgrave, Jonathan
1990 Dust and Damn'd Oblivion: A Study of Cremation in Ancient Greece. *The Annual of the British School at Athens* 85:271–299.

Nakase-Richardson, Risa, et al.
2011 Utility of Post-Traumatic Amnesia in Predicting 1-Year Productivity Following Traumatic Brain Injury: Comparison of the Russell and Mississippi PTA Classification Intervals. *Journal of Neurology, Neurosurgery, and Psychiatry* 82(5):494–499.

Narváez Vargas, Alfredo
2009 *Arqueología y conservación.* Vol. 1 of *Proyecto de emergencia para la investigación, conservación, y acondicionamiento turístico de la fortaleza de Kuelap Etapa V.* MinceBtur, Plan Copesco Nacional, Gobierno Regional de Amazonas, Instituto Nacional de Cultura, Chachapoyas.

Nerlich, Andreas, G., O. Peschel, Albert Zink, and Friedrich W. Rösing
2003 The Pathology of Trepanation: Differential Diagnosis, Healing, and Dry Bone Appearance in Modern Cases. In *Trepanation: History, Discovery, Theory,* edited by Robert Arnott, Stanley Finger, and C. U. M. Smith, pp. 43–51. Swets and Zeitlinger, Lisse.

Nerlich, Andreas G., Albert Zink, Ulrike Szeimies, Hjalmar G. Hagedorn, and Friedrich W. Rösing
2005 Perforating Skull Trauma in Ancient Egypt and Evidence for Early Neurosurgical Therapy. In *Trepanation: History, Discovery, Theory,* edited by Robert Arnott, Stanley Finger, and C. U. M. Smith, pp. 191–201. Swets and Zeitlinger, Lisse.

Netter, Frank H.
1977 *The Ciba Collection of Medical Illustrations.* Vol. 1 of *Nervous System.* CIBA/Case-Hoyt, Rochester.

Niles, Susan A.
1999 *The Shape of Inca History: Narrative and Architecture in an Andean Empire.* University of Iowa Press, Iowa City.

Nystrom, Kenneth C.
2004 Trauma y identidad entre Los Chachapoya. *Sian* 9(15):20–21.
2007 Trepanation in the Chachapoya Region of Northern Peru. *International Journal of Osteoarchaeology* 17(1):39–51.

Nystrom, Kenneth C., and J. Marla Toyne
2014 "Place of Strong Men": Skeletal Trauma and the (Re)construction of Chachapoya Identity. In *The Routledge Handbook of the Bioarchaeology of Human Conflict,* edited by Christopher Knüsel and Martin J. Smith, pp. 371–388. Routledge, London and New York.

Oakley, K. P., Winifred M. A. Brooke, A. Roger Akester, and D. R. Brothwell
1959 Contributions on Trepanning or Trephination in Ancient and Modern Times. *Man* 59:93–96.

Oliver, Thomas
1888 Notes on a Case of Traumatic Epilepsy Successfully Treated by Trephining. *British Medical Journal* 1:236–237.

Orlove, Benjamin
1994 Sticks and Stones: Ritual Battles and Play in the Southern Peruvian Andes. In *Unruly Order: Violence, Power, and Identity in the Southern High Provinces of Peru,* edited by Deborah A. Poole, pp. 133–164. Westview Press, Boulder, Colo.

Orman, J. A., D. Geyer, J. Jones, E. B. Schneider, J. Grafman, M. J. Pugh, and J. Dubose
2012 Epidemiology of Moderate to Severe Penetrating Versus Closed Traumatic Brain Injury in the Iraq and Afghanistan Wars. *Journal of Trauma and Acute Care Surgery* 73(6), supplement 5.

Ortner, Donald J.
2003 *Identification of Pathological Conditions in Human Skeletal Remains.* 2nd ed. Academic Press, San Diego.

Pahl, Wolfgang M.
1992 A Singular Case of Craniotomy from Al-Kōm Al-Ahmar/Šārūna: New Light on the Medical Practice of Ancient Egypt. In *Proceedings of the First World Congress on Mummy Studies,* edited by Conrado Rodriguez-Martín, pp. 387–393. Museo Arqueológico y Etnográfico de Tenerife, Tenerife.

Panourias, Ioannis G., Panayiotis K. Skiadas, Damianos E. Sakas, and Spyros G. Marketos
2005 Hippocrates: A Pioneer in the Treatment of Head Injuries. *Neurosurgery* 57(1):181–189.

Papagrigorakis, Manolis J., Panagiotis Toulas, Manolis G. Tsilivakos, Antonis A. Kousoulis, Despina Skorda, George Orfanidis, and Philippos N Synodinos

2014　Neurosurgery During the Bronze Age: A Skull Trepanation in 1900 BC Greece. *World Neurosurgery* 81(2):431–435.

Parry, T. Wilson

1936　Three Skulls from Palestine Showing Two Types of Primitive Surgical Holing; Being the First Skulls Exhibiting This Phenomenon that Have Been Discovered on the Mainland of Asia. *Man* 36:170.

Patt, Stephan, and Michael Brodhun

1999　Neuropathological Sequelae of Traumatic Injury in the Brain: An Overview. *Experimental and Toxicologic Pathology* 51(2):119–123.

Paul, Anne

1990　*Paracas Ritual Attire: Symbols of Authority in Ancient Peru.* University of Oklahoma Press, Norman.

Paul, Anne (editor)

1991　*Paracas Art and Architecture: Object and Context in South Coastal Peru.* University of Iowa Press, Iowa City.

Pelling, Margaret

1998　*The Common Lot: Sickness, Medical Occupations, and the Urban Poor in Early Modern England; Essays.* Longman, New York.

Pendleton, Courtney, S. M. Raza, G. L. Gallia, and Alfredo Quiñones-Hinojosa

2014　Harvey Cushing's Early Operative Treatment of Skull Base Fractures. *Journal of Neurological Surgery* 75(1):27–34.

Pendleton, Courtney, Jallo George I., and Alfredo Quiñones-Hinojosa

2012　Early Multimodality Treatment of Intracranial Abscesses. *World Neurosurgery* 78(6):712–714.

Peters, Ann

1987　Chongos: Sitio Paracas en el valle de Pisco. *Gaceta arqueológica andina* 16:30–34.

n.d.　Paracas Archaeology Research Resources. Electronic document, http://www.arqueologia-paracas.net/, accessed June 1, 2014.

Pezzia Assereto, Alejandro

1968　*Ica y el Perú precolombino.* Vol. 1 of *Arqueología de la provincia de Ica.* Editora Ojeda, Ica.

1969　*Guía al mapa arqueológico-pictográfico del departamento de Ica.* Editorial Italperu, Lima.

Piggott, Stuart

1940　A Trepanned Skull of the Beaker Period from Dorset and the Practice of Trepanning in Prehistoric Europe. *Proceedings of the Prehistoric Society* 6:112–132.

Pozo Flórez, C. Auturo del

1988　*Guia de antropología física.* Vol. 1 of *Paracas.* Museo Nacional de Antropología y Arqueología, Lima.

Prescott, William Hickling

1847　*History of the Conquest of Peru, with a Preliminary View of the Civilization of the Incas.* Harper, New York.

Protzen, Jean-Pierre

1993　*Inca Architecture and Construction at Ollantaytambo.* Oxford University Press, New York.

Prunières, Barthélémy

1874　Sur les crânes perforés et les rondelles crâniennes de l'époque Néolithique. *Compte rendu de la association français pour l'avancement des sciences* 3:597–635.

Quevedo, Sergio A.

1941　Los antiguos pobladores del Cuzco (región de Calca). *Revista del Museo Nacional* 10:282–307, and 11:59–96.

1943a　La trepanación incana en la región de Cuzco. *Revista universitaria* 84:1–197. Universidad Nacional del Cuzco.

1943b　La trepanación incana en la región del Cuzco. *Revista del Museo Nacional* 12–14.

1970　Un caso de trepanación craneana en vivo, realizado con instrumentos pre-colombinos del Museo Arqueológico. *Revista del Museo e Instituto Arqueológico* 22:1–73.

Qureshi, Mubashir Mahmood, and David Oluoch-Olunya

2010　History of Neurosurgery in Kenya, East Africa. *World Neurosurgery* 73(4):261–263.

Rawlings III, Charles E., and Eugene Rossitch Jr.

1994　The History of Trephination in Africa with a Discussion of Its Current Status and Continuing Practice. *Surgical Neurology* 41(6):507–513.

Reichlen, Henry, and Paulette Reichlen

1950　Recherches archéologiques dans les Andes du Haut Utcubamba. *Journal de la Société de Américanistes* 39:219–251.

Richards, Gary D.

1995 Brief Communication: Earliest Cranial Surgery in North America. *American Journal of Physical Anthropology* 98:203–209.

Rifkinson-Mann, Stephanie

1988 Cranial Surgery in Ancient Peru. *Neurosurgery* 23:411–416.

Risdon, D. L.

1939 A Study of the Cranial and Other Human Remains from Palestine Excavated at Tell Duweir (Lachish) by the Wellcome-Marston Archaeological Research Expedition. *Biometrika* 31(1–2):99.

Roberts, Charlotte, and Keith Manchester

1995 *The Archaeology of Disease.* 2nd ed. Cornell University Press, Ithaca, N.Y.

Rocca, Julius

2003 Galen and the Uses of Trepanation. In *Trepanation: History, Discovery, Theory*, edited by Robert Arnott, Stanley Finger, and C. U. M. Smith, pp. 253–271. Swets and Zeitlinger, Lisse.

Rogers, Spencer L.

1938 The Healing of Trephine Wounds in Skulls from Pre-Columbian Peru. *American Journal of Physical Anthropology* 23(3):321–340.

Romero, Julio

1970 Dental Mutiltation, Trephination, and Cranial Deformation. In *Physical Anthropology,* edited by T. D. Stewart, pp. 50–67. Vol. 9 of *Handbook of Middle American Indians,* edited by Robert Wauchope. Unversity of Texas Press, Austin.

Rose, F. Clifford

2003 An Overview from Neolithic Times to Broca. In *Trepanation: History, Discovery, Theory*, edited by Robert Arnott, Stanley Finger, and C. U. M. Smith, pp. 347–363. Swets and Zeitlinger, Lisse.

Rostworowski de Diez Canseco, María

1999 *History of the Inca Realm.* Translated by Harry B. Iceland. Cambridge University Press, Cambridge.

Rowe, John H.

1946 Inca Culture at the Time of the Spanish Conquest. In *Handbook of South American Indians*, vol. 2, edited by Julian H. Steward, pp. 183–330. Government Printing Office, Washington, D.C.

1990 Machu Picchu a la luz de documentos de siglo XVI. *Historica* 14(1):139–154.

Rowe, John H., and Max Uhle

1954 *Max Uhle, 1856–1944: A Memoir of the Father of Peruvian Archaeology.* University of California Press, Berkeley.

Rubini, M.

2008 A Case of Cranial Trepanation in a Roman Necropolis (Cassino, Italy, 3rd Century BC). *International Journal of Osteoarchaeology* 18:95–99.

Ruffer, Marc Armand

1918 Studies in Palaeopathology: Some Recent Researches on Prehistoric Trephining. *Journal of Pathology and Bacteriology* 22:90–104.

Ruisinger, Marion Maria

2003 Lorenz Heister (1683–1758) and the "Bachmann Case": Social Setting and Medical Practice of Trepanation in Eighteenth-Century Germany. In *Trepanation: History, Discovery, Theory*, edited by Robert Arnott, Stanley Finger, and C. U. M. Smith, pp. 273–288. Swets and Zeitlinger, Lisse.

Ruiz Estrada, Arturo

2013 *La trepanación prehispánica en Amazonas, Perú.* Fondo Editorial de la Universidad Nacional Mayor de San Marcos, Lima.

Salomon, Frank

1995 "The Beautiful Grandparents": Andean Ancestor Shrines and Mortuary Ritual as Seen through Colonial Records. In *Tombs for the Living: Andean Mortuary Practices*, edited by Tom D. Dillehay, pp. 315–353. Dumbarton Oaks Research Library and Collection, Washington, D.C.

2004 *The Cord Keepers: Khipus and Cultural Life in a Peruvian Village.* Duke University Press, Durham.

Sanan, Abhay, and Stephen J. Haines

1997 Repairing Holes in the Head: A History of Cranioplasty. *Neurosurgery* 40:588–603.

Sauer, Norman J., and Samuel Strong Dunlap

1985 The Assymmetrical Remodelling of Two Neurosurgical Burr Holes: A Case Study. *Journal of Forensic Sciences* 30(3):953–957.

Savoy, Gene

1970 *Antisuyu: The Search for the Lost Cities of the Andes.* Simon and Schuster, New York.

Schjellerup, Inge

1997 *Incas and Spaniards in the Conquest of the Chachapoyas: Archaeological and Ethnohistorical Research in the North-Eastern Andes of Peru.* Doctoral thesis, Göteborg University, Göteborg, Sweden.

2005   *Incas y españoles en la conquista de los Chachapoya.* Pontificia Universidad Católica del Perú, Lima.

Silverman, Helaine
1991   The Paracas Problem, Archaeological Perspectives. In *Paracas Art and Architecture: Object and Context in South Coastal Peru*, edited by Anne Paul, pp. 349–415. University of Iowa Press, Iowa City.

Smitherman, Todd A., Rebecca Burch, and Loder Elizabeth Sheikh Huma
2013   The Prevalence, Impact, and Treatment of Migraine and Severe Headaches in the United States: A Review of Statistics from National Surveillance Studies. *Headache* 53(3):427–436.

Spencer, Frank
1997   Hrdlička, Aleš (1869–1943). In *History of Physical Anthropology*, vol. 1, edited by Frank Spencer, pp. 503–504. Garland, New York.

Springer, Martin F. B., and Frank J. Baker
1988   Cranial Burr Hole Decompression in the Emergency Department. *The American Journal of Emergency Medicine* 6(6):640–646.

Squier, Ephraim George
1877   *Peru: Incidents of Travel and Exploration in the Land of the Incas.* Macmillan, London.

Stanish, Charles, and Brian S. Bauer
2004   *Archaeological Research on the Islands of the Sun and Moon, Lake Titicaca, Bolivia: Final Results of the Proyecto Tiksi Kjarka.* Cotsen Institute of Archaeology, University of California, Los Angeles.

Starkey, J. L.
1936   Discovery of Skulls with Surgical Holing at Tell Duweir, Palestine. *Man* 36:169.

Steinbock, R. Ted
1976   *Paleopathological Diagnosis and Interpretation: Bone Diseases in Ancient Human Populations.* Charles C. Thomas, Springfield, Ill.

Stevens, G. C., and J. Wakely
1993   Diagnostic Criteria for Identification of Seashell as a Trephination Implement. *International Journal of Osteoarchaeology* 3:167–176.

Stewart, T. Dale
1943   Skeletal Remains from Paracas, Peru. *American Journal of Physical Anthropology* 1:47–63.
1950   Deformity, Trephining, and Mutilation in South American Indian Skeletal Remains. In *Handbook of South American Indians*, vol. 6, edited by Julian H. Steward, pp. 43–47. Bureau of American Ethnology, Washington, D.C.
1956   Significance of Osteitis in Ancient Peruvian Trephining. *Bulletin of the History of Medicine* 30:293–320.
1958   *Stone Age Skull Surgery: A General Review, with Emphasis on the New World.* Smithsonian Institution Publication no. 4314. Smithsonian Institution, Washington, D.C.
1975   Cranial Dysraphism Mistaken for Trephination. *American Journal of Physical Anthropology* 42(3): 435–437.
1976   Are Supra-Inion Depressions Evidence of Prophylactic Trephination? *Bulletin of the History of Medicine* 50:414–434.
1981   Aleš Hrdlička, 1869–1943. *American Journal of Physical Anthropology* 56(4):347–351.

Stiles, Joan
2012   The Effects of Injury to Dynamic Neural Networks in the Mature and Developing Brain. *Developmental Psychobiology* 54(3):343–349.

Stone, James L., and Javier Urcid
2003   Pre-Columbian Skull Trepanation in North America. In *Trepanation: History, Discovery, Theory*, edited by Robert Arnott, Stanley Finger, and C. U. M. Smith, pp. 237–24. Swets and Zeitlinger, Lisse.

Stübel, Alphons, and Max Uhle
1892   *Die Ruinenstaette von Tiahuanaco im Hochlande des Alten Perú: Eine Kulturgeschichtliche Studie auf Grund Selbstaendiger Aufnahmen.* Verlag von K. W. Hiersemann, Leipzig.

Su, Thung-Ming, Tsung-Han Lee, Wu-Fu Chen, Tao-Chen Lee, and Ching-Hsiao Cheng
2008   Contralateral Acute Epidural Hematoma after Decompressive Surgery of Acute Subdural Hematoma: Clinical Features and Outcome. *The Journal of Trauma* 65(6):1298–1302.

Tello, Julio C.
1909   *La antigüedad de la sífilis en el Perú.* Sanmarti y Ca, Lima.
1913   Prehistoric Trephining among the Yauyos of Peru. In *Proceedings of the 18th Session of the International Congress of Americanists*, vol. 1, pp. 75–83. Harrison and Sons, London.
1929   *Antiguo Perú, primera epoca.* Comisión Organizadora del Segundo Congreso Sudamericano de Turismo, Lima.

Tello, Julio C., and César W. Astuhuamán Gonzáles

2005 *Paracas.* 2nd ed. Universidad Alas Peruanas; Corporación Financiera de Desarrollo; Fondo Editorial, Universidad Nacional Mayor de San Marcos; Centro Cultural de San Marcos; Museo de Arqueología y Antropología UNMSM, Lima.

Tello, Julio C., and Toribio Mejía Xesspe

1959 *Paracas.* Institute of Andean Research, New York.

1979 *Paracas, segunda parte: Cavernas y necrópolis.* Universidad Nacional Mayor de San Marcos, Lima.

Temkin, Nancy R., Sureyya Dikmen, and H. Richard Winn

1991 Management of Head Injury: Posttraumatic Seizures. *Neurosurgery Clinics of North America* 2(2):425–435.

Thurman, David J., Clinton Alverson, Kathleen A. Dunn, Janet Guerrero, and Joseph E. Sniezek

1999 Traumatic Brain Injury in the United States: A Public Health Perspective. *Journal of Head Trauma Rehabilitation* 14(6):602–615.

Tiesler, Vera

2012 *Transformarse en maya: El modelado cefálico entre los mayas prehispánicos y coloniales.* Universidad Nacional Autónoma de Mexico, Instituto de Investigaciones Antropológicas, Universidad de Yucatán, México.

Titelbaum, Anne R., Naji S. Ibarra Bebel, O. L. Azàldegui, and Zhu M. Valladares K.

2013 Challenges of Terrain and Human Interaction: Fracture Patterns from a Late Intermediate Highland Sample from Marcajirca, Department of Ancash, Peru. Poster presented at the 40th Annual Meeting of the Paleopathological Association, Knoxville, Tenn.

Torres-Rouff, Christina

2013 Human Skeletal Remains from Bandelier's 1895 Expedition to the Island of the Sun. In *Advances in Titicaca Basin Archaeology*, vol. 2, edited by Alexei Vranich and Abigail R. Levine, pp. 181–187. Cotsen Institute of Archaeology, University of California, Los Angeles.

Toyne, J. Marla

2011 Análisis osteológico de los restos humanos de Etapa VI del Proyecto Especial de Kuélap, Chachapoyas, Perú. Report on file with Alfredo Narváez, Chiclayo, Peru.

2014 You Can Trepan If You Want To or You Can Leave Your Skull Alone: Patterns in Ancient Cranial Surgery at Kuélap, Chachapoyas, Peru.

Paper presented at the 83rd Annual Meting of the American Association of Physical Anthropologists, Calgary, Alberta Canada. *American Journal of Physical Anthropology,* supplement 58:255.

Toyne, J. Marla, and Alfredo Narváez Vargas

2014 The Fall of Kuelap: Bioarchaeological Analysis of Death and Destruction on the Eastern Slopes of the Andes. In *Embattled Bodies, Embattled Places: War in Pre-Columbian Mesoamerica and the Andes,* edited by Andrew K. Scherer and John W. Verano, pp. 341–364. Dumbarton Oaks Research Library and Collection, Washington, D.C.

Toynbee, Jocelyn M. C.

1971 *Death and Burial in the Roman World: Aspects of Greek and Roman Life.* Cornell University Press, Ithaca.

Tullo, E.

2010 Trepanation and Roman Medicine: A Comparison of Osteoarchaeological Remains, Material Culture and Written Texts. *The Journal of the Royal College of Physicians of Edinburgh* 40(2):165–171.

Tung, Tiffiny A.

2007 Trauma and Violence in the Wari Empire of the Peruvian Andes: Warfare, Raids, and Ritual Fights. *American Journal of Physical Anthropology* 133:941–956.

2008 Violence after Imperial Collapse: A Study of Cranial Trauma among Late Intermediate Period Burials from the Former Huari Capital, Ayacucho, Peru. *Ñawpa Pacha* 29:101–117.

2012 *Violence, Ritual, and the Wari Empire: A Social Bioarchaeology of Imperialism in the Ancient Andes.* University Press of Florida, Gainesville.

Turner, Bethany L.

2009 Insights into Immigration and Social Class at Machu Picchu, Peru, Based on Oxygen, Strontium, and Lead Isotopic Analysis. *Journal of Archaeological Science* 36(2):317–332.

Turner, Bethany L., and George J. Armelagos

2012 Diet, Residential Origin, and Pathology at Machu Picchu, Peru. *American Journal of Physical Anthropology* 149(1):71–83.

Turner, Christopher

2007 Like a Hole in the Head. *Cabinet,* no. 28. Electronic document, http://www.cabinet magazine.org/issues/28/turner.php, accessed May 20, 2014.

Tyson, Rose A., and Elizabeth S. Dyer Alcauskas (editors)

1980 *Catalogue of the Hrdlička Paleopathology Collection.* San Diego Museum of Man, San Diego.

Ubelaker, Douglas H.

1999 Aleš Hrdlička's Role in the History of Forensic Anthropology. *Journal of Forensic Sciences* 44(4):724–730.

Uhle, Max

1903 *Pachacamac. Report of the William Pepper, M.D.LL.D. Peruvian Expedition of 1896.* Department of Archaeology, University of Pennsylvania, Philadelphia.

Unkel, Ingmar, Bernd Kromer, Markus Reindel, Lukas Wacker, and Guenther Wagner

2007 A Chronology of the Pre-Columbian Paracas and Nasca Cultures in South Peru Based on AMS C-14 Dating. *Radiocarbon* 49(2):551–564.

Urton, Gary

1993 Moieties and Ceremonialism in the Andes: The Ritual Battles of the Carnival Season in Southern Peru. In *El mundo ceremonial andino*, edited by Luis Millones and Yoshio Onuki, pp. 117–142. National Museum of Ethnology, Osaka, Japan.

Valenstein, Elliot S.

1997 History of Psychosurgery. In *A History of Neurosurgery in Its Scientific and Professional Contexts*, edited by Samuel H. Greenblatt, T. Forcht Dagi, and Mel H. Epstein, pp. 499–516. American Association of Neurological Surgeons, Park Ridge, Ill.

Vega, Garcilaso de la (El Inca)

1960 *Obras completas del Inca Garcilaso de la Vega.*
[1604] Ediciones Atlas, Madrid.

Velasco-Suarez, Manuel, Josefina Bautista Martinez, Rafael Garcia Oliveros, and Philip R. Weinstein

1992 Archaeological Origins of Cranial Surgery: Trephination in Mexico. *Neurosurgery* 31(2):313–319.

Verano, John W.

2003a Trepanation in Prehistoric South America: Geographic and Temporal Trends over 2000 Years. In *Trepanation: History, Discovery, Theory*, edited by Robert Arnott, Stanley Finger, and C. U. M. Smith, pp. 223–236. Swets and Zeitlinger, Lisse.

2003b Human Skeletal Remains from Machu Picchu: A Reexamination of the Yale Peabody Museum's Collections. In *The 1912 Yale Peruvian Scientific Expedition Collections from Machu Picchu: Human and Animal Remains*, edited by Richard L. Burger and Lucy C. Salazar, pp. 65–117, and Appendix A. Yale University Division of Anthropology, Peabody Museum of Natural History, New Haven, Conn.

Verano, John W., and Valerie A. Andrushko

2010 Cranioplasty in Ancient Peru: A Critical Review of the Evidence, and a Unique Case from the Cuzco Area. *International Journal of Osteoarchaeology* 18:1–11.

Verano, John W., and Stanley Finger

2010 Ancient Trepanation. In *History of Neurology*, edited by Stanley Finger, François Boller, and Kenneth L. Tyler, pp. 3–14. Handbook of Clinical Neurology 95, 3rd series. Elsevier, B. V., Amsterdam.

Verano, John W., and Tania Delabarde

2013 A Possible Trephination from the North Coast of Peru and the Challenges of Differential Diagnosis of Healed Cranial Defects. Paper presented at the 40th Annual Meeting of the Paleopathology Association, Knoxville, Tenn.

Verano, John W., and J. Michael Williams

1992 Head Injury and Surgical Intervention in Pre-Columbian Peru. *American Journal of Physical Anthropology*, supplement 14:167–168.

Von Hagen, Adriana

2002 People of the Clouds. In *Chachapoyas: El reino perdido*, edited by Elena Gonzáles and Rafo León, pp. 24–265. INTEGRA AFP, Lima.

Von Hagen, Adriana, and Craig Morris

1993 *The Inka Empire and Its Andean Origins.* Abbeville Press, New York.

Voorhees, Jennifer R., Aaron A. Cohen-Gadol, and Dennis D. Spencer

2005 Early Evolution of Neurological Surgery: Conquering Increased Intracranial Pressure, Infection, and Blood Loss. *Neurosurgery Focus* 18(4):1–5.

Wadley, J. P., G. T. Smith, and C. Shieff

1997 Self-Trephination of the Skull with an Electric Power Drill. *British Journal of Neurosurgery* 11(2):156–158.

Walker, Alan E.

1951 *A History of Neurological Surgery.* Williams and Wilkins, Baltimore.

Walker, Phillip L.

1997　Wife Beating, Boxing, and Broken Noses: Skeletal Evidence for the Cultural Patterning of Violence. In *Troubled Times: Violence and Warfare in the Past*, edited by Debra L. Martin and David W. Frayer, pp. 145–179. Gordon and Breach, Amsterdam.

2008　Sexing Skulls Using Discriminant Function Analysis of Visually Assessed Traits. *American Journal of Physical Anthropology* 136(1):39–50.

Wassén, Henry, and Wolmar Bondeson

1972　*A Medicine-Man's Implements and Plants in a Tiahuanacoid Tomb in Highland Bolivia.* Göteborgs Etnografiska Museum, Göteborg.

Wehrli, G. A.

1939　Trepanation in Former Centuries. *Ciba Symposia* 1:178–186.

Weiss, Pedro

1932　Restos humanos de Cerro Colorado. Exploracion en Cerro Colorado. *Revista del Museo Nacional* 2:90–102.

1949　*La cirugia del craneo entre los antiguos peruanos.* Tipografía peruana, Lima.

1953　Las trepanaciones peruanas estudiadas como técnica y en sus relaciones con la cultura. *Revista del Museo Nacional* 22:17–34.

1958　*Osteologia cultural: Prácticas cefálicas*, vol. 1. Universidad Nacional Major de San Marcos, Lima.

Wintzen, Axel R.

1980　The Clinical Course of Subdural Haematoma: A Retrospective Study of Aetiological, Chronological, and Pathological Features in 212 Patients and a Proposed Classification. *Brain* 103(4):855–67.

Wilkinson, Richard G.

1975a　Techniques of Ancient Skull Surgery. *Natural History* 84:94–101.

1975b　Trephination by Drilling in Ancient Mexico. *Bulletin of the New York Academy of Medicine* 51:838–850.

Wilkinson, Richard G., and Marcus C. Winter

1975　Cirugía craneal en Monte Albán. *Boletín INAH*, época II, 12:21–26.

Williams, J. Michael, Francisco Gomes, Owen W. Drudge, and Marc Kessler

1984　Predicting Outcome from Closed Head Injury by Early Assessment of Trauma Severity. *Journal of Neurosurgery* 61(3):581–585.

Wilms, G., W. Van Roost, J. Van Russelt, and J. Smits

1983　Biparietal Thinning: Correlation with CT Findings. *Radiologe* 23(8): 385–386.

Winter, Marcus

1989　*Oaxaca, the Archaeological Record.* Minutiae Mexicana, Mexico City.

Wölfel, D. J.

1925　Die Trepanation. *Anthropos* 20:1–50.

Woodall, John

1639　*The Surgeon's Mate, or, Military and Domestic Surgery.* Rob Young, for Nicholas Bourne, London.

World Health Organization (WHO)

2012　Headache Disorders, Fact Sheet no. 277. Electronic document, http://www.who.int/mediacentre/factsheets/fs277/en/, accessed April 8, 2014.

Yacovleff, Eugenio, and Jorge Muelle

1932　Una exploración en Cerro Colorado. *Revista del Museo Nacional* 1:30–59. Lima.

Zevallos Quiñones, Jorge

1994　*Huacas y huaqueros en Trujillo durante el virreinato, 1535–1835.* Editora Normas Legales, Trujillo.

CONTRIBUTORS

Bebel Ibarra Asencios is an archaeologist who specializes in the prehistory of highland Ancash, Peru. He earned his bachelor's degree and licenciatura in archaeology at the Universidad Nacional Mayor de San Marcos. He went on to do graduate studies at the University of Paris 1, and then entered the doctoral program in anthropology at Tulane University in 2013. He has conducted archaeological excavations in highland Ancash since 2004, and has directed the Proyecto Arqueológico Huari-Ancash since 2007. He has published numerous articles, book chapters, and books on the archaeology of northern highland Peru, including two edited volumes and one single-authored book: *Arqueología de la sierra de Ancash: Propuestas y perspectivas, segunda edición* (2004); *Cien años de la arqueología en la sierra de Ancash* (2014); and *Arqueología de la sierra de Ancash: Evidencias y cronología* (in press).

David Kushner, MD, is board certified in neurology by the American Board of Psychiatry and Neurology and currently serves as an associate professor of physical medicine and rehabilitation at the University of Miami Miller School of Medicine. He has served on the faculty at the University of Miami since 1994. His academic career continues to involve patient care, teaching, writing, and research. In addition to neurosurgical patients with craniectomies, his patients include those having traumatic brain injury, stroke, spinal cord injury, and multiple trauma, as well as other neurological disorders and conditions; he also treats patients needing rehabilitation for geriatric, orthopedic, post-surgical, and general medical conditions and burns. Dr. Kushner teaches medical students and medical residents in neurology and rehabilitation. He is the author of peer-reviewed articles, books, and chapters on topics that include traumatic brain injury, stroke, trauma, burns, and neurologic rehabilitation. His interests include the history of neurology and neurosurgery. Dr. Kushner's clinical research interests include topics involving craniectomy patient outcomes, traumatic brain injury, stroke, and quality-improvement issues in rehabilitation.

MELLISA LUND VALLE is a forensic anthropologist and bioarchaeologist who has conducted extensive field and laboratory research in Peru and on international missions investigating human rights violations. She has participated in and organized forensic anthropology and bioarchaeology workshops in Peru, Nepal, Colombia, and Venezuela. From 2001–2011, she was a member of the Equipo Peruano de Antropología Forense (EPAF), where she participated in investigations of human rights violations and the excavation of mass graves. In 2014, she accepted a position with the International Committee of the Red Cross as a forensic advisor for Bolivia, Ecuador, and Peru, providing guidance in the investigation of missing persons and the recovery and identification of victims of mass disasters. Lund Valle earned her bachelor's degree in archaeology at the Universidad Nacional Mayor de San Marcos in 2000, and a master's degree in forensic anthropology and bioarchaeology from the Pontificia Universidad Católica del Perú in 2009. She has published articles on bioarchaeology and forensic anthropology, and has presented papers at a number of international scientific meetings.

ANNE R. TITELBAUM is a biological anthropologist who specializes in human osteology, paleopathology, and bioarchaeology. Her primary research area is Andean South America, with research interests that include pathology in ancient skeletal remains, developmental anomalies, trauma, musculoskeletal stress, and mortuary practices. She has participated in a number of archaeological projects in Peru, including the Proyecto Arqueológico Huaca de La Luna, the Proyecto Arqueológico Complejo El Brujo, the Huaca Prieta Archaeological Project, and the Proyecto Arqueológico Huari-Ancash. She is currently an assistant professor in the Department of Basic Medical Sciences at the University of Arizona College of Medicine-Phoenix. Titelbaum is the author of multiple peer-reviewed journal articles and book chapters on paleopathology and bioarchaeology in ancient Peru.

JOHN W. VERANO is a biological anthropologist who specializes in human osteology, paleopathology, bioarchaeology, and forensic anthropology. His primary research area is Andean South America, where he has conducted fieldwork and museum research for more than thirty years. His research interests include pathology in ancient skeletal and mummified remains, trepanation and other ancient surgery, warfare, human sacrifice, and mortuary practices. A two-time Fulbright Lecturer in Peru, he is currently a professor of anthropology at Tulane University. He is coeditor of *Disease and Demography in the Americas* (1992, with Douglas Ubelaker) and *Embattled Bodies, Embattled Places: War in Pre-Columbian Mesoamerica and the Andes* (2014, with Andrew Scherer).

J. MICHAEL WILLIAMS graduated from the doctoral program in clinical psychology with a specialty in Neuropsychology from the University of Vermont. Following clinical and academic research positions at Memphis State University and Hahnemann Medical University, he now serves as an associate professor of Drexel University. His research has focused on clinical prediction models and clinical trials in the treatment of traumatic brain injury, memory disorder, sensory neglect, and other neurological disorders. Functional MRI studies of the hippocampus, memory and emotion, Diffusion Tensor Imaging of brain development, and connectivity modeling are the focus of his current studies. His clinical practice included neuropsychological assessment and rehabilitation services for patients with traumatic brain injuries. On a hunch that cranial trepanation practiced by the Peruvians may have led them to knowledge about brain function, he called the Smithsonian Museum of Natural History in 1987 and was eventually connected with John Verano, a research associate in the Department of Anthropology. Thereafter followed an exotic adventure in examining skulls. Although evidence that the Peruvians developed knowledge of brain function proved elusive, he was instrumental in encouraging Verano to continue his research on cranial trepanation, one of the most fascinating medical crafts of prehistoric culture.

INDEX

at Paracas, 113, *113–115*, 265; postoperative care and support, social network for, 288–289; on south coast, 265; in southern highlands, 181, 193, 221, 224–225, 228, 265

Sudan, 240

suprainion lesions, 31–34, *32, 33*

supratentorial lesions, 254

sutures, cranial, surgical avoidance or non-avoidance of, 36–38, 59, 105, 133, *165*, 194, 203, *205, 206, 215*, 216

suturing of wounds, 108–109, 240

swallowing function, 261

T

Taforalt Cave, Morocco, 283

Tama Tam chullpa, 230, *232, 233*

Tanzania, Tende of, 241

taphonomic damage, postmortem, 34, *35–37*

techniques. *See* tools and techniques

Tell Dueir (Lachish), Israel, 66

Tello, Julio César, and Tello collection skulls: *Antiguo Peru, primera epoca* (1929), 101, 108; from central highlands, ix, *42*, 42–43, 47–48, 51, 52–53, *54*, 68, 77, 82; contextualization of, 289; experimentation with cadavers, 248; from Paracas, 48, 52, 89, 91–102, *103*, 108, 109, 116, 132, 133; *Paracas: Primera parte* (1959), 108; on south-coast crania, 135–140

Tende of Tanzania, 241

terraza tombs, 97

Tibesti, 240

Tibu, 240

Titelbaum, Anne R., 141, 253, 288, 310

Titicaca (Lake), 14, 194, 229–230, *231*, 234, 235

Tiwanaku, 14, 229–230, 235

Tolai, 238–239

tombs. *See* burials

tools and techniques, 1–3; on Altiplano, 230; in central highlands, 66–77, *67*, *69–76*, 264–265; comparative models, 3, *4*, 238, 239, 240, *241*, 242–245, *244*, *246*, 247–248, 285–286, *286*; "crown" trephine or trepan, 1–3, *2*, 241, 285; etymology of trepanation/trephination and, 1; healing process affecting identification of, 68, *69*; modern experimentation on living patients, 76–77, 237, 248–251; neurosurgery, modern, 253, 256, *257, 258*, 264–265; in northern highlands and cloud forest, 151, *152*, 160, *161, 167, 168*, 169; Paracas, 97, 106–109, *107, 108*, 110–112, 242, 264; southern highlands, 177, 186–193, *188, 189, 191, 192*, 219, 227–228, 265; Woodall's instruments, 1, *2. See also specific techniques and tool types and fabrics*

Topará, 99, 135

Torontoy, 176, 177, 178, 181, *185, 187*

Torres-Rouff, Christina, 230

trauma: Chachapoyas, variable incidence of head trauma at, 170, 173–174; differential diagnosis of, 27–31, *29–31*; high risk of head injury in central highlands, 53, 85–88, *87*; at Machu Picchu, 175; Marcajirca, high incidence of head trauma at, 144, *148, 149*, 151; non-trepanned skulls from central highlands with, 82–88, *83–87*; in southern highlands, 175

trauma, association of trepanation with, ix, 3–4; on Altiplano, 230–234, *231–233*; in central highlands, 53, *54, 57–59*, 77–82, *78–82*; in comparative models, 238, 239, 240, 242, 247; continuation into modern times, 234–235; location of trepanations indicating, *82*, 220; neurosurgical perspective on, 253, 258–260; in northern highlands and cloud forest, 153–160, *154–159*, 170, 173–174; Paracas, 116–122, *119–125*; in southern highlands, 178–185, *180–185*, 196–201, *197–200*, 214, 216–219, *217, 218*, 219–221, 220, 228

traumatic brain injury, 267–282; cognitive and behavioral consequences, 262, 271–275, *272*; modern closed head injuries versus Pre-Columbian blunt-force or penetrating wounds, 267–268, 275, 276; modern preneuroimaging case studies, 275–280; neurosurgical perspective on, 260–263, *264*, 265–266; reconstruction of Pre-Columbian case from southern highlands skull, 280–282, *281*; recovery process, 273–275, 288–289; skull fracture and impact on brain tissue, 268. *See also* hematoma; neurosurgical perspective on trepanation

trepanation in Pre-Columbian Peru, xi–xii, 1–9; Altiplano, *8, 9*, 229–235, *231–233*; anthropological/archaeological discovery of, 11–19 (*See also* anthropological/archaeological discovery of Pre-Columbian trepanation); bones of skull and anatomical landmarks, map of, *291*; central highlands, 39–88 (*See also* central highlands trepanned crania); comparative models, ix, 237–252 (*See also* comparative models); continuation into modern times, 1, 88, 234–235, 237, 289; data-recording methodology, 34–38; defined, 1; differential diagnosis of, 21–38 (*See also* differential diagnosis); geographic patterning and regional clustering of, 286–287; map of principle geographic areas, *8*; motives for, ix, 3–4, 288 (*See also* motives for trepanning); neurosurgery differentiated, 3, 3–4; neurosurgical perspective on, 253–266 (*See also* neurosurgical perspective on trepanation); northern highlands and cloud forest, 141–174 (*See also* northern highlands and cloud forest); origins and history of, viii–ix, 6–9, *9*, 89–90, 140; Paracas, 89–140 (*See also* Paracas); reasons for common use of trepanning in Peru, 288–289; south coast, 134–140 (*See also* south coast); southern highlands, 175–229 (*See also* southern highlands); spread of surgical knowledge, 288; terms for, 1–3; tools and

techniques, 1–3 (*See also* tools and techniques);
trauma, association with, ix, 3–4 (*See also* trauma,
association of trepanation with); traumatic brain
injury and, 267–282 (*See also* traumatic brain injury);
trephination differentiated, 1
trephination differentiated from trepanation, 1
tumi knives, 76–77, 249, 250
túmors and cancerous lesions, 27, *28*, *130–132*, 131, 235, 253,
254, 263, 288
Tuna (central highlands site), *58*, *73*, *74*, *75*
Tunga, 135

U
Uareg Berbers, 240
Uhle, Max, 32, 225–227, *226*, *227*, 289

V
Valcárcel, Luis, 97
venous-arterial malformations, 263
Verano, John, vii, viii–ix, xii, 141, 170, 310
Virgins of the Sun, 175

W
Wakely, Jennifer, 239
Wambu Chaka, *63*
Wari culture, 135, 140, 143, 151
Wari Kayan, Necropolis of, 96, 99–101, *100*, 103, 134

Wata, 224
Weiss, Amalia, vii
Weiss, Anita Barker de, vii
Weiss, Pedro, vii, viii*, *31*, 97, 101, 102, 109, 132, 133;
Osteologica cultural: Prácticas cefálicas (1958), vii, 106
Wernicke, Karl, and Wernicke's aphasia, 272
West Africa, cranium with saber wound from, *31*
Whitaker, D., 24
Wiener, Charles, 162
Wilkinson, Richard, 285–286
Williams, J. Michael, xi, 267, 288, 310–311
Wilson, O. R. L., 279
Winter, Marcus, 285–286
Wölfel, D. J., 238
women. *See* females
Woodall, John, 1

X
x-rays, 38

Y
Yacovleff, Eugenio, 102
Yale expedition discoveries in southern highlands, 175,
176–186, *179–185*
Yanamanchi, 176, 178
Yauyos province. *See* central highlands
Yucay/Yucay Valley, 14, 186, *187*, 190

STUDIES IN PRE-COLUMBIAN ART AND ARCHAEOLOGY

Published by Dumbarton Oaks Research Library and Collection, Washington, D.C.